Radiology in Surgical Practice

Edited by

Susan J. Neuhaus MBBS PhD FRACS
Consultant Surgeon, the Queen Elizabeth Hospital,
Woodville and the Royal Adelaide Hospital,
South Australia

Peter G. Devitt MBBS MS FRACS
Associate Professor,
University of Adelaide, Royal Adelaide Hospital,
South Australia

Kirsten L. Gormly MBBS FRANZCR
Consultant Radiologist,
Royal Adelaide Hospital,
South Australia

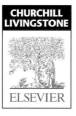

EDINBURGH LONDON NEW YORK OXFORD PHILADELPHIA
ST LOUIS SYDNEY TORONTO 2006

CHURCHILL
LIVINGSTONE
ELSEVIER

First published 2006

ISBN 10: 0-443-10016-0
ISBN 13: 978-0-443-10016-1

British Library Cataloguing in Publication Data
A catalogue record for this book is available from the British Library

Library of Congress Cataloging in Publication Data
A catalog record for this book is available from the Library of Congress

Notice
Knowledge and best practice in this field are constantly changing. As new research and experience broaden our knowledge, changes in practice, treatment and drug therapy may become necessary or appropriate. Readers are advised to check the most current information provided (i) on procedures featured or (ii) by the manufacturer of each product to be administered, to verify the recommended dose or formula, the method and duration of administration, and contraindications. It is the responsibility of the practitioner, relying on their own experience and knowledge of the patient, to make diagnoses, to determine dosages and the best treatment for each individual patient, and to take all appropriate safety precautions. To the fullest extent of the law, neither the Publisher nor the Authors assume any liability for any injury and/or damage to persons or property arising out or related to any use of the material contained in this book.

The Publisher

The publisher's policy is to use **paper manufactured from sustainable forests**

Printed in China

Contents

Preface

Over recent years, radiology and ancillary investigations have assumed an increased importance in clinical medicine – particularly in the practice of surgery. In the management of surgical problems a radiological investigation is now almost the rule rather than the exception. Similarly, radiological intervention is gaining increased importance in the management of many conditions and often replaces surgical intervention.

These changes have many implications for surgeons, not the least being the increased importance of knowing what radiological investigations are available. Surgeons also need to know which investigation or investigations would be most applicable in a given situation, the limitations and risks of the procedure and how to interpret the results, and be able to read and understand the images.

This book is aimed at addressing some of these issues. It is not an atlas of radiology. Rather, we have sought to bring together all the areas of radiology that the general surgeon is likely to encounter, to describe the radiological techniques and to elaborate on their role in the different fields within general surgery.

Chapter 1 discusses a number of issues such as the need for evidence-based studies, cost–benefit analysis of the new technology and some of the ethical dilemmas now being faced. The rest of the first section of the book describes the standard radiological investigations such as contrast studies, CT scanning, nuclear medicine and ultrasound. The second, and larger, section of the book is devoted to description of radiological investigations and interventions in the different surgical disciplines. We have aimed to describe the place of particular procedures, their advantages and shortcomings and what should be looked for, with each investigation. The chosen images are meant to do no more than highlight a point or provide an example, rather than cover the subject exhaustively.

When we set out to write this book, our selected target was those training in surgery. However, the more we became involved in the project, the more we realised that as practising surgeons (Peter Devitt and Susan Neuhaus), we knew a reasonable amount about radiology in our own field, a comfortable amount on the radiology of our sister disciplines, but frighteningly little of the advances being made around us. Thus, we realised that this should be a book aimed not just at the trainee but also at the practising surgeon who, like the editors, are in constant danger of being left behind.

Radiology is changing rapidly and this book can be no more than a step in the march of progress. We have been only able to touch on some areas – such as co-registered PET-CT, virtual colonography and microbubble contrast ultrasonography – which may well be standard practice and commonplace in a few years time.

Adelaide 2006

SJ Neuhaus
PG Devitt
KL Gormly

Contributors

Ahmad Aly FRACS
Anstior Hospital, Heidelberg, Victoria, Australia

Justin R Bessell MBBS MD FRACS
Consultant Surgeon, Flinders Medical Centre, Bedford Park, South Australia

Barry E Chatterton
Director, Department of Nuclear Medicine, Royal Adelaide Hospital, South Australia

Andrew Chew BMBS FRACS
Consultant Surgeon, Repatriation Hospital, Daw Park, South Australia

Peter G Devitt MBBS MS FRACS
Associate Professor, University of Adelaide, Royal Adelaide Hospital, South Australia

Robert Fitridge MBBS FRACS
Senior Lecturer in Vascular Surgery, Queen Elizabeth Hospital, Woodville, South Australia

Paul Gallagher MD FRCSEd (Gen Surg)
Consultant, Upper Gastro-intestinal and Laparoscopic Surgeon, Northumbria Healthcare Trust, Northumberland, UK

Mary Gabb FRANZCR
Emeritus Consultant Radiologist, Royal Adelaide Hospital, South Australia

Kirsten L Gormly MBBS FRANZCR
Consultant Radiologist, Royal Adelaide Hospital, South Australia

Nigel R Jones MBBS DPhil FRACS
Clinical Professor of Neurosurgery, University of Adelaide, Royal Adelaide Hospital, South Australia

Jonathon Heysen MBBS FRANZCR
Consultant Radiologist, Royal Adelaide Hospital, South Australia

Ian D Kirkwood MBBS FRACP
Consultant in Nuclear Medicine, University of Adelaide, Royal Adelaide Hospital, South Australia

Guy J Maddern MBBS PhD MS MD FRACS
RP Jepson Professor of Surgery, University of Adelaide, Queen Elizabeth Hospital, Woodville, South Australia

Peter Malycha MBBS FRACS
Consultant Surgeon, Royal Adelaide Hospital, South Australia

Villis Marshall FRACS
Consultant Urological Surgeon, Royal Adelaide Hospital, South Australia

Ian Martin FRACS
Consultant Surgeon, Princess Alexandra Hospital, Woolloongabba, Queensland, Australia

Jo Morgan BM FRACS
Peter MacCallum Cancer Centre, East Melbourne, Australia

Mark Muhlmann MBBS
Surgical Registrar, Sir Charles Gairdner Hospital, Nedlands, Western Australia

Susan J Neuhaus MBBS PhD FRACS
Consultant Surgeon, the Queen Elizabeth Hospital, Woodville and the Royal Adelaide Hospital, South Australia

Philippa Rabbitt MBBS
Senior Registrar, Flinders Medical Centre, Bedford Park, South Australia

Nicholas A Rieger MBBS MS FRACS
Senior Lecturer in Surgery, University of Adelaide, Queen Elizabeth Hospital, Woodville, South Australia

Denise Roach MBBS DDU FRACS
Consultant Surgeon and Sonologist, Department of Surgery, Queen Elizabeth Hospital, Woodville, South Australia

Susie Saloniklis BMBS FRANZCR
Consultant Radiologist, Royal Adelaide Hospital, South Australia

Ruben Sebben FRANZCR
Consultant Radiologist, Queen Elizabeth Hospital, Woodville, South Australia

James L Sweeney MBBS FRACS
Consultant Surgeon, Flinders Medical Centre, Bedford Park, South Australia

D James Taylor FRANZCR
Director of Radiology, Royal Adelaide Hospital, South Australia

Michelle Thomas MBBS FRACS
Research Fellow, Department of Surgery, Royal Adelaide Hospital, South Australia

William Thompson MBBS FRANZCR
Consultant Radiologist, Fremantle Hospital, Western Australia

David Walsh MBBS FRACS
Senior Lecturer in Surgery, Queen Elizabeth Hospital, Woodville, South Australia

Melissa Lea FRANZCR
Consultant Radiologist, Queen Elizabeth Hospital, Woodville, South Australia

David Walters DDU FRACS
Lecturer in Surgery, Queen Elizabeth Hospital, Woodville, South Australia

Randolph S Williams MBBS FRACS
Consultant Surgeon, Modbury Public Hospital, Modbury, South Australia

Philip J Worley MBBS FRACS
Consultant Surgeon, Modbury Public Hospital, South Australia

Acknowledgements

Production of a multiauthor book invariably means the collaboration and cooperation of many individuals; some wholeheartedly and some slightly less so, but all with a common purpose. We would like to acknowledge all those who have been involved in this book.

We are grateful for the help given, not only by our colleagues who sat down and wrote the chapters, but also those whose contributions involved proofreading and finding images.

We also wish to thank those no less important, but perhaps more peripherally involved, particularly family members who tolerated authors spending their precious free time huddled over a computer. Peter and Grace Neuhaus saw less of Susan than they would have wished, and the same must be said of the families of the other contributors.

We would particularly like to thank Laurence Hunter of Elsevier for giving us the opportunity to produce this work and then having the patience and tolerance to accept our excuses as to why the manuscript would not quite get there on time.

Apart from the images provided by the individual authors, we are indebted to others who have kindly found and provided material. In particular, we would like to thank Matthew Clark, Justin Lee, Eleanor Moskovic, Angela Ridell, Cheryl Richardson, Bhuey Sharma and Meirion Thomas (Royal Marsden Hospital), Vicki Warbey (Royal Brompton Hospital), Matthew Lawrence (St Mark's Hospital), John Harper, Eric Sclavos and Peter Sharwood (Princess Alexandra Hospital), Glyn Jamieson (Royal Adelaide Hospital), and Michael Sage (Flinden Medical Centre).

Adelaide 2006

SJ Neuhaus
PG Devitt
KL Gormly

List of commonly used abbreviations

Abdominal aortic aneurysm	AAA
Ankle–brachial pressure index	ABPI
Adrenal cortical thyrotropic hormone	ACTH
Anteroposterior	AP
Arteriovenous malformation	AVM
Abdominal X-ray	AXR
Barium	Ba
Becquerel unit	Bq
Common bile duct	CBD
Craniocaudal view (mammography)	CC
Contrast enhanced computed tomography	CECT
Chemical shift images	CSI
Computed tomography	CT
Computed tomography angiography	CTA
Computed tomography arterial portography	CTAP
Chest X-ray	CXR
Double contrast barium enema	DCBE
Dimercaptosuccinic acid	DMSA
Diagnostic peritoneal lavage	DPL
Digital subtraction angiography	DSA
Deep venous thrombosis	DVT
Indium-111-diethylene triamine penta-acetic acid (DTPA)-octreotide	DTPA
Endoanal ultrasound	EAS

Extradural haematoma	EDH
Endoscopic retrograde cholangiopancreatography	ERCP
Endorectal magnetic resonance imaging	ERMRI
Endorectal ultrasound	ERUS
Endoscopic ultrasound	EUS
Focused abdominal sonography in trauma	FAST
Fluorine-18 fluorodeoxyglucose (FDG)	FDG
Fluorine-18 fluorodeoxyglucose postitron emission tomography	FDG-PET
Fine needle aspiration	FNA
Fine needle aspiration cytology	FNAC
Fibronodular hyperplasia	FNH
Gastrointestinal stromal tumour	GIST
Gastrointestinal tract	GIT
Gray (measure of radiation dose: 1 Gy = 100 rad)	Gy
Hepatocellular carcinoma	HCC
High-resolution computed tomography	HRCT
High-resolution ultrasound	HRUS
Hounsfield units	HU
Image intensifier	II
Inferior vena cava	IVC
Intraoperative cholangiogram	IOC
Intraoperative ultrasound	IOUS
Intravenous	IV
Intravenous urography	IVU
Kidney–ureter–bladder	KUB
Longitudinal section	LS
Mega Hertz	MHz
Metaiodobenzylguianidine	MIBG
^{99m} technetium hexakis-2-methoxyisobutylisonitrile	MIBI
Minimal invasive parathyroidectomy	MIP
Medial–lateral–oblique view (mammography)	MLO

Mammogram	MMG
Magnetic resonance angiography	MRA
Magnetic resonance cholangiopancreatography	MRCP
Mean short axis diameter	MSAD
Multislice computed tomography	MSCT
Motor vehicle accident	MVA
National Health and Medical Research Council of Australia	NHMRC
Noriodocholesterol (NP-59)	NP-59
Non-small-cell lung cancer	NSCLC
Picture archiving and communication system	PACS
Phase contrast	PC
Pulmonary embolism	PE
Percutaneous endoscopic gastrostomy	PEG
Positron emission tomography	PET
Peripherally inserted central catheter	PICC
Percutaneous radiological gastrostomy	PRG
Percutaneous transhepatic cholangiography	PTC
Peripheral vascular disease	PVD
Measure of radiation dose (1 Gy = 100 rad)	Rad
Renal artery stenosis	RAS
Renal cell cancer	RCC
Radiofrequency electromagnetic waves	RF
Radiofrequency ablation	RFA
Radionuclide imaging	RNI
Sagittal	Sag
Subdural haematoma	SDH
Squamous cell carcinoma	SCC
Solitary pulmonary nodule	SPN
Single photon emission computed tomography	SPECT
Superparamagnetic oxide	SPIO
Superior vena cava	SVC
Sieverts (biological-equivalent measure of radiation exposure)	Sv

T1-weighted relaxation time	T1
T2-weighted relaxation time	T2
Transarterial chemoembolisation	TACE
Thoracic aortic injury	TAI
Tuberculosis	TB
Time gain compensation	TGC
Transjugular intrahepatic portosystemic shunt	TIPS
Transoesophageal echocardiography	TOE
Total parenteral nutrition	TPN
Transrectal ultrasound	TRUS
Tranverse section	TS
Transvaginal ultrasound	TV-US
Ultrasound	US
Ultrasmall paramagnetic iron oxide	USPIO
Videoassisted thoracoscopy	VAT
Ventilation/perfusion	V/Q
Whole-body bone scan	WBBS

Section one

Radiological investigations

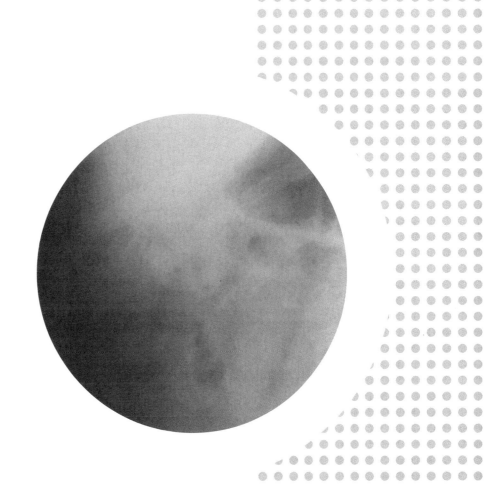

Current radiological practice

1

P.G. Devitt

THE CHANGING FACE OF RADIOLOGY

Among the many recent developments in medicine, perhaps the most spectacular have been in imaging. The contemporary practice of surgery is heavily reliant on imaging for the diagnosis, screening and staging of disease, for predicting resectability, for detecting complications and – increasingly – for therapeutic interventions such as abscess drainage and vascular stenting. Current imaging modalities provide accurate anatomical localisation and definition, which has extended surgical resection options into new areas.

Radiology has progressed from being a mere provider of diagnostic information based on plain two-dimensional radiography, sometimes supplemented with contrast. Today, radiology is moving forwards rapidly, both in terms of technological advances and in the ability of the radiologist to provide a therapeutic service, the latter often in place of the surgeon. This book describes the place of radiology in surgical prac-

tice and focuses on some of the advances as they apply to the general surgeon.

THE SURGEON–RADIOLOGIST RELATIONSHIP

To provide optimum care for their patients, surgeons need to understand the principles, indications and interpretation of the ever-increasing array of images that form part of their day-to-day management decisions. Apart from keeping up with the changes in radiological practice, it is vitally important that surgeons are aware of the diagnostic and therapeutic options available and their potential risks and benefits.

Advances and sophistication in imaging technology make the relationship between the surgeon and radiologist an increasingly important component of overall patient care. With a plethora of imaging techniques available, it is important that imaging is placed into an appropriate clinical context. Imaging must not be seen as an alternative to appropriate history and clinical examination or good surgical judgement. Neither should imaging be sought as part of 'defensive practice'. All imaging carries a risk to the patient and it is imperative that the number of inappropriate investigations is kept to a minimum. Inappropriate radiology carries individual patient risk, as well as being a drain on the health dollar.

Good communication between the surgeon and radiologist becomes ever more important. With the rapid technological changes now occurring, the surgeon might not always know what radiological investigations or procedures are available for a particular problem, or the limitations of an investigation that might have been requested. Similarly, the radiologist will not always be armed with sufficient clinical information to determine how best to approach a diagnostic problem. On its simplest level, this communication relies on adequate provision of clinical data to the radiologist on the request form. For example, patients on metformin must be identified because they are at increased risk of lactic acidosis if given contrast as part of a computed tomography (CT) series. It is obvious that the more clear and full the information provided by the surgeon, the more likely the radiologist will be able to provide a satisfactory answer. By necessity, surgeons and radiologists view the same images in a different manner. For the radiologist, diagnosis is the principal aim of reporting. The surgeon, however, must interpret the imaging findings in the light of overall clinical care and appropriately weight the report with the results of other investigations such as blood tests and pathology.

RADIOLOGY IN THE DIGITAL AGE

As in many other areas of everyday life, digital technology has had a major impact on technology in radiology. In its most obvious form there has been a massive shift from 'hard copy' X-ray films to digitised images. This change has facilitated image acquisition, data storage, distribution and data retrieval. No longer dependent on finding space to store bulky and heavy films, large amounts of digital data can be acquired and stored on hard drives, CDs, DVDs and a variety of other storage devices. Apart from the hardware advances that allow increased storage of data, sophisticated software programs now facilitate the acquisition, interpretation and display of data in a manner not even imagined a decade ago. These digitised images are often best viewed on workstations, where 3-D modelling of images can be undertaken. For the convenience of the end-user, much of this digitised information is still translated into hard copy, but it is increasingly made available through downloads to personal computers, whether on the specialist's desk or on the ward. It is likely the traditional film and heavy packet of X-rays will soon be a thing of the past.

The term 'teleradiology' is sometimes used to describe the process of sending large blocks of radiological data in electronic format to a remote site for diagnostic purposes. In practice, the format can vary from an image grabbed off a viewing box by a simple digital camera and sent by e-mail, to a sophisticated arrangement of digitisation equipment and automatic transfer to a dedicated workstation. The latter facility is frequently used for reporting CT scans from remote sites. In all cases the diagnostic accuracy will be largely dependent on the quality and resolution of the images transferred. Hard copy that needs to be digitised and compressed before being sent down a telephone line to a low-resolution monitor will be of lesser quality than CT scans sent directly from source to a nearby workstation.

Teleradiology has several potential advantages and some possible problems. Such a facility will allow better access for patients and practitioners based in remote areas and may reduce the need for referral to specialist centres. This is well reported from areas such as South Africa, where the distances to specialist centres can be considerable and such travel is not practical for many patients.

Radiological consultations can be undertaken on an intercontinental basis, when the global day–night differences can provide cost-savings. For example, a busy emergency department in the USA might choose to direct its out-of-hours CT scan images for interpretation overseas. In addition to the convenience of being able to get a report back in less than 90 minutes, the process might save money by minimising delay in the emergency room and saving on consultant fees. A major potential problem with such systems will be the issue of liability with respect to diagnostic accuracy. Who will bear the responsibility for mis-diagnosis and how will the laws related to malpractice in one country relate to those of another?

A more positive use of teleradiology will be the ability of such systems to enable expert advice to be provided at a distance. For example, a neurosurgeon will be able to give advice to non-experts in a remote area of the management of head injury, where interpretation of the CT scan may be pivotal and the transfer of the patient impractical.

In addition to image quality, other problems include confidentially, clinicians' computer skills and availability of hardware to display the images. While data is kept within hospital intranets, the use of 'firewalls' can ensure reasonable degrees of confidentially of patient information. However, with downloading of radiological data on to practitioners' home or office computers, such security is less likely to be ensured.

Current issues over poor image resolution will lessen as digital hardware improves and, as with digital cameras rapidly coming abreast of film-based cameras, so the quality of digital radiology will match and overtake that of film-screen. In addition, the digital image can be manipulated to display different aspects of the image (e.g. lung, mediastinum or bone on a chest image) – something that could never be done on a single radiograph. Likewise, individuals' computer skills and the availability of computers will cease to be issues as digital technology becomes ever more part of our lives.

AN EVIDENCE-BASED APPROACH

The introduction of any new drug requires extensive animal and clinical trials, documentation of the results of these trials, consideration of the results of these trials by a specialist in that area, a recommendation by that specialist on the safety and efficacy of that drug and finally approval by the appropriate government regulating body. Unfortunately the same rigor has not always been applied to the introduction of new therapeutic techniques, such as using medical imaging by interventional radiologists or indeed, surgeons. Sometimes the safety and efficacy of the technique might not be accredited by the institution in which it is undertaken. These issues need to be addressed by the profession, to ensure that there is a rigid assessment of the clinical benefit of new techniques as they are developed. Although efforts are frequently made to report the new technologies, the studies are all too often based on observational data rather than case-controlled or prospective, randomised trials. As issues surface with respect to the cost-effectiveness of new radiological techniques, so it will become more important to be able to show the clinical efficacy of a particular procedure. This is particularly relevant in screening (Chapter 23).

Although it is often difficult to identify and document appropriate outcomes such as reduction in symptoms, avoidance of unnecessary (interventional) procedures, cost-savings, some endpoints such as time in hospital and long-term survival can be measured. In one such prospective randomised study it has been shown that CT assessment and planned pleural biopsy will improve the diagnostic accuracy of standard pleural biopsy and reduce the need for unnecessary biopsy. Similarly judicious use of CT might reduce the need for other invasive procedures, such as bronchoscopy, in patients with possible carcinoma of the lung. Such positive outcomes are countered by reports that suggest that CT imaging is of no practical value in the early assessment of acute ischaemic stroke. Unfortunately, relatively little information in the literature looks critically at the clinical effectiveness of the new technologies.

COST BENEFITS OF THE NEW TECHNOLOGY

Apart from a need to show the clinical efficacy of any new diagnostic and therapeutic tools in radiology, a further requirement must be their cost-effectiveness. There are several different comparisons that might be made. These include:

- radiological procedure versus clinical judgement
- one radiological procedure versus another radiological procedure
- radiological procedure versus surgical intervention.

One argument used to justify the use of CT scanning is a perceived reduction in waiting time in emergency departments and prevention of unnecessary admission of patients with undiagnosed and clinically insignificant abdominal pain (see Chapter 10). In other words, can the CT scan be superior and more cost effective than clinical assessment? The answer to this might never be forthcoming as medicolegal issues and liability often cloud decision-making.

An endpoint that is rather easier to measure is disease recurrence. Several studies have shown that routine CT scanning is not cost effective in the detection of Hodgkin's disease or colorectal cancer. The pick-up rate of recurrent disease is low and most patients with recurrence either develop symptoms or have the disease found on clinical review.

Comparisons of the cost effectiveness of different radiological procedures show that newer is not necessarily better. It has been suggested (and is often practised) that it might be more cost effective to perform CT as the initial investigation of trauma patients than to waste time and money on clinical evaluation and plain radiology. Whereas CT scanning of patients with suspected spinal injuries appears to be more reliable and time-saving than plain radiological assessment, the same instruments applied to the assessment of chest trauma does not show any cost-effective advantage for CT.

It has been suggested that positron emission tomography (PET) scanning might reduce the overall cost of management of recurrent colorectal cancer. Enthusiasts for the new technology claim that PET will detect recurrent disease, not picked up by CT, and thus avoid the costs of unnecessary surgical intervention. However, claims of superior sensitivity of PET over CT might be difficult to substantiate when histological evidence of the alleged recurrence disease is not obtained or the standards of CT not defined. Whereas PET might eventually be shown to provide a cost–benefit advantage, this will have to be made on the basis that PET (or any investigation) is not only more sensitive and specific in achieving the desired information, but that the investigative tool replaces and does not merely add to, the pre-existing procedure. Other factors that must be considered in the global cost–benefit analysis include the costs involved with chemotherapy or other treatments if the radiological investigation has determined that surgery in inappropriate.

Whereas some of the new technology, such as magnetic resonance (MR) scanning might have extremely high set-up costs, these could eventually be off-set if the new test replaces (rather than adds to) an existing test that is invasive, risky and costly in terms of consumables. For example, it has been suggested that MR angiography is more cost effective than conventional angiography in the assessment of medication-resistant hypertension. The proponents for the introduction of new technologies will often state that the so-called cost–benefit of the procedure lies in its ability to be performed on an outpatient basis, so minimising all the costs associated with admission and occupying a hospital bed. What tends to be conveniently forgotten is the cost of consumables used. For example, the cost of an endovascular aortic stent might be significantly more than the cost of a conventional aortic graft. Likewise, the cost (and clinical outcome) of a transjugular intrahepatic portasystemic shunt, both in terms of consumables and manpower, might be no different from a conventional surgical shunt. Any interpretation of such data needs to take all the hidden costs into account.

If a radiological procedure can avoid unnecessary surgical intervention, it might be cost effective. For example, CT and biopsy of solitary pulmonary nodules might obviate the need for thoracotomy for benign lesions. Similarly, accurate radiological staging of malignant disease might be cost effective in the prevention of unnecessary laparotomy or thoracotomy for unresectable disease. As yet there is no good evidence that CT and/or PET has sufficient sensitivity to replace laparoscopy or thoracoscopy in the assessment of aerodigestive tract carcinomas, particularly for tumour deposits less than 1 cm in size.

Diagnostic and therapeutic radiology claims a substantial proportion of any health budget and without care this proportion may continue to increase. It therefore behoves the users and proponents of these technologies to demonstrate their place in clinical medicine, their efficacy and ability to provide an overall saving to the community.

TRAINING AND EDUCATION IN RADIOLOGY

There is little argument that diagnostic radiology is, at present, the domain of the radiologist. The rapid advancement and development of many different interventional and therapeutic radiological procedures has raised questions of who should be trained in interventional techniques and how training should be undertaken and recognised. The boundaries between radiology and certain components of surgery have become blurred. Similar overlaps now exist in other fields such as radiology and interventional cardiology. Colleges and training organisations need to look at the needs of the future specialist and perhaps move beyond traditional training practices. For example, should the trainee radiologist who plans a career in interventional radiology undergo some formal surgical training? Should the surgical trainee who wants to be a vascular surgeon be required to spend a proportion of training in radiology units? Things are already moving in this direction, albeit often on an ad-hoc basis. In Australia, many surgeons training in vascular or breast surgery elect to undertake the Diploma of Diagnostic Ultrasound, under supervision of the Royal Australasian College of Radiologists. Rather than be overtaken by events, the colleges, hospitals and credentialing committees need to develop programmes, fellowships and accredited specialist positions to meet these needs.

ETHICAL DILEMMAS

Advances in imaging have raised several ethical dilemmas. Advertising and self-promotion is now viewed as ethically acceptable in medicine and is used widely, most noticeably in the fields of cosmetic surgery and ophthalmology. Advertising varies from a discrete listing in a medical directory to blatant, full-page, colour advertisements in weekend newspapers. A profusion of internet sites promotes practitioners and their particular services. Some of the promotion is aimed directly at the patient and some at the medical practitioner. Examples of contentious medical practice include the encouragement of self-referral for whole body imaging and the performance of unnecessary or superfluous radiological investigations for conditions that are readily diagnosed on clinical grounds.

Currently, some medical imaging facilities are promoting CT scanning of the whole body as a means of screening asymptomatic people for disease. This has been referred to as 'whole body CT scanning' or 'whole body CT screening'. This differs from the normal use of CT, which is usually undertaken to identify a cause for a patient's symptoms. In this situation, CT imaging is targeted to the area of clinical concern. Whole body CT scanning is a non-targeted examination, and its application is controversial. Some of the concerns raised by health professionals include:

- Exposing healthy individuals to unnecessary radiation.
- Discovering incidental findings that might warrant invasive procedures or follow-up. Any additional radiological examinations would increase total radiation exposure and, if contrast agents are administered, produce the risk of an adverse reaction.
- The false reassurances of a normal study, as not all diseases may be detected by this method.
- The issue of 'informed consent.' Adequate information regarding the efficacy of the CT screening procedure and potential impact of positive test results might not be given to the individual prior to the scan.
- No specific age groups are targeted by this procedure. Young people who are at an increased risk of radiation-induced cancers might be exposing themselves unnecessarily to radiation. There is no evidence to support the screening of

persons younger than 40, given the low likelihood of significant disease in this age group.

At present, the American College of Radiology (ACR) believes there is insufficient evidence showing that 'whole body CT screening' prolongs life or is cost effective. The US Food and Drug Administration (FDA) concurs that 'whole body CT' provides uncertain benefit with potential for some risks.

CT screening subjects healthy individuals to radiation exposure from X-rays. The dose received from a typical CT study is significantly greater compared with conventional radiographs (see Appendix, p. 313). For a person with a medical indication for the procedure, the possibility of developing a radiation-induced cancer is considered negligible. For an individual without symptoms, the radiation from periodic CT screening exams might exceed upper limits or expose that person to an increased risk of cancer later in life. This could become a public health concern if large numbers of the population undergo regular CT screening procedures. Facilities performing screening CT scans can adjust the radiation dose, and this has been called 'low-dose CT scans'. By reducing radiation dose, image quality can be degraded and this might, in turn, impact on disease detection.

Practitioners themselves are often put under pressure to undertake radiological procedures. This pressure may come from the patient ('wouldn't an X-ray show the cause?') or the radiologist's report ('further information might be gained from doing a CT scan'). It is becoming commonplace for clinical examination to be accompanied or supplanted by the radiological investigation. Patients with obvious lipomas and inguinal hernias are often referred for ultrasound examination. Whether this represents poor medical diagnostic skills, patient pressure or fear of litigation is unclear. How much these practices reflect zealous radiological practice or zealous business practice is also a matter for speculation.

LEGAL ASPECTS

Defensive medicine has become part of the clinician's life. Although it is often tempting to retreat behind the shield of diagnostic imaging and other investigations, sound clinical judgement should govern patient management and any radiological investigation or intervention should be performed on the basis of clinical effectiveness. The clinician should make these decisions based on knowledge and understanding of what radiology can and cannot provide, the effectiveness or efficacy of the investigation or intervention and what are the risks to which the patient will be subjected.

The radiologist has new responsibilities, some of which are enshrined in law, particularly with regard to the use of ionising radiation. The recent introduction of legal statutes in Europe requires radiologists to justify a procedure before using ionising radiation, and makes an offence to use ionising radiation when a non-ionising technique would provide comparable information. Although this statute might appear draconian, it reflects the development and availability of radiological techniques and changes of practice not imagined ten years ago. In the foreseeable future, clinicians ordering radiology are likely to be required to advise the patient of the expected radiation dose (and to justify this dose). Never has the need for evidence-based practice to be more closely applied, and for both radiologists and surgeons to undertake objective and trial-based evaluation of new procedures, been greater.

Further reading

Brandt MM, Wahl WL, Yeom K et al. Computed tomographic scanning reduces cost and time of complete spine evaluation. J Trauma 2004; 56:1022–6

Carlos RC, Axelrod DA, Ellis JH et al. Incorporating patient-centered outcomes in the analysis of cost-effectiveness: imaging strategies for renovascular hypertension. AJR Am J Roentgenol 2003; 181:1653–61

Dippel DW, Du Ry van Beest Holle M, van Kooten F, Koudstaal PJ. The validity and reliability of signs of early infarction on CT in acute ischaemic stroke. Neuroradiology 2000; 42:629–33

Dohrmann PJ. Low-cost teleradiology for Australia. Aust N Z J Surg 1991; 61:115–17

Dryver ET, Jernstrom H, Tompkins K et al. Follow-up of patients with Hodgkin's disease following curative treatment: the routine CT scan is of little value. Br J Cancer 2003; 89:482–6

Esses D, Birnbaum A, Bijur P et al. Ability of CT to alter decision making in elderly patients with acute abdominal pain. Am J Emerg Med 2004; 22:270–2

Fenton JJ, Deyo RA. Patient self-referral for radiologic screening tests: clinical and ethical concerns. J Am Board Fam Pract 2003; 16:494–501

Gilbert FJ, Grant AM, Gillan MG et al; Scottish Back Trial Group. Low back pain: influence of early MR imaging or CT on treatment and outcome – multicenter randomized trial. Radiology 2004; 231:343–51

Hare WS. Teleradiology. Aust N Z J Surg 1991; 61:89

Jithoo R, Govender PV, Corr P, Nathoo N. Telemedicine and neurosurgery: experience of a regional unit based in South Africa. J Telemed Telecare 2003; 9:63–6

Kalyanpur A, Weinberg J, Neklesa V et al. Emergency radiology coverage: technical and clinical feasibility of an international teleradiology model. Emerg Radiol 2003; 10:115–18

Kalyanpur A, Neklesa VP, Pham DT et al. Implementation of an international teleradiology staffing model. Radiology 2004; 232:415–19

Kelly RF, Tran T, Holmstrom A et al. Accuracy and cost-effectiveness of [18F]-2-fluoro-deoxy-D-glucose-positron emission tomography scan in potentially resectable non-small cell lung cancer. Chest 2004; 125:1413–23

Laroche C, Fairbairn I, Moss H et al. Role of computed tomographic scanning of the thorax prior to bronchoscopy in the investigation of suspected lung cancer. Thorax 2000; 55:359–63

McEwan CN, Fukuta K. Recent advances in medical imaging: surgery planning and simulation. World J Surg 1989; 13:343–8

Maskell NA, Gleeson FV, Davies RJ. Standard pleural biopsy versus CT-guided cutting-needle biopsy for diagnosis of malignant disease in pleural effusions: a randomised controlled trial. Lancet 2003; 19(361):1326–30

Renton J, Kincaid S, Ehrlich PF. Should helical CT scanning of the thoracic cavity replace the conventional chest x-ray as a primary assessment tool in pediatric trauma? An efficacy and cost analysis. J Pediatr Surg 2003; 38:793–7

Rosen MP, Siewert B, Sands DZ et al. Value of abdominal CT in the emergency department for patients with abdominal pain. Eur Radiol 2003; 13:418–24

Schoemaker D, Black R, Giles L, Toouli J. Yearly colonoscopy, liver CT, and chest radiography do not influence 5-year survival of colorectal cancer patients. Gastroenterology 1998; 114:7–14

Stormo A, Sollid S, Stormer J, Ingebrigtsen T. Teleconsultations in northern Norway. J Telemed Telecare 2004; 10:135–9

Szot A, Jacobson FL, Munn S et al. Diagnostic accuracy of chest X-rays acquired using a digital camera for low-cost teleradiology. Int J Med Inf 2004; 73:65–73

Tsushima Y, Endo K. Analysis models to assess cost effectiveness of the four strategies for the work-up of solitary pulmonary nodules. Med Sci Monit 2004; 10:65–72

Valk PE, Abella-Columna E, Haseman MK et al. Whole-body PET imaging with [18F]-fluorodeoxyglucose in management of recurrent colorectal cancer. Arch Surg 1999; 134:503–11

Plain radiography

K.L. Gormly, S.J. Neuhaus, P.G. Devitt, M. Thomas

INTRODUCTION

K.L. Gormly

The majority of radiological examinations involve the use of X-rays, which are a type of ionizing electromagnetic radiation. The production of the plain film is the simplest form and a brief description of the process of obtaining an image is described.

An X-ray tube consists of two electrodes within a vacuum. Electrons are emitted from a heated tungsten filament (cathode) and accelerated by a high potential difference (voltage) across the tube to hit a metal target in the anode. The sudden deceleration of the fast moving stream of electrons causes energy conversion, with 99% converted into heat, and 1% converted into X-rays. By using collimation and filtration, a relatively uniform beam of X-rays is emitted from the X-ray tube and passes through the patient.

The body consists of tissues of different density, thickness and atomic number and it is these factors that will affect the absorption of the X-ray beam as it travels through the patient. Reduction in the intensity of an X-ray beam as it passes through matter is termed attenuation. Differential absorption of X-rays by different tissues is reflected in the intensity of the beam leaving the patient, it continues on to the screen, carrying with it a 'memory' of the tissue through which it has passed. Once the X-rays reach the intensifying screen they are converted into light photons, which can be used to expose a conventional film. This film is developed and viewed, or converted into a latent image that is read by a laser beam, producing a signal that is processed and stored in a computer (digital radiography).

The exposure of an X-ray film produces blackening, with varying shades of grey produced by different intensities. For example, in an X-ray of a hand, the bone absorbs most of the X-rays, soft tissues only mildly attenuate the beam, and air surrounding the hand transmits the X-ray beam, resulting in an image with areas that are white, grey and black, respectively.

The beam emitted from an X-ray tube is cone shaped, and therefore any object within the beam will be magnified on the image. The greater the distance between the structure and the film, the greater will be the degree of magnification. This is shown by the difference between the PA and AP chest X-rays, where in a PA projection the anterior mediastinum sits almost against the plate, but in the AP projection it is further away from the plate and will be magnified. If an object sits obliquely within the beam it will be distorted due to unequal magnification, with the amount of distortion greatest at the edge of the film. This is seen on a lateral spine film, where the vertebral bodies at the superior and inferior aspects of the film often appear distorted. Due to these factors it is ideal to centre an image over the area of interest, and keep the structure as parallel to the beam as possible to minimise distortion.

Fluoroscopy is direct viewing of an X-ray image in real time. Initial fluoroscopes involved direct viewing of light emitted by a fluorescent screen. This was of extremely low intensity and required dark vision adaptation by the radiologist, who had to wear red goggles for 20–30 minutes prior to an examination. The development of the image intensifier (II), means the emitted light can be intensified to a level visible to normal photopic vision. Modern fluoroscopy units use a closed circuit TV chain, whereby the image can be seen on a monitor and captured on video. Focal spot images may also be obtained during the procedure.

THE CHEST RADIOGRAPH

S.J. Neuhaus

Background

The chest X-ray (CXR) has historically been one of the most frequently used forms of radiology. Because of the large amount of information that can be obtained from a CXR, it is important to have a systematic approach to its interpretation.

ANATOMY AND TYPES OF CHEST X-RAY

Anatomy

An understanding of the radiological anatomy of the chest is important if the radiograph is to be interpreted accurately. Key anatomical landmarks include the pleural fissures, diaphragm and outlines of the heart and major vessels (Figs 2.1 and 2.2).

AP versus PA films

The types of CXR available are:

- posteroanterior (PA)
- anteroposterior (AP)
- lateral
- lordotic
- tangential.

Posteroanterior films

Routine chest films are taken in PA and lateral positions. In the PA position the beam passes from back to front with the plate at the front of the patient. The patient is erect, with the elbows lifted to the side, moving the scapulae laterally. The anterior part of the patient is closest to the film resulting in relatively little magnification.

Anteroposterior films

AP films are generally used in trauma patients and for portable X-rays. The X-ray beam passes from front to back and the anterior structures such as the heart and anterior mediastinum are magnified as the diverging X-ray beam reaches the film. The patient is often sitting in a 'hunched' position and this can impede inspiration and 'crowd' the lung markings. AP films should be labelled as such, but can be identified by the fact that the scapula blade is projected over the lungs. The major disadvantages of the AP film are:

- Crowding of lung markings which may mimic pulmonary disease.
- The heart and mediastinum appear relatively larger, mimicking a widened mediastinum.
- If supine, air-fluid levels will not be apparent and pleural collections, e.g. a haemothorax, can be missed.

Lateral films

The majority of lesions are visible on the PA film. CT is frequently the most appropriate means of further evaluation. The main benefit of lateral films is in assessing the posterior pleural space and lobar collapse. Specific rib views can assist in assessing rib fractures, although the anterior rib is cartilaginous and not visible on plain films.

Lordotic films

These are occasionally used to obtain a better view of pathology in the apex of the lung as the clavicles are

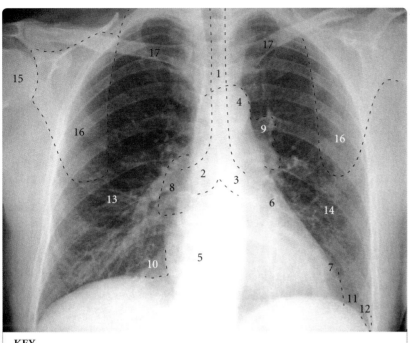

Fig. 2.1 Normal AP chest X-ray.

KEY

1	Trachea	10	Inferior vena cava
2	Right main bronchus	11	Cardiophrenic angle
3	Left main bronchus	12	Lateral costophrenic angle
4	Aortic arch (knuckle)	13	Right lung
5	Heart	14	Left lung
6	Left atrial appendage	15	Humerus
7	Left ventricular border	16	Scapula
8	Right pulmonary artery	17	Clavicle
9	Left pulmonary artery		

moved off the lung tissue by the projection. Lordotic films have now been largely been superseded by CT.

Tangential films

Tangential views are predominantly used for assessing the chest wall, in particular identification of foreign bodies.

SYSTEMATIC APPROACH TO THE CHEST RADIOGRAPH

The chest radiograph in surgical practice is usually undertaken to provide information about cardiorespi-

ratory comorbidity rather than an investigation into primary surgical disease. It is also often a routine first-line examination in the trauma patient. When looking at a CXR it is often easiest to divide the assessment into:

- mediastinum
- hilum
- lungs.

Box 2.1 is a guide to abnormalities that should be systematically looked for when assessing a CXR. More detail on the assessment of the mediastinum, hilum and lungs is provided below.

Fig. 2.2 Normal lateral chest X-ray.

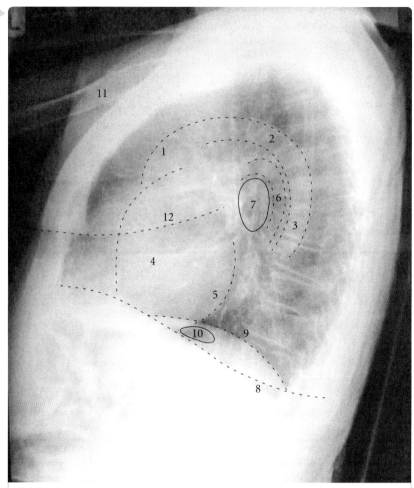

KEY

1	Ascending aorta	7	Left main bronchus
2	Aortic arch	8	Right hemidiaphragm
3	Descending thoracic aorta	9	Left hemidiaphragm
4	Heart	10	Gastric gas bubble
5	Left atrial border	11	Humeral shaft
6	Left main pulmonary artery	12	Lower border of arm

Mediastinal abnormalities

The right paratracheal stripe is the soft tissue between the trachea and right lung; it should measure less than 5 mm. If enlarged, this is usually due to lymphadenopathy. This should not be confused with the normal density due to the SVC and right brachiocephalic vein, which lie more anteriorly (Fig. 2.3).

Cardiac outline

The cardiac outline should normally occupy less than one half of the maximum diameter of the thoracic

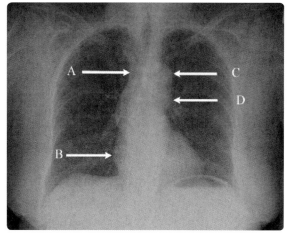

Fig. 2.3 A normal chest radiograph showing the SVC (A), border of the right atrium (B), aortic arch (C) and the pulmonary trunk (D).

cavity on CXR. This only applies to a PA film, as the cardiac outline will be variably enlarged on an AP view. Enlargement of the cardiac outline can be due to:

- cardiomegaly, e.g. cardiac failure
- distended pericardium, e.g. post-traumatic blood or pericarditis.

Great vessels
Enlargement of the outline of the great vessels can occur with:

- fusiform aneurysm (calcification may also be present)
- aortic dissection.

Widening of the mediastinum
Widening of the mediastinum following trauma usually indicates aortic trauma and is covered in Chapter 25. In a non-trauma setting the 'rule of T's' applies and the following conditions should be considered:

- teratoma
- thyroid mass (Fig. 2.4)
- thymic lesions
- 'terrible' lymphoma

Mediastinal air
The presence of air in the mediastinum is usually associated with trauma or oesophageal perforation (Chapter 11). Air might track up into the neck, where it can be detected most sensitively on a lateral cervical film. The presence of a concomitant pneumothorax should be looked for.

Hilar abnormalities
Enlargement of the hila
Bilateral hilar enlargement is most commonly due to an inflammatory condition, e.g. sarcoidosis (Fig. 2.5). Unilateral hilar enlargement is often more sinister, e.g. underlying carcinoma of the lung, metastases or lymphoma.

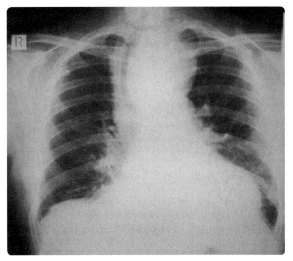

Fig. 2.4 A large retrosternal goitre with displacement of the trachea to the right.

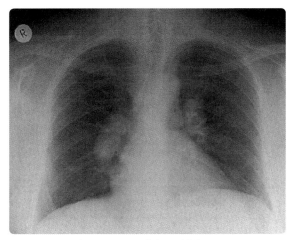

Fig. 2.5 CXR demonstrating bilateral hilar lymphadenopathy. This patient had sarcoidosis.

Table 2.1 'Things' causing alveoli to appear white in CXR	Substance	Suspect
	Water	Alveolar pulmonary oedema (cardiac failure, drowning or noxious gases) (Fig. 2.6)
	Pus	Pneumonia (Fig. 2.7)
	Blood	Trauma
	Tissue	Tumour (alveolar cell carcinoma)
	Protein	Alveolar proteinosis

Abnormalities of the lungs

Air spaces (alveoli)

Air spaces in the lungs normally appear 'black' but become whiter when the alveoli are filled with 'something'; examples are given in Table 2.1. This appears as 'consolidation' on the CXR, with white areas containing black air-bronchograms, representing the air-filled bronchi surrounded by alveoli full of 'something'.

Occasionally, the pattern of consolidation might suggest a diagnosis. Acute pulmonary oedema is classically perihilar, bilateral and symmetrical; features also seen in acute respiratory distress syndrome. Focal consolidation might be due to pneumonia, haematoma, pulmonary haemorrhage following pulmonary embolism or bronchoalveolar cell carcinoma. The same features are demonstrated on CT. As the imaging features are so non-specific, the patient's history and any other findings are crucial in determining the diagnosis.

Abnormal air distribution

Abnormalities of air distribution include bullae, diffuse hyperinflation, hypoinflation including poor respiratory effort and pneumothorax (Figs 2.8 and 2.9).

Bronchi and interstitium

Bronchi are usually too thin walled to be visible, except end-on, when they appear as thin-walled 'circles' approximately the same size as the adjacent blood vessel. Bronchi can become visible when dilated in bronchiectasis, or when the walls become thickened, for example in:

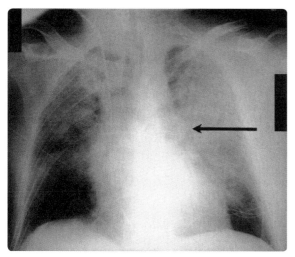

Fig. 2.6 Acute pulmonary oedema with air bronchograms visible in the left lung (arrow).

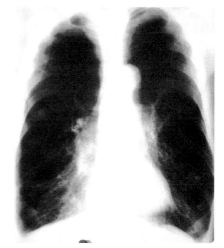

Fig. 2.8. Emphysema with bullae. The lungs are hyperinflated with depression of the diaphragms and large air-filled spaces (bullae) in the apices, devoid of vascular markings.

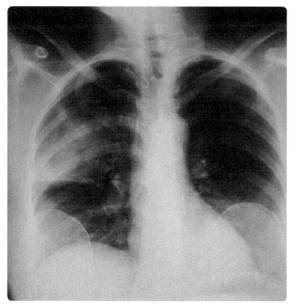

Fig. 2.7 Right upper lobe pneumonia. The patient also happens to have bilateral breast prostheses.

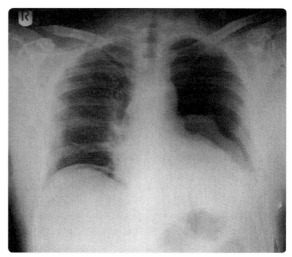

Fig. 2.9. A large left pneumothorax. This occurred after a laparoscopic fundoplication. Also note the free air under the right hemidiaphragm.

- acute inflammation (acute asthma, viral pneumonia)
- chronic inflammation (smoking, chronic bronchitis).

Interstitial septa become visible when thickened. Table 2.2 lists examples of materials that can cause this thickening.

A detailed description of interstitial lung disease is beyond the scope of this text. However, important conditions to include in the differential diagnosis of this radiological pattern are:

Table 2.2 Thickening of insterstitial septa

Material	Example
Water	Smooth thickening of interlobular septa in interstitial pulmonary oedema, e.g. Kerley B lines extending medially from the pleural surface
Tumour	Smooth or nodular thickening of interstitium due to lymphangitic spread of tumour (see lymphangitis carcinomatosis, below)
Fibrosis	Thickened interstitium with associated volume loss

- sarcoidosis
- collagen vascular disease
- intersitial pneumonia
- interstitial pulmonary oedema
- pneumoconiosis
- metastatic tumour.

Pulmonary vasculature

Vessels in the central two-thirds of the lungs can normally be clearly seen (see Fig. 2.3) and the upper lobe vessels are smaller than the lower lobe vessels when the patient is in the upright position. In acute pulmonary oedema there is increased distension of the upper lobe veins (evident on an erect film, as this is normal on a supine film).

Pulmonary vessels become blurred in conditions giving rise to increased interstitial opacity e.g. interstitial pulmonary oedema (see Fig. 2.6). Hypovascular areas due to pulmonary embolus are usually only identified in very large emboli, and even then changes might be subtle or absent. Occasionally there might be enlargement of the pulmonary artery central to the thrombus due to increased pressure. A normal chest X-ray does not exclude even a major pulmonary embolus.

CLINICAL SURGICAL PROBLEMS

- Pleural effusions.
- Atelectasis.
- Lymphangitis carcinomatosis.
- Pulmonary nodules.
- Trauma.
- Pneumothorax.
- Elevated hemidiaphragm.

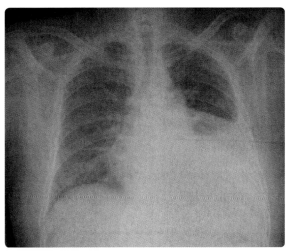

Fig. 2.10 A left side pleural effusion. The costophrenic angle has been blunted.

Pleural effusions

Fluid in the pleural cavity is usually recognised as homogeneous increased density with a characteristic meniscus and blunting of the costophrenic angles (Fig. 2.10). A lateral chest radiograph is more sensitive than a PA film as small amounts of fluid will collect posteriorly. Occasionally fluid will collect within the oblique fissure, giving a 'pseudotumour' appearance on the PA film, which is easily resolved on the lateral projection.

Loculation of pleural fluid is suggested by the presence of a convex border and a non dependant location. If suspected, this is best confirmed with ultrasound or CT.

Bilateral effusions

The most common cause of bilateral pleural effusions is cardiac failure. Other conditions to be considered include:

- hypoproteinaemia
- metastatic tumour
- collagen vascular disease
- ascites.

Unilateral effusion

There are multiple causes of unilateral pleural effusions. The important causes to identify in surgical practice include:

- pneumonia
- malignant disease (particularly carcinoma of the breast, ovary or lung)
- sympathetic effusion secondary to intra-abdominal disease (e.g. pancreatitis, subphrenic abscess)
- pulmonary embolus/infarction
- iatrogenic (e.g. leak from oesophageal anastomosis).

Atelectasis

Atelectasis is common in the postoperative patient. It ranges from linear bands of subsegmental atelectasis, to collapse of an entire lobe (Fig. 2.11). It appears as a

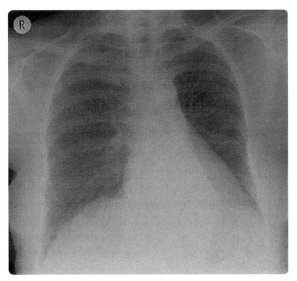

Fig. 2.11 CXR demonstrating left lower lobe collapse.

dense opacity with no air bronchograms. Secondary signs include shift of the hilum, elevation of the ipsilateral hemidiaphragm and shift of the mediastinum towards the side of collapse in severe cases. Collapse of the left upper lobe is hardest to identify as the lobe collapses against the anterior chest wall and gives only a subtle veiling opacity. Any evidence of a central obstructing foreign body or mass should be sought.

Lymphangitis carcinomatosis

Lymphangitis carcinomatosis is typically associated with carcinoma of the lung, breast and pancreas. The characteristic finding is thickened interstitial markings, which is best seen peripherally. In comparison with acute pulmonary oedema they are often unilateral and extend into the upper one third of the hemithorax. Early diagnosis of lymphangitis carcinomatosis is important as it indicates tumour dissemination and/or the need for chemotherapy.

Pulmonary nodules

Pulmonary nodules are classified as solitary or multiple. Multiple pulmonary nodules almost invariably represent metastatic tumour. However, solitary nodules can present a significant diagnostic challenge; 30% are malignant and suspicious factors include increasing size, lack of calcification and spiculation. Accurate CT density and volume measurements are increasingly used to assess pulmonary nodules.

The further investigation of a solitary lung nodule is outlined in Chapter 4. The most important diagnosis to exclude is bronchial carcinoma. Some of the differential diagnoses to consider are listed in Table 2.3. An important feature to look for is the presence of calcification. If present, this usually indicates a benign cause such as a calcified granuloma.

Trauma and the chest X-ray

The place of the radiograph in the assessment of chest trauma is detailed in Chapter 25. A normal chest X-ray does not exclude significant injury.

In one study of patients presenting to a major trauma centre, 29% of patients had significant chest injuries (most commonly pneumothorax, haemothorax, spinal and sternal injuries) that were not diagnosed on the plain chest X-ray. The current philosophy

Table 2.3 Examples of solitary pulmonary nodules

Cause	Example(s)
Congenital	Bronchogenic cyst
Vascular	Arteriovenous malformation, haematoma
Inflammatory	Tuberculosis, fungal infection (Fig. 2.12)
Immune disease	Wegener's granulomatosis
Tumour	Hamartoma, primary lung tumour, lymphoma or solitary metastasis

---

WHAT TO LOOK FOR — Box 2.2

on the CXR in suspected pneumothorax

- Radiolucent air peripherally, with loss of vascular markings
- White line indicating the visceral pleura
- Displacement of mediastinal structures (e.g. tracheal deviation)
- Associated injuries (e.g. fractured ribs) (Fig. 2.13)
- Associated sequelae of trauma (e.g. haemothorax, subcutaneous emphysema)

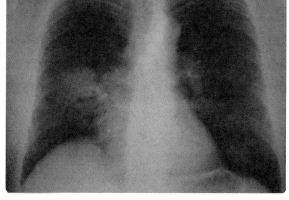

Fig. 2.12 A solitary pulmonary nodule in the right mid-zone in a 46-year-old man. This eventually proved to be inflammatory in origin.

is to perform a CT scan in patients who are thought to have significant chest injury.

Things that should be looked for specifically in immediate assessment of a trauma CXR include:

- pericardial effusion
- mediastinal widening (beware of the AP film)
- fractured ribs
- ruptured diaphragm
- haemopneumothorax (best seen on an erect film).

Pneumothorax

The most common cause of pneumothorax in a hospital environment is iatrogenic trauma (e.g. secondary to insertion of central lines). A small pneumothorax can easily be missed unless looked for carefully (Box 2.2). The sensitivity for detection of a small pneumothorax is greater with CT. This is generally not clinically relevant unless the patient is to undergo anaesthesia with intermittent positive pressure ventilation (IPPV).

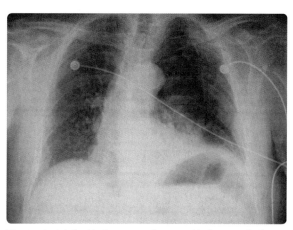

Fig. 2.13 A left sided pneumothorax with fractured ribs.

It must be emphasised that if the patient has any signs of a tension pneumothorax, a chest radiograph is not an appropriate investigation and will only delay treatment of what is a life-threatening emergency. The chest should be decompressed as an emergency procedure prior to obtaining radiological confirmation.

The occult pneumothorax

The increasing use of CT for the evaluation of blunt abdominal trauma has diagnosed undetected pneumothoraces in many patients. In one study, up to 8% of patients had a pneumothorax demonstrated on a CT scan that was not seen on the plain film. The clinical significance of the occult and asymptomatic pneumothorax is doubtful.

Elevated hemidiaphragm

An elevated hemidiaphragm might be secondary to trauma or to thoracic or abdominal pathology. If possible, a previous radiograph should be reviewed because it might be a longstanding finding. Phrenic nerve palsy resulting in paradoxical movement of the diaphragm with respiration occurs in up to 6% of the population.

Common causes of elevation of the diaphragm are listed in Table 2.4.

Ultrasound or CT might be required to further assess suspected thoracic or abdominal pathology.

SPECIFIC SURGICAL ISSUES

Value of the preoperative radiograph

The routine use of a preoperative chest X-ray in patients undergoing elective surgery is controversial. Several studies suggest that a routine X-ray is unlikely to influence the decision to operate or the choice of anaesthetic. In healthy women aged less than 60 undergoing standard surgery, the probability of a useful preoperative chest radiograph ranges from 0.2% to 3.5%. The probability increases in men or elderly subjects, in the presence of coexisting respiratory diseases, or in ASA class 3.

Routine chest X-ray in intensive care units

The use of routine daily chest X-rays is a widespread practice in many intensive care units. A review of this practice in surgical units found that only 12% (89 of 775) showed new findings, of which 3 of 89 (0.4% of all CXRs) had any potential clinical impact (pneumothorax in two, effusion in one). These data show that there is an extremely low yield of clinically significant and unsuspected new findings or device malposition on routine screening.

THE PLAIN ABDOMINAL RADIOGRAPH
P.G. Devitt, M. Thomas

Background

In everyday clinical practice the plain abdominal radiograph has been largely supplanted by ultrasound and CT. However, this investigation remains an important component of the management of many surgical conditions, particularly the patient with acute abdominal pain. In such circumstances the radiographs often vary in quality, might not be supervised by a radiologist and their interpretation will often be undertaken by a

Above the diaphragm	Diaphragmatic	Below the diaphragm
Phrenic nerve palsy (mediastinal tumour, iatrogenic)	Traumatic rupture	Subphrenic collection
Splinting secondary to trauma	Eventration	Other abdominal pathology, e.g. gaseous colonic distension
Pulmonary collapse/ consolidation	Hernia	

Table 2.4 Common causes of elevation of the diaphragm

junior member of the surgical team. However, much information can be obtained from the plain abdominal film, particularly when it is examined in a systematic manner.

In practice, the plain radiograph has most value in delineation of the conditions listed in Table 2.5.

To understand where the plain abdominal radiograph is of most use, it is necessary to appreciate what the investigation will and will not show. The investigation is best suited to show the extremes of tissue density, i.e. bone and air. If time, money and irradiation were no concern, then all the information that can be derived from the plain film could be gleaned from a CT scan. However, this is not practical in most surgical departments.

THE RADIOGRAPHIC PROJECTION AND ANATOMY

The typical plain abdominal radiograph is taken in the anterior-to-posterior projection, with the patient lying supine on the X-ray plate. In most adults the whole abdominopelvic cavity will not be displayed on a single film. The clinician must state what is required on the request form. Problems related to the genitourinary tract will require the pelvis to be seen clearly ('kidneys, ureters, bladder; KUB') (Fig. 2.14), whereas patients with upper abdominal problems will require an X-ray that includes views of the diaphragm. Sometimes it is most convenient to request a chest X-ray to obtain views of the diaphragm accompanied by an abdominal film showing the pelvis.

Traditionally, there are two components to plain imaging of the abdomen; the erect and the supine film. Whereas the erect view will show gas–fluid interfaces in patients with intestinal obstruction, it is doubtful that these views add much further useful diagnostic information to the supine film (see Chapter 10). If a pneumoperitoneum is suspected, free gas under the diaphragm is best seen on an erect radiograph of the chest or upper abdomen (Fig. 2.15). Lateral projections tend to be reserved for the study of ill patients, who are unable to sit or stand.

A SYSTEMATIC APPROACH TO THE PLAIN ABDOMINAL RADIOGRAPH

Preliminary inspection should include:

- name and age of patient
- orientation of film (erect, supine, lateral decubitus)
- extent of film (adult films will include full views of either the diaphragms or pelvis, but not both).

Although it is tempting to focus immediately on a particular part of the film, most is to be learned (or less is to be missed) if the observer examines each radiograph in a standard, systematic fashion.

First, the observer is advised to stand back from the viewing box and to absorb the radiograph as a whole. An organised examination of the radiograph is then undertaken. This involves the study of five components:

- bony structures
- soft tissue shadows
- gas patterns
- calcification
- miscellaneous.

Bony structures

The main objective in assessing the bony structures is to look for fractures, deformities and changes in bone density (either localised or generalised). In particular look at the:

Table 2.5 Abnormalities for which plain abdominal radiograph is most useful

Gas patterns	Calcified sites
In the gastrointestinal tract	Renal tract
In other structures (particularly the liver)	Vascular system
Outside the gastrointestinal tract (e.g. pneumoperitoneum)	Chronic infection (e.g. TB)
Changes in gas patterns with time	Biliary system

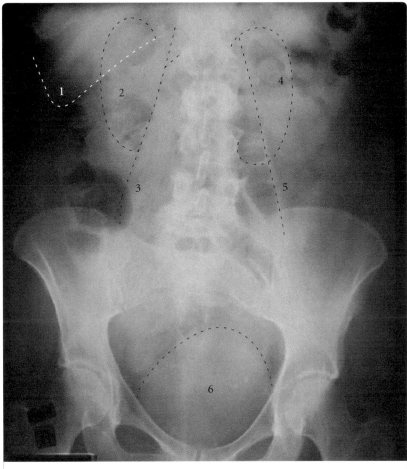

Fig. 2.14 Normal abdominal film demonstrating anatomical features of the soft tissue outlines.

KEY

1	Inferior liver edge	4	Left renal outline
2	Right renal outline	5	Left psoas shadow
3	Right psoas shadow	6	Bladder

- ribs and costal margins
- spine
- pelvis
- hip joints
- femoral necks and proximal shafts (Fig. 2.16).

Soft tissue shadows

This is the most difficult and unreliable part of interpretation of the plain abdominal radiograph. Soft tissue densities constitute a 'grey zone' and structures of interest are often obscured by overlying gas shadows.

Abnormal masses might be visible as a soft tissue density or be evident by displacement of (gas filled) loops of intestine. Assessment should include the:

- kidneys
- liver, spleen
- psoas muscles (Fig. 2.17)
- (full) bladder (Fig. 2.18)
- (full) stomach.

In gross ascites there is a generalised increase in density in the region of the peritoneal cavity. The inferior liver

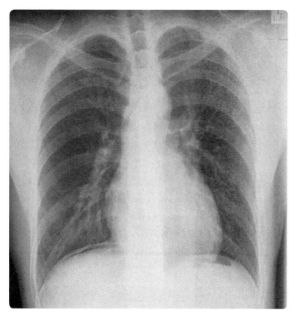

Fig. 2.15 Free gas under the right hemidiaphragm in a 22-year-old man with a perforated duodenal ulcer.

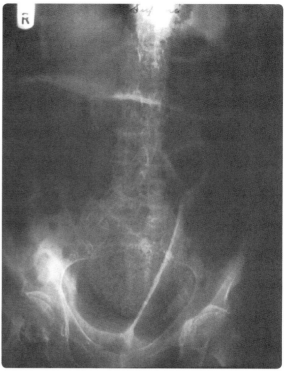

Fig. 2.16 A fractured neck of the right femur nearly missed in a patient who presented with abdominal pain and constipation. The patient had developed pseudo-obstruction secondary to the fracture.

edge will not be seen because it has fluid rather than fat next to it. The bladder is often seen as a compressed structure within the pelvis with a fat plane over the dome of the bladder, between it and the ascitic fluid.

Gas patterns

The presence of normal or abnormal gas patterns is one of the most valuable aspects of a plain radiograph. Gaseous distension of small and large bowel produces characteristic radiological appearances. This is discussed further in Chapter 10. Gas in a structure other than the gut might indicate a fistulous communication with the gut or the presence of gas-forming organisms (Box 2.3).

Free intraperitoneal air Large volumes of air in the peritoneal cavity are usually clearly evident on the erect plain radiograph or lateral decubitus film. A number of more subtle findings can be seen with smaller volumes of air. It is also possible to accurately diagnose pneumoperitoneum on a supine film if it is carefully looked for. Some of these signs are of esoteric interest only but are listed in Table 2.6.

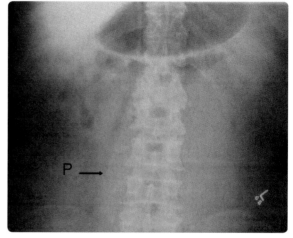

Fig. 2.17 Obliteration of the lateral margin of the left psoas muscle in a patient with a leaking abdominal aortic aneurysm. The lateral margin of the right psoas muscle is identified (P).

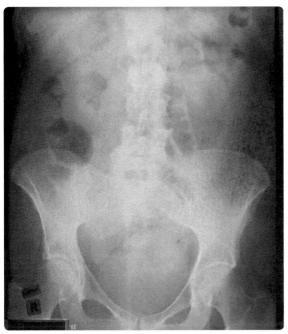

Fig. 2.18 A full bladder outlined on a plain abdominal radiograph.

WHAT TO LOOK FOR	Box 2.3

Gas in the plain abdominal radiograph

Normal distribution
- Stomach
- Small intestine (small volumes)
- Colon and rectum

Abnormal distribution
- Obstruction:
  - proximal distension (Fig. 2.19)
  - distal absence of gas (Fig. 2.20)
  - narrowing of gut lumen
- Within structures outside the gut:
  - biliary tree
  - portal vein
  - liver
  - bladder
  - wall of the intestine
  - peritoneal cavity
  - retroperitoneum
  - abscess cavity

Table 2.6 Signs of pneumoperitoneum visible on a supine abdominal radiograph

Bowel	Right upper quadrant	Peritoneal ligament
Rigler's sign (bowel wall highlighted due to presence of gas on both sides of wall)	Gas in Morrison's pouch (subhepatic triangular lucency)	Football sign (upper abdominal lucency transected by falciform ligament, resembling a football)
Triangle sign (gas trapped between three adjacent loops of bowel or two loops and parietal peritoneum)	Ovoid lucency in the right upper quadrant (highlighted by the homogenous nature of the liver)	Lateral umbilical ligaments, visualised as an inverted 'V'
	Liver edge silhouette (crescentic shadow)	Urachus sign (density between umbilicus and bladder)
	Ligamentum teres (slit-like lucency of trapped air along line of liver fissure)	

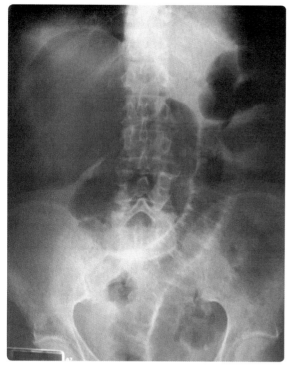

Fig. 2.19 Abnormal gas pattern of dilated caecum and small bowel caused by a band adhesion obstructing the transverse colon.

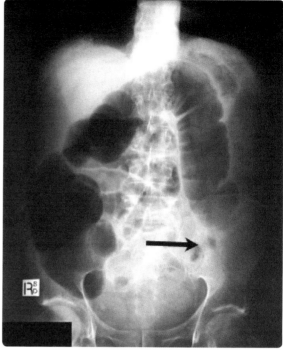

Fig. 2.20 An obstructing carcinoma of the sigmoid colon. There is an abrupt cut-off in intestinal gas at this point, with very little gas in the sigmoid and rectum. The tumour is identified by the abnormal gas pattern (arrow).

Rigler's sign is only evident with 750–1000 mL of air and may be simulated by two adjacent loops or a fat pad between loops (Fig. 2.21). The triangle sign is more sensitive. Anterior peritoneal ligament signs are only seen with massive pneumoperitoneum. The ligamentous teres fissure sign is relatively insensitive as the X-ray beam runs parallel to the fissure.

A chest radiograph is more sensitive than the erect abdominal radiograph in the detection of free gas. If radiological confirmation of free gas is important, the sensitivity of the investigation is greatly increased by placing the patient in the left lateral position (i.e. right side up) for 20 minutes, then upright for 10 minutes. This will encourage any free air to move to the right side of abdomen and then up under the right hemidiaphragm, where it will be more easily seen against the homogenous liver. By careful attention to technique, it is possible to detect as little as 1–2 mL of free gas on plain films. If the patient is too unwell to sit upright,

a left lateral decubitus film can be diagnostic. In this position the free gas is visualised between the liver and the lateral abdominal wall.

Signs suggestive of free intraperitoneal gas can be confused with:

- bowel gas shadow under the diaphragm (Fig. 2.22)
- subphrenic fat (1% patients), peripherally but not below the dome
- basal lung linear atelectasis
- translucent fat pad on decubitus film
- large amount of subserosal fat
- giant diverticula appearing as gas shadow (Fig. 2.23).

Gas within the retroperitoneum can be easily distinguished from intraperitoneal gas as it outlines the kidneys and tracks along the psoas muscles.

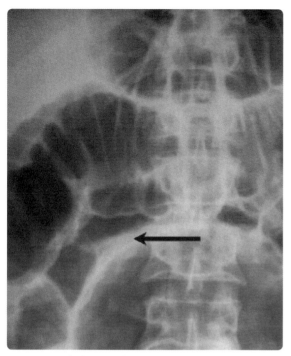

Fig. 2.21 Rigler's sign. The radiograph shows free gas between the loops of bowel (arrow). Gas is visible on both sides of the bowel wall.

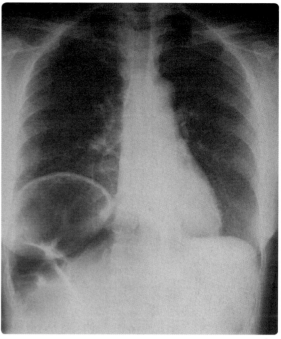

Fig. 2.22 Apparent free gas under the right hemidiaphragm. Closer inspection shows that the gas is contained with loops of bowel.

Air in the biliary tree Air in the biliary tree is often an incidental finding in patients who have undergone insertion of a biliary stent or formation of a chole-dochoenterostomy. It is an occasional finding in patients with small bowel obstruction and can suggest a fistulous communication between the gall bladder and intestine particularly if large stones can be seen (Figs 2.24 and 2.25). Air in the biliary tree is also seen in acute cholangitis (see Chapter 12).

Portal venous gas Portal venous gas can be seen as branching lucencies in the liver and is usually periph-eral following the flow of the portal venous blood (Fig. 2.26). This is in contrast to gas in the biliary tree, which is more prominent centrally (see Figs 2.24 and 2.25).

Calcification

Calcification in sites other than bone (ectopic calcifi-cation) is a common finding on a plain abdominal radiograph. Calcification is a frequent sequela of many degenerative and chronic healing conditions. This is particularly the case in older patients and those from parts of the world where diseases such as tuber-culosis and hydatid are endemic. Whereas most foci of calcification will be incidental and can be ignored, some may deserve further thought. These include:

- renal tract stones (long-standing obstruction and renal failure)
- gall bladder (increased risk of malignancy)
- abdominal aortic aneurysm (risk of rupture).

Calcification can be classified pathologically as out-lined in Table 2.7.

Miscellanous

See Table 2.8.

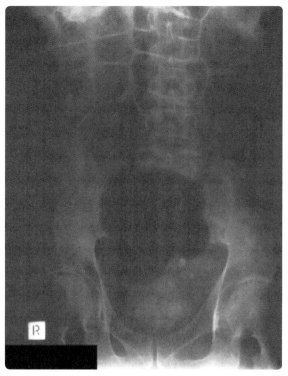

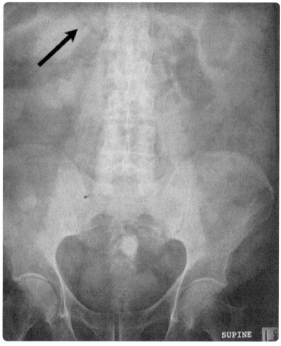

Fig. 2.24 Gas in the biliary tree (arrow) and a laminated gallstone. This patient has a biliary fistula.

Fig. 2.23 A large collection of apparently free air in the lower abdomen. A contrast study showed this to be a giant sigmoid diverticulum.

Table 2.7 Pathological classification of calcifications

Cause	Example(s)
Congenital	Medullary sponge kidney
Degenerative	Aorta Visceral vessels (e.g. splenic artery) (Fig. 2.27) Pelvic veins (phleboliths) Fibroids
Chronic inflammation	Pancreatitis Porcelain gall bladder (Chapter 12)
Chronic infection	Tuberculosis Hydatid Biliary and renal tract stones (Fig. 2.28)
Metabolic	Gallstones Renal tract stones
Neoplasia	Dermoid cyst (Fig. 2.29)
Miscellaneous	Appendicolith (Fig. 2.30)

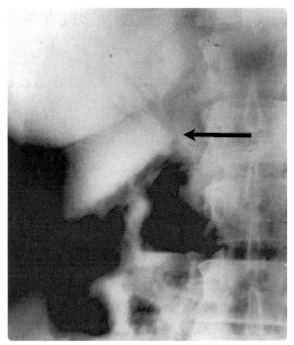

Fig. 2.25 Gas in the biliary tree. The common bile duct (arrow) and main ducts are outlined. The patient had undergone a biliary–enteric anastomosis.

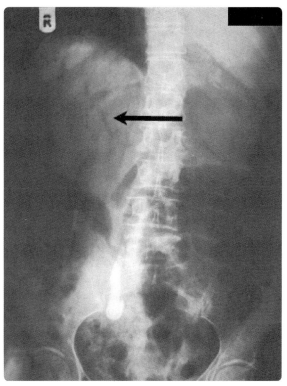

Fig. 2.26 Gas in the portal vein associated with ischaemic gut. Gas in the portal venous system tends to be peripheral in comparison with the more central distribution of gas in the biliary tree. This patient succumbed to overwhelming sepsis and at autopsy the portal vein (arrow) was found to be full of gas.

Table 2.8 Miscellaneous objects on the abdominal radiograph

Iatrogenic	Patient-related	Intraluminal	Missiles
Stents (vascular, biliary, gut)	Buttons, etc.	Rectum	Shrapnel
Clips	Piercings	Stomach	Bullets (Fig. 2.31)
Nasogastric tubes		Bladder	Nails or staples from power tools
Overlying lines, e.g. ECG leads		Uterus	

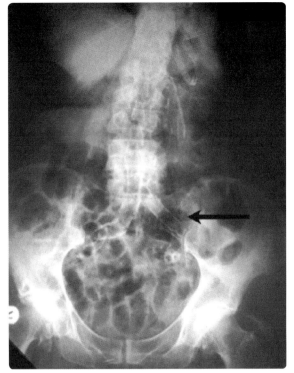

Fig. 2.27 Widespread arterial calcification in an elderly patient. The calcified iliac vessels (arrow) are particularly noticeable.

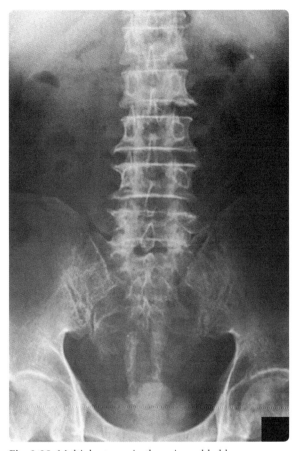

Fig. 2.28 Multiple stones in the urinary bladder.

SPECIFIC SURGICAL USES OF THE PLAIN ABDOMINAL RADIOGRAPH

The emergency department

The mainstay of the plain film has been its use in the emergency department in the management of the patient with acute abdominal pain. For a number of reasons, this is changing. First, there is a relatively poor rate of diagnostic return. This is probably through overuse of the investigation to include most patients attending with acute abdominal pain. At least 20% of patients attending the emergency department with abdominal pain are discharged with a diagnosis of non-specific pain. A selective approach to the use of the plain radiograph is likely to have better yields. For example, specific radiological findings are most unlikely in acute appendicitis and the finding of an appendicolith or localised ileus must be considered fortuitous rather than diagnostic. A plain radiograph is most unlikely to provide any useful

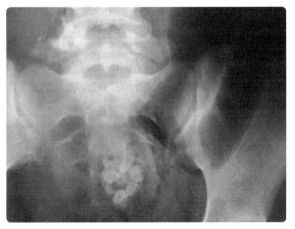

Fig. 2.29 A young woman with an ovarian dermoid cyst. Teeth can be seen within the cyst.

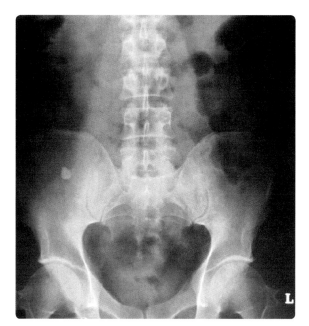

Fig. 2.30 A young man with appendicitis and an appendicolith visible on the plain radiograph.

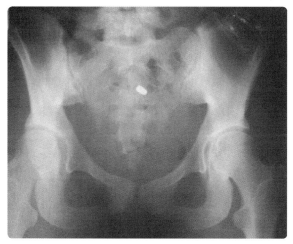

Fig. 2.31 Missile injury. The point of entry was well away from the site where this missile eventually lodged. The plain radiograph served to help guide the surgeons where to look for the bullet.

information in patients whose acute abdominal pain is the result of inflammation, whereas conditions in which the pain is due to gaseous distension of the gut might well have diagnostic features visible on the abdominal X-ray.

Another reason for the diminishing importance of the plain abdominal radiograph in the emergency department is the increasing availability of ultrasound and CT. As discussed in the chapters on biliary disease and acute abdominal pain, these two modalities can be highly sensitive and specific in the diagnosis of some of the common problems seen in emergency departments, such as gallstone disease and renal tract stone disease.

A plain radiograph should be considered in the initial management of:

- suspected intestinal perforation (see Chapter 10)
- intestinal obstruction (see Chapter 10)
- missile injuries (see Fig. 2.31).

Obstruction and perforation

A plain radiograph does not diagnose intestinal obstruction. It merely confirms a clinical suspicion. The dilated loops of intestine might be the result of ileus rather than mechanical obstruction, and the distinction between the two conditions is made on clinical and not radiological grounds. The role of the plain radiograph in cases of intestinal obstruction is to:

- define the site and extent of any obstruction
- observe the changes in the degree of obstruction with time.

The assessment of the site of intestinal obstruction, and whether the obstruction is complete or incomplete, should be a clinical one backed up with radiological investigation. The plain radiograph may be supplemented by a contrast study or CT (see Chapter 10). Plain abdominal film features of bowel obstruction are usually chararacteristic. This topic is covered in detail in Chapter 10.

SUMMARY

In summary, given the availability of ultrasound and CT and their increasing use, the value of the plain abdominal radiograph will diminish. However, used appropriately, this simple and cheap radiological investigation will continue to help the surgeon with the initial management of many patients, particularly when resources are limited and expert advice is not close at hand.

Further reading

Ahn SH, Mayo-Smith WW, Murphy BL et al. Acute nontraumatic abdominal pain in adult patients: abdominal radiography compared with CT evaluation. Radiology 2002; 225:159–64

Bouillot JL, Fingerhut A, Paquet JC et al. Are routine preoperative chest radiographs useful in general surgery? A prospective, multicentre study in 3959 patients. Eur J Surg 1996; 162:597–604

Curry TS, Dowdey JE, Murray RC. Christensen's physics of diagnostic radiology, 4th edn. Lea & Febiger, Philadelphia, 1990

Farr RF, Allisy-Roberts PJ. Physics for medical imaging. WB Saunders, London, 1998

Feyler S, Williamson V, King D. Plain abdominal radiographs in acute medical emergencies: an abused investigation? Postgrad Med J 2002; 78:94–6

Flower CDR, Verschakelen JA. The diaphragm. In: Grainger RG, Allison D (eds) Grainger and Allison's diagnostic radiology: a textbook of medical imaging, 3rd edn. Churchill Livingstone, London, 1997, p 270–7

Hill SL, Edmisten T, Holtzman G, Wright A The occult pneumothorax: an increasing diagnostic entity in trauma. Am Surg 1999; 65:254–8

Ikezoe J, Godwin JD, Hunt KJ, Marglin SI. Pulmonary lymphangitic carcinomatosis: chronicity of radiographic findings in long-term survivors. AJR 1995; 165:49–52

Kerr IH. The preoperative chest X-ray. Br J Anaesth 1974; 46:558–63

Millar WT. Introduction to clinical radiology. Macmillan, New York, 1982

Nagurney JT, Brown DF, Novelline RA et al. Plain abdominal radiographs and abdominal CT scans for nontraumatic abdominal pain-added value? Am J Emerg Med 1999; 17:668–71

No authors listed. Preoperative chest radiology. National study by the Royal College of Radiologists. Lancet 1979 14 2(8133):83–6

Oikarinen H, Paivansalo M, Tikkakoski T, Saarela A. Radiological findings in biliary fistula and gallstone ileus. Acta Radiol 1996; 37:917–22

Rao PM, Rhea JT, Rao JA, Conn AK. Plain abdominal radiography in clinically suspected appendicitis: diagnostic yield, resource use, and comparison with CT. Am J Emerg Med 1999; 17:325–8

Robinson PJ, Wilson D, Coral A et al. Variation between experienced observers in the interpretation of accident and emergency radiographs. Br J Radiol 1999; 72:323–30

Silverstein DS, Livingston DH, Elcavage J et al. The utility of routine daily chest radiography in the surgical intensive care unit. J Trauma 1993; 35:643–6

Silvestri L, Maffessanti M, Gregori D et al. Usefulness of routine pre-operative chest radiography for anaesthetic management: a prospective multicentre pilot study. Eur J Anaesthesiol 1999; 16:749–60

Suri S, Gupta S, Sudhakar PJ et al. Comparative evaluation of plain films, ultrasound and CT in the diagnosis of intestinal obstruction. Acta Radiol 1999; 40:422–8

Tan BB, Flaherty KR, Kazerooni EA, Iannettoni MD. The solitary pulmonary nodule. Chest 2003; 123(1 Suppl):89S–96S

Triebel HJ, Jessel A, Reuter M. Roentgenologic diagnosis and differential diagnosis of carcinomatous lymphangiosis of the lungs. Rontgenblatter 1987; 40:57–63

Contrast studies 3

K.L. Gormly, M. Gabb

INTRODUCTION

K.L. Gormly

Background

Historically, contrast media were limited to investigation using X-ray and fluoroscopy. Recent advances in imaging have led to the development of contrast agents for CT, ultrasound and MRI. In addition, new contrast agents are now available with tissue-specific contrast enhancement capability.

IODINATED CONTRAST AGENTS

Iodine is the most useful element for providing radio-opacity in radiological examinations and is used for X-ray, fluoroscopic and CT procedures. It can be injected intra-arterially, intravenously, or into any orifice. Initial ionic iodinated contrast agents have a higher risk of allergic reaction and renal nephrotoxicity, compared with the newer low-osmolar and iso-osmolar non-ionic iodinated contrast media (Table 3.1).

Clearance

Intravenous contrast is cleared rapidly by the kidneys, with approximately 50% excreted within 2 hours, 75% within 4 hours and 98% within 24 hours in patients with normal renal function. Less than 1% is normally excreted by extrarenal routes such as the biliary system. Accumulation of large amounts of contrast in the gall-bladder should prompt checking of renal function.

Allergic reactions

There is a risk of allergic reaction to iodine based contrast agents, which is increased in patients with known iodine allergy and asthma. Anaphylactoid contrast reactions range from urticaria and itching to severe bronchospasm, cardiovascular collapse and potential death. Commonly seen dose-related reactions include nausea and vomiting. In patients with previous moderate or severe reaction, intravascular injection is contraindicated. Patients with asthma or previous mild urticaria should be premedicated with steroids for 12 hours.

Nephrotoxicity

Contrast-induced nephrotoxicity is a significant problem in patients with pre-existing renal impairment, with an incidence of 12–27% in prospective trials. It is usually self-limiting, resolving in 1–2 weeks, but increases the risk of developing severe non-renal complications and extended hospital stay. Checking the patient's serum creatinine before intravascular injection of contrast, and avoiding contrast adminis-

Table 3.1 Iodinated contrast media

	Compound	Trade name
Ionic (high osmolar)	Metrizoate	Isopaque 350®
	Diatrizoate	Urografin®
	Diatrizoate	Gastrografin®
Non-ionic monomer (low osmolar)	Iohexol	Omnipaque®
	Iopromide	Ultravist®
	Iopamidol	Isovue®
	Ioversol	Optiray®
Non-ionic dimer (iso-osmolar)	Iodixanol	Visipaque®
	Iotrolan	Isovist®

Table 3.2 MRI contrast agents

	Compound	Trade name
IV and extracellular	Gadolinium chelates	Magnevist®
Reticuloendothelial specific	Superparamagnetic iron oxide	Resovist®
Hepatocyte specific	Mangafodipir trisodium	Teslascan®
	Gadobenate dimeglumine	MultiHance®

tration in patients with poor renal function is recommended. Adequate hydration of patients will also decrease the risk. In diabetic patients on metformin, contrast-induced nephrotoxicity can lead to accumulation of biguanide within the tissues, and development of potentially fatal lactic acidosis. Metformin should therefore be ceased for 48 hours following contrast injection and renal function rechecked prior to restarting.

NON-IODINATED CONTRAST AGENTS

Barium sulphate

This lipid-soluble contrast agent is used for gastrointestinal procedures. Allergic reactions are very rare but have been reported in the literature.

MRI contrast agents

Gadolinium chelates have an intravascular and extra-cellular distribution similar to iodine. Allergic reactions are rare and there is no cross-reactivity between iodine allergy and reaction to gadolinium.

Tissue specific contrast agents include superparamagnetic iron oxide particles, taken up by the reticuloendothelial system and mangafodipir trisodium, a manganese chelate with hepatocyte biliary uptake and excretion (Table 3.2).

Ultrasound contrast agents

Microbubbles

Microbubbles are intravenous contrast agents comprising gas (air or perfluorocarbon) stabilised by denatured albumin, phospholipids, surfactant or cyanoacrylate, e.g. Levovist®, Sonovist® (Table 3.3). Some agents have a hepatosplenic specific parenchymal phase and can be used for liver imaging. Allergic reactions are rare.

CLINICAL APPLICATIONS AND SAFETY CONSIDERATIONS

Biliary procedures (ERCP, cholangiogram, T-tubogram)

Biliary procedures generally use ionic iodinated contrast. Although renal excretion of contrast following

ERCP has been documented, and several sensitivity reactions have been described, the risk of reaction is much lower than for intravascular injection. In a patient with a history of severe allergic reaction to intravascular iodine or asthma, it might be prudent to use non-ionic iodinated contrast to decrease the risk even further. Some clinicians will also premedicate the patient with oral steroids.

Intravenous cholangiography uses iodinated contrast such as Biligrafin®. Contrast is administered both orally and intravenously. Biliary contrast agents stimulate gall bladder contraction. They should be given after fasting to reduce enterohepatic circulation. Allergic reactions have been described and can be severe. These agents require a functioning liver to concentrate the contrast. They are therefore not used in the presence of jaundice.

Gastrointestinal procedures (swallow, meal, small bowel series, enema)

Barium is the most frequently used contrast agent, but is generally avoided if there is a risk of leak into the peritoneal cavity. Gastrografin® is the agent of choice in the clinical setting of perforation. The hyperosmolarity of Gastrografin® induces a chemical pneumonitis and so should be avoided if there is risk of aspiration. This property is utilised in paediatric enemas to both diagnose and treat meconium plug syndrome.

Urological procedures

Direct visualisation: cystogram, nephrostogram, retrograde pyelogram

Ionic iodinated contrast such as Urografin® is the contrast of choice.

Indirect visualisation: intravenous urogram

As this involves intravenous injection non-ionic iodinated contrast is used to minimse the risk of reaction and renal nephrotoxicity.

Computed tomography

Oral contrast

A dilute barium or iodinated contrast agent is generally used to opacify the bowel (see Chapter 4), although with the advent of multislice CT, many centres are now using water as an oral contrast agent instead. While there is a debatable benefit of using oral contrast in the trauma patient, elective scans of the abdomen and pelvis do benefit from the use of some form of oral contrast. There is a theoretical risk of anaphylactic reaction to iodine absorbed from the gastrointestinal tract, however only two cases have been reported.

Intravenous contrast

Intravenous contrast uses non-ionic iodinated contrast. For concerns regarding contrast allergy, renal failure and potentially fatal lactic acidosis in patients on metformin, see above.

Magnetic resonance imaging

Intravenous gadolinium chelates are the most frequently used contrast agent and have a low risk of reaction (see Chapter 5). They can also be used for MR angiography. There is no cross-reactivity with iodinated contrast. Newer tissue-specific contrast agents are constantly developing (Table 3.2).

Use	Compound	Trade name
Vascular	Air	Levovist®
	Sulphur hexafluoride	Sonovue®
Liver specific	Air	Levovist®
	Air	Sonavist®

Table 3.3 Microbubble ultrasound contrast agents

Conventional Angiography

Intra-arterial and intravenous injections use non-ionic iodinated contrast. In the setting of contrast allergy or renal impairment it is possible to use carbon dioxide (see Chapter 21). Investigation is continuing into the use of gadolinium, but this is not currently recommended. Intra-arterial injection is more nephrotoxic than intravenous injection.

GASTROINTESTINAL CONTRAST STUDIES

M. Gabb

Background

Contrast studies typically refer to the use of a contrast agent with plain film radiography or fluoroscopy. The double-contrast study has historically been the investigation of choice to provide information on mucosal patterns and pathology. In this context, current endoscopic and CT scanning practices have tended to relegate the contrast study to a back-up role. However, contrast studies still have an important role in the assessment of patients with suspected obstruction or perforation. Whereas contrast studies are increasingly combined with CT scanning, this section of the chapter covers the conventional planar imaging procedures used to examine the digestive tract.

CONTRAST MATERIALS

A number of different contrast agents can be used in gastrointestinal studies. Contrast can be administered orally, rectally or via a stoma. Single-agent contrast can be used, although it is more common to use a 'double-contrast' technique by combination with a negative contrast agent such as air (see below). Single-contrast studies with barium or iodine are more likely to be used when perforation is suspected or when anatomical detail is of secondary importance, such as where the study is used to confirm small or large bowel obstruction.

For an optimum study the choice of contrast will vary with the clinical situation. For example, barium is viscous and will stick to serosal surfaces, so is not the agent of choice if there is intestinal perforation (see below).

Barium

Modern barium sulphate products are formulated for use in specific situations. The larger the particle size, the more rapid the sedimentation and barium of relatively large particle size is favoured for procedures with a short examination time (e.g. oesophagogram). For examination of the small and large bowel, a smaller barium particle is used. This is more likely to remain in suspension for the duration of a longer examination and produce a homogenous pattern to the contrast material. Barium is lipid soluble and sticks to the mucosa, providing good mucosal definition.

Allergic reactions to barium sulphate preparations are rare, although they have been reported. Oral barium can lead to constipation and in an effort to avoid this, patients are recommended to increase their water intake following a procedure.

Barium should be avoided if there is a plan to proceed directly to surgery or if there is evidence of free intestinal perforation, to avoid abdominal contamination with lipid-soluble contrast material.

Iodine

Iodine-based contrast agents are water soluble and are preferred when there is a possible or proven perforation of the digestive tract. The most commonly used iodinated agent in gastrointestinal contrast studies is Gastrografin®, which is a high osmolar, ionic compound. In other circumstances the hygroscopic and irritant effects of Gastrografin® may be used to stimulate small bowel peristaltic activity (see Chapter 10) but fluid shifts into the bowel lumen can induce serious hypovolaemic changes, particularly in children and infants. These same properties mean that Gastrografin® must be used with care if aspiration is a possibility as it can spread rapidly in the bronchial tree to dependent portions of the lungs, where it may cause pulmonary oedema and chemical pneumonitis.

Negative agents

Gas and air are negative contrast agents, which may be useful by themselves, but are more frequently used in conjunction with positive contrast agents to perform a 'double-contrast' examination. The aim of a double-contrast study is to thinly coat the mucosal surface with a positive contrast agent such as barium, with additional gaseous distension enabling mucosal surface details to be more clearly visualised. Air (swallowed or by insufflation) or carbon dioxide (produced from interaction of an alkali and a food acid) can be used to produce a double-contrast study.

CONTRAST PROCEDURES

Upper digestive tract series

Examination of the upper tract includes a contrast swallow and meal. Although the barium meal has been largely replaced by endoscopy for assessment of ulcer disease and malignancy, barium swallow may still be used in the primary assessment of dysphagia (see Chapter 11).

Contrast swallow

The contrast swallow is particularly useful for the assessment of motility disorders and deglutition, and is often used in conjunction with a speech pathologist in the assessment of postoperative patients. A swallow is best performed with the patient in the erect position, using barium. It is particularly important to avoid Gastrografin® if there is a risk of aspiration (see above). Double-contrast studies are used in the setting of possible malignancy, whereas single-contrast studies are used for obstruction, motility disorders and the assessment of anastomotic integrity following surgery. In possible oesophageal perforation a water-soluble agent is usually used initially, although if no obvious leak is seen, small volumes of barium will provide better opacification. Box 3.1 outlines the features to look out for.

Contrast meal

A double-contrast meal for assessment of the gastric mucosa uses gas as a negative contrast agent, and the stomach is imaged in various positions to avoid blind spots from pools of contrast. This examination includes visualisation of the proximal duodenum. If a meal is performed to assess gastric outlet obstruction, a single agent is used, usually barium because of the potential risk of vomiting and aspiration.

 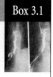

WHAT TO LOOK FOR Box 3.1

on the contrast swallow —

- Luminal narrowing:
  - benign type (long, smooth tapered ends)
  - malignant type (irregular, ulcerating)
- Mucosal abnormality:
  - ulceration
  - varices
- Fistula
- Contrast leak

Small bowel series

The small bowel is assessed by barium. A traditional small bowel follow through involves oral ingestion of barium and assessment as it transits through the small bowel. Enteroclysis (small bowel enema) involves insertion of a nasojejunal tube and injection of barium and methyl cellulose to produce a double contrast examination. The various merits of these two examinations are debated by radiologists and largely depend on local expertise and preferences.

The small bowel contrast examination is helpful in the detection and assessment of:

- mucosal disease, e.g. coeliac disease, gluten enteropathy and ischaemia
- developmental and acquired abnormalities, e.g. bands, malrotation, diverticula
- mass lesions, e.g. tumours, intussusception, Crohn's disease.

The examination will provide information on the mucosal pattern of the bowel and any focal lesions, which are recorded on spot films. Normal jejunal mucosa is 'feathery' whereas ileal mucosa is much smoother. The examination also includes observations regarding motility and pliability. This latter aspect involves observing the motion of the bowel on fluoroscopy, rather than relying on spot films. Pliability relates to the inherent softness of normal tissues which can be deliberately deformed by compression, but

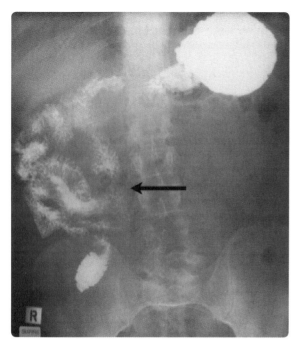

Fig. 3.1 Malrotation of the small bowel. The duodenojejunal flexure (arrow) is to the right of the midline. This abnormality was only found after a colonoscopy revealed the caecum to be lying in the right upper quadrant.

regain normal shape on release of the compression. A stiffened, infiltrated segment loses its compressibility and pliability.

In the adult, congenital structural abnormalities of the small bowel are not common and are usually incidental findings (see Fig. 3.1, Box 3.2).

Large bowel contrast studies

Large bowel contrast studies are performed as either a double-contrast study for the assessment of the bowel mucosa, or as a single-contrast enema in the setting of obstruction or suspected perforation.

Double-contrast barium enema (DCBE)

Before the 1950s, single-contrast studies were routinely used. Double-contrast studies using both barium and air have shown superiority in the detailed examination of the colon. Preliminary preparation of the colon by means of low residue diets and laxatives is required to remove faecal material. A rectal tube is inserted and barium is run in under pressure of gravity. In order to coat the entire colon it is necessary for the patient to be continent, and to be able to roll around on the narrow X-ray table to aid the flow of barium through the colon to the caecum. The procedure is difficult to perform adequately in the obese, immobile, acutely unwell, uncooperative or incontinent patient. The positive contrast is then drained and the bowel insufflated with air. These are dynamic investigations which are assessed while the images are being obtained using fluoroscopy. Multiple films are taken in different positions to ensure adequate bowel visualisation. As barium tends to pool in the dependant portions, acquiring images in supine and both decubitus positions helps to decrease the number of blind spots. If a patient has a very redundant colon it is necessary to take a number of images in different positions in an attempt to unwind the bowel and minimise overlapping loops.

Advances in endoscopic techniques and CT scanning have relegated this modality to a more supportive role. However, the barium enema is a cost-effective procedure and does not require any sedation. It is limited by having only a diagnostic role. The role of barium enema in screening for colorectal cancer is discussed in Chapter 23.

Box 3.3 lists features that might be found in a DCBE. The classic 'apple core' appearance of a tumour appears as irregular shouldering (Fig. 3.2), while a benign stricture will appear smooth (Fig. 3.3). Focal or segmental changes in calibre and/or contours may indicate stiffening due to an infiltrative process. This may be circumferential or partial, for example involving only the posterior haustra at the attachment of the transverse mesocolon, indicating extension of disease from the stomach or pancreas (Fig. 3.4).

The normal small bowel shows a prominent fold pattern of valvulae conniventes, which diminish with distance from the duodenum. Colonic mucosa is smooth and barium coating should produce a continuous, pencil-sharp white line. A disturbance of the mucosal pattern such as thickening, irregularity, flattening and ulceration can be identified compared with normal adjacent segments.

Diverticula and polyps are most frequently seen on colonic imaging. A diverticulum may be seen projecting away from the bowel lumen, but if seen *en-face* it is difficult to differentiate from a polyp. Typically, a polyp should have a ring of barium around its base with a clearly defined inner border (Fig. 3.5) whereas a diverticulum will have a clearly defined outer margin with a graduated inner edge, as contrast coats the inner surface (Fig. 3.6). A pedunculated polyp may be seen in different positions on the varying films due to the effect of gravity. In the colon it is necessary to have good bowel preparation in order to differentiate small mucosal lesions from residual faeces.

Single contrast enema

For a single-contrast enema a water-soluble contrast is used. Contrast is run in as far as necessary to demonstrate a leak or obstructing lesion and this is a much shorter procedure. The most common use is to confirm the presence and level of obstruction in mechanical large bowel obstruction (see Chapter 13).

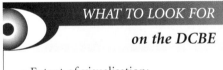

WHAT TO LOOK FOR Box 3.3

on the DCBE

- Extent of visualisation:
  - trace entire colon
  - note any blind areas due to pooled barium and overlapping segments
- Luminal calibre:
  - normal distension of entire colon
  - focal strictures of spasm
  - irregular 'apple core' lesion typical of malignancy
  - extrinsic compression
  - distortion of contour due to adjacent pathology
- Mucosal abnormality:
  - ulceration
  - polyps
  - diverticula
- Contrast leak

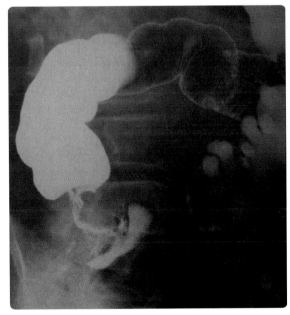

Fig. 3.2 Carcinoma of the ascending colon. Note the narrowed, irregular mucosa within the tumour and the shouldered margins.

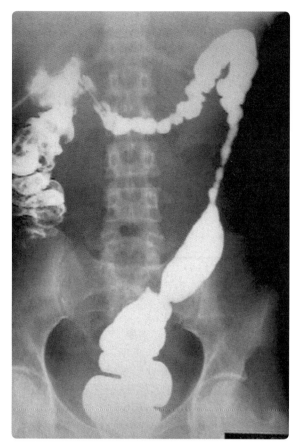

Fig. 3.3 A benign (ischaemic) stricture of the descending colon. Note the smooth and tapered margins to the stricture.

CLINICAL APPLICATION OF CONTRAST STUDIES

Specific applications of contrast studies are discussed in the relevant clinical chapters. The section below outlines the general principles of using contrast in obstruction, perforation, motility assessment and postoperatively.

Obstruction

Assessment of upper and lower gastrointestinal tract obstruction is principally reliant on clinical findings and plain radiology. Contrast studies have largely been superseded by CT but are useful when clinical and radiological findings are equivocal. The role of contrast studies in obstruction is to demonstrate:

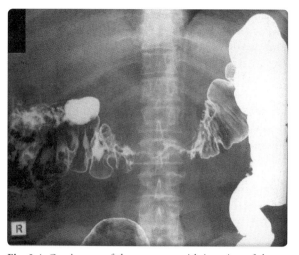

Fig. 3.4 Carcinoma of the pancreas with invasion of the transverse colon. There has been circumferential infiltration of the colon.

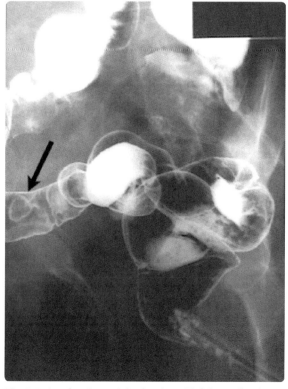

Fig. 3.5 A polyp (arrow) in the sigmoid colon. It has been outlined by a fine coat of barium.

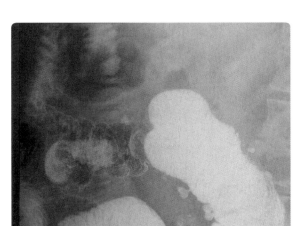

Fig. 3.6 Diverticulosis of the sigmoid colon. Contrast has coated the inner surfaces of the diverticulae.

- the presence of obstruction
- the level of obstruction
- if the obstruction is partial or complete
- identify any mucosal abnormality that may suggest a cause.

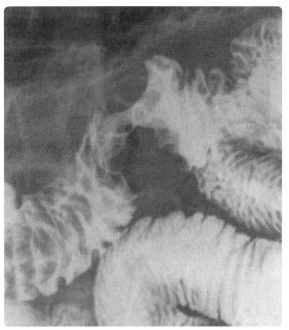

Fig. 3.7 A primary tumour of the third part of the duodenum. The contrast outlines the shouldered appearances of the tumour.

Upper gastrointestinal obstruction

Long, complex oesophageal strictures may be best assessed radiologically, as are patients with adynamic obstruction (e.g. achalasia) and this is described in more detail in Chapter 11. Barium is the preferred contrast agent in obstruction affecting the upper digestive tract. Contrast studies are rarely diagnostic in gastric outlet obstruction. The fluid-filled stomach may be visible on the plain radiograph, and more information is likely to be obtained from an endoscopy or CT scan.

Duodenal obstruction is an uncommon form of small bowel obstruction and is often better defined radiologically than endoscopically. Most often contrast is used to define the nature of an acute obstruction (Fig. 3.7). In small bowel adhesion obstruction, dilute (50%) Gastrografin® may be given to define the site of obstruction and the likely need for surgical intervention (see Chapter 10). If it is thought that the cause of the obstruction may be a mass lesion, a CT scan may be more appropriate. Gastrografin has also been advocated as a therapeutic agent in partial small bowel obstruction due to adhesions (see below).

Large bowel obstruction

Radiological assessment remains an important component of the management of large bowel obstruction. The plain abdominal radiograph is used to confirm the diagnosis, if not the cause (see Chapter 10) and to provide a comparative picture of the progress or resolution of obstruction. Increasingly, the CT scan is used in the assessment of colonic obstruction, where it can provide information not obtainable from a pure contrast study, such as gas in the bowel wall and mass lesions outside the gut lumen.

Perforation

Perforation of the oesophagus may be emetogenic (rare) or, most often, the result of an endoscopic dilatation. Iatrogenic injury in the pharyngeal region is most often due to blind passage of an instrument, producing posterior damage, involving the apex of the pyriform sinus (see Chapter 11). Without delay, once the diagnosis of perforation has been considered, a contrast examination should be performed (Fig. 3.8).

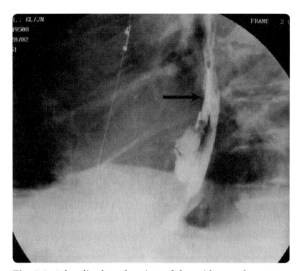

Fig. 3.8 A localised perforation of the mid-oesophagus, sustained after dilatation of a peptic stricture. The arrow points to the site of the perforation, with contrast pooled below and along side the oesophagus.

Free intraperitoneal perforation of a part of the gut does not require any form of contrast imaging, provided that the decision has already been made that the patient requires operative intervention. If not, and the plain radiological findings are inconclusive, a CT is likely to be more useful than a contrast study. Although the CT might not localise the site of perforation, it will avoid the risk of contamination of the peritoneal cavity with contrast (see Chapter 10).

Perforations are best identified with a small volume (5–10 mL) of water-soluble contrast or diluted barium and with the patient first in the lateral and then the frontal position. Contrast may track for a variable distance down the posterior mediastinum. Thin barium is cleared surprisingly quickly. However, the patient may refuse to swallow an amount sufficient for adequate examination; 10 mL of diluted barium (e.g. Polibar®) is more acceptable and does not compromise the respiratory tract. Instrumental perforations are usually treated conservatively and in such circumstances it is preferable to use water-soluble contrast. If it is likely the patient is going to require surgical intervention, the use of barium is more acceptable, as it will be surgically cleared from the already contaminated mediastinum and pleural surface.

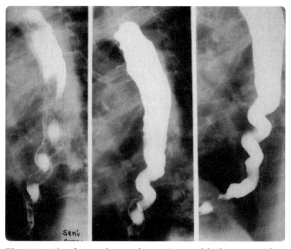

Fig. 3.9 A 'corkscrew' oesophagus in an elderly man with a long history of dysphagia.

Gut motility

Apart from manometric and radioisotopic procedures, contrast studies are often performed to look at functional gut problems. Deglutition and oesophageal peristaltic disorders can be well documented and the procedure is often captured on video to enable review in slow motion. While some appearances such as the 'bird-beak' of achalasia or the 'corkscrew' of tertiary contractions are captured on spot films (Fig. 3.9), focal delays or disordered deglutition need to be assessed on real time imaging. Assessment of the time taken for gastric emptying and transit through the small bowel provide indications of motility, although nuclear medicine transit studies may also be used (Chapter 7). Fluoroscopic observation of the small bowel during a small bowel series will provide information of peristaltic activity but, due to the frequent use of antispasmodics during an enema, large bowel activity is not usually assessed.

Postoperative use of contrast studies

Contrast studies are used in the postoperative setting of:

- anatostomotic dehiscence
- stents
- post-fundoplication, adjustable gastric banding devices.

Contrast studies may be undertaken to look at the integrity of an anastomosis when there is:

- clinical suspicion of leakage (Fig. 3.10)
- a high risk of leakage because of the nature of the procedure (e.g. pharyngogastric anastomosis).

Contrast studies are sometimes used to check the correct positioning of a fundoplication wrap or adjustable gastric banding device to confirm the absence of obstruction prior to the patient recommencing oral intake. Contrast studies are also useful to assess stent patency and positioning (see Chapter 9).

Therapeutic uses of contrast

Gastrografin® has been used in small bowel obstruction to accurately define complete obstruction and predict the need for surgery. More controversially, it has also been advocated as a therapeutic tool for patients with partial small bowel obstruction secondary to adhesions. Theoretically, this may result in earlier resolution of bowel obstruction although results from studies are conflicting. Gastrografin® is thought to exert an irritative peristaltic effect and osmotic effect on the bowel, drawing fluid into the lumen and decreasing oedema of the bowel wall. It is probable that these properties confer an ability to hasten resolution of adhesion–obstruction in terms of:

- shorter time to first bowel action
- more rapid resumption of diet
- shorter hospital stay.

Care must be taken to avoid respiratory aspiration when delivering Gastrografin®, which may cause pulmonary oedema. A volume of 100 mL given orally or by nasogastric tube (subsequently clamped) is sufficient. A supine film is taken three to four hours later. This helps to gauge the need for, and the timing of, the next film (Figs 3.11 and 3.12). Serial radiographs are used to monitor the progress of contrast through the bowel. If contrast reaches the caecum by 24 hours (usually earlier) then operative intervention is unlikely to be required, but conversely, if contrast fails to reach the caecum then 90% of patients will require surgery.

These therapeutic effects of Gastrografin® apply only in incomplete obstruction. The ability of Gastrografin® to avert the need for surgery in adhesive bowel obstruction is difficult to quantify. Protocols and defi-

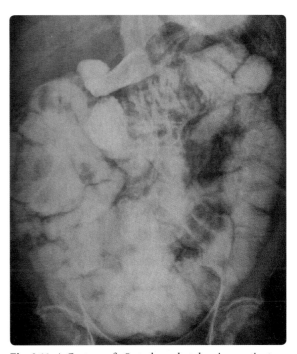

Fig. 3.11 A Gastrografin® study undertaken in a patient with adhesion-obstruction. This film was taken 3 hours after ingestion of the contrast and already shows material throughout the small bowel, suggestive that any obstruction is only partial.

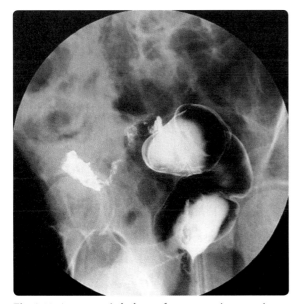

Fig. 3.10 Anastomotic leakage after an anterior resection of the rectum.

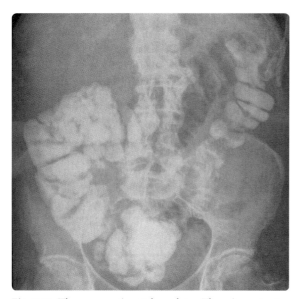

Fig. 3.12 The same patient 1 hour later. There is contrast in the colon. Any obstruction that was present has now resolved and no underlying cause has been identified.

nitions on the timing and need for surgery differ between studies making it difficult to determine the impact of Gastrografin® studies, but it seems unlikely that in the presence of complete mechanical obstruction anything other than surgery would relieve the obstruction.

Most patients with small bowel obstruction can be successfully managed without contrast radiology. Gastrografin® can be used where there is diagnostic uncertainty or where it is desirable to hasten the efficacy of conservative management. It should be stressed that such an approach is only indicated in adhesion-obstruction where laparotomy is not otherwise indicated. While the radiological investigation may incur costs, these are easily offset by the savings in bed-days brought about by earlier decision-making based on the results of the imaging.

Further reading

Assalia A, Schien M, Kopelman D et al. Therapeutic effect of oral gastrografin in adhesive partial small bowel obstruction: a prospective randomised trial. Surgery 1994; 115:433–7

Biondi S, Pares D, Mora L et al. Randomized clinical study of gastrografin administration in patients with adhesive small bowel obstruction. Br J Surg 2003; 90;542–6

Choi HK, Chu KW, Law WL. Therapeutic value of Gastrografin in adhesive small bowel obstruction after unsuccessful conservative treatment: a prospective randomised trial. Ann Surg 2002; 236:1–6

Chung CC, Meng WCS, Yu SCH et al. A prospective study on the use of water soluble contrast follow through radiology in the management of small bowel obstruction. Aust N Z J Surg 1996; 66:598–601

Coffin CM, Diche T, Mahfouz A-E et al. Benign and malignant hepatocellular tumours: evaluation of tumoural enhancement after magnafodipir trisodium injection on MR imaging. Eur Radiol 1999; 9:444–9

Draganov P, Cotton PB. Iodinated contrast sensitivity in ERCP. Am J Gastroenterol 2000; 95(6):1398–401

Evers K, Kressel HY. Principles of performance and interpretation of double-contrast gastrointestinal studies. Radiol Clin N Am 1982; 20(4):667–85

Fan ST, Lau WY, Yip WC et al. Limitations and danger of gastrograph in swallow after esophageal and upper gastric operations. Am J Surg 1988; 155; 495–7

Gore RM, Levine MS, Laufer I (eds). Textbook of gastrointestinal radiology, vol 1. WB Saunders, Philadelphia, 1994

Grainger RG, Allison DJ, Adam A, Dixon AK. Diagnostic radiology. A textbook of medical imaging, vol 2, 4th edn. Churchill Livingstone, New York, 2001

Harvery CJ, Pilcher JM, Eckersley RJ et al. Advances in ultrasound. Clin Radiol 2002; 57:157–77

Hopper KD, Wegert SJ, Hallgren SE. Renal excretion of endoscopic retrograde cholangiopancreatography injected contrast. A common phenomenon. Invest Radiol 1989; 24:394–6

Joyce WP, Delaney PV, Gorey TF, Fitzpatrick JM. The value of water soluble contrast radiology in the management of acute small bowel obstruction. Ann R Coll Surg Engl 1992; 74:422–5

Laufer I. Barium studies: principles of double contrast diagnosis. In: Gore RM, Levine MS, Laufer I (eds) Textbook of gastrointestinal radiology, vol 1. WB Saunders, Philadelphia, 1994

Marik PE, Patel SY. Anaphylactoid reaction to oral contrast agent. AJR 1997; 168:1623

Miller SH. Anaphylactoid reaction after oral administration of diatrizoate meglumine and diatrizoate sodium solution. AJR 1997; 168:959–61

Rubesin SE, Levine MS. Radiologic diagnosis of gastrointestinal perforation. Radiol Clin N Am 2003; 41:1095–115

Seymour PC, Kesack CD. Anaphylactic shock during routine upper gastrointestinal series. AJR 1997; 168:957–8

Tanomkiat W, Galassi W. Barium sulfate as contrast medium for evaluation of postoperative anastomotic leaks. Acta Radiol 2000; 41:482–5

Thompson JJ. Contrast radiology and intestinal obstruction. Ann Surg 2002; 236:7–8

Thomsen HS, Morcos SK. Contrast media and the kidney: European Society of Urogenital Radiology (ESUR) Guidelines. BJR 2003; 76:513–18

Computed tomography 4

K.L. Gormly, N. Jones, A. Chew, P. Gallagher, G. Maddern

INTRODUCTION

K.L. Gormly

Background

When CT was first introduced in 1972 it revolutionised imaging due to the ability to obtain information about soft tissues. Continuous technical developments since the first scanners have sped up acquisition times from imaging the brain in 15 minutes to imaging the chest, abdomen and pelvis in 15 seconds. In 1989 spiral (helical) scanners were introduced which provided many significant improvements, and the more recent introduction of multi-detector or 'multislice' CT scanners has revolutionised the capabilities of CT still further.

COMPUTED TOMOGRAPHY SCANNERS

In a modern spiral scanner the patient moves through a continuous beam at a fixed rate and a volume of data is acquired in the shape of a helix. The initial spiral scanners were 'single slice' spiral scanners, with a single row of detectors acquiring a single slice per rotation. Advancements in detector technology have enabled the implementation of multiple rows of detectors, which can acquire multiple slices per rotation and allow much smaller slice thicknesses. These scanners are called 'multislice' spiral scanners and while the majority of scanners in clinical use have 4–16 rows of detectors, new scanners have up to 64 rows. The high speed and narrow slice thicknesses in multislice spiral scanners allow high-quality reconstructions and the ability to scan in a specific vascular phase. The amount of data acquired requires extensive post processing, with sophisticated software systems and large amounts of computer memory. Hundreds of images are routinely acquired for a scan of the chest, abdomen and pelvis and these need to be viewed on a workstation, where the images may be reconstructed in any plane or into 3D images.

The modern multislice spiral CT scanner has allowed the expansion of CT into many areas which were previously imaged with other modalities. These include the use of CT angiography for pulmonary, coronary and peripheral vessels, and the development of virtual colonoscopy and bronchoscopy which may rival traditional endoscopic procedures in the future.

VIEWING THE COMPUTED TOMOGRAPHY SCAN

Traditionally, images obtained by CT examination were printed on sheets of film for reporting. The advent of multislice technology and the resultant large number of images now means that a workstation is necessary to view all the acquired data. The printed images are representative images, which are printed as thicker slices than those viewed on the workstation, and they will not necessarily best demonstrate any abnormalities that have been detected. If PACS (picture archiving and communication system) is available then no film will be printed and images are viewed directly on a computer monitor, however these may still be limited to thicker slice reconstructions. Images are displayed as if viewed from the feet, with the patient's left on the right of the film and vice versa.

Each pixel within the image has a CT number, which reflects the attenuation of the tissue (i.e. its density) expressed as a Hounsfield unit (HU) (Table 4.1). Water has an HU of 0, air of −1000 and dense bone has an HU of greater than +1000. Therefore tissues of lower attenuation than water appear darker (e.g. fat) and structures of higher attenuation appear brighter (e.g. muscle).

Although > 2000 different HUs can be detected by the scanner, the human eye can distinguish far fewer shades of grey. It is therefore necessary to 'window' the image to see the tissues of interest. A window level (WL) is set at the midrange of interest, and the window width (WW) determines the range of CT numbers to be displayed. These will be different for different tissues, for example bone (WL 350, WW 2000),

soft tissue (WL 40, WW 350) and lung (WL −500, WW 1500). The large WW for lung and bone means there is less differentiation between tissues, whereas the relatively small WW for soft tissue viewing means small changes in density will be appreciated as different shades of grey. For example, an image of the chest on soft tissue windows will differentiate vessels, nodes, fluid and mediastinal fat while the lungs look black. The same image on lung windows will show details of the lung parenchyma, but the mediastinal structures will appear white. The process of windowing alters the visualisation of an image but the original data remains unchanged (Box 4.1).

COMPUTED TOMOGRAPHY CONTRAST

Intravenous contrast

The addition of intravenous contrast to a CT scan aids in assessment of soft tissues as different structures

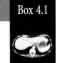

WHAT TO LOOK FOR | Box 4.1
on any CT

- Patient's left on the right of the image
- View the appropriate window settings for the structure of interest
- Assess the use of contrast media and timing of the scan
- Use a methodical approach to assess all organs and systems
- If necessary view reconstructions or different windows on the CT workstation

Table 4.1 Hounsfield units (HU) for different structures

Structure	CT number (Hounsfield unit)
Dense bone	> +1000
Soft tissue	+20–80
Water	0
Fat	−100
Air	−1000

enhance differently, visualised as different shades of grey. Contrast travels through the vessels, moves into the extracellular space (except in the brain where it is prevented by the blood–brain barrier) and is predominantly excreted renally. The contrast is iodine based, with a higher density than unenhanced soft tissue, and structures that contain contrast appear brighter. The amount of contrast within a structure determines its attenuation value (HU). Intravascular contrast carries a risk of allergic reaction and may induce contrast nephrotoxicity. The latter is critical in patients on the biguanide metformin as accumulation of the drug can lead to potentially fatal lactic acidosis. Further descriptions are included in Chapter 3.

Contraindications to use of intravascular contrast:

- renal failure
- known iodine allergy (e.g. previous severe contrast reaction).

Relative contraindications (require premedication with steroids):

- history of significant asthma
- previous mild reaction such as urticaria.

Patients on metformin:

- drug withheld for 48 hours following injection
- restart following normal renal function test
- if abnormal renal function, metformin should also be withheld for 48 hours before the injection.

In some circumstances, CT scans are performed without administration of intravenous contrast. Examples of this include the assessment of calcification or acute haemorrhage, because on postcontrast images it can be difficult to differentiate these from contrast. Abdominal scans termed 'non-contrast' due to the lack of intravenous contrast often have oral contrast administered.

The different phases of imaging following intravenous injection have greatest impact in the abdomen and pelvis.

Other contrast

In scans of the abdomen and pelvis oral contrast is often administered, which aids the differentiation of bowel loops from other structures. Oral contrast may be dilute barium, an iodine based contrast, or water.

Occasionally rectal contrast is inserted in cases of pelvic pathology and dilute iodinated contrast may be injected into the bladder or a fistulous tract for further definition.

IMAGING OF THE BRAIN
N. Jones

Background

Non-contrast CT remains the investigation of choice in head trauma. It provides more information than plain radiographs, is relatively widely available and can be performed rapidly. Contrast is not helpful in the acute trauma situation and may cause diagnostic difficulties. The bright appearance of an acute intracranial bleed may be easily confused with contrast given as part of another investigation (e.g. body CT or cerebral angiogram). MRI is not useful in acute head trauma (except rarely for possible arterial dissection). This is fortunate because it is a much greater technical challenge to take a multiply injured, monitored and ventilated patient into the magnet than to the CT room.

With suspected tumour or infection, contrast is always used with CT except if there is a strong contraindication (e.g. allergy or renal failure). Gliomas, metastases, meningiomas and abscesses can all be missed on a non contrast CT scan. MRI is extremely useful in neuro-oncology and provides valuable information regarding the anatomical location and most likely pathological diagnosis.

PET scanning has a much more limited role in neurosurgery. It is sometimes helpful to distinguish between radiation necrosis and tumour recurrence in malignant gliomas but is also used in specialised units in the preoperative workup for epilepsy surgery and neurovascular surgery.

TRAUMA

Indications for computed tomography head scan

The indications for a CT head scan in acute neurotrauma in a regional or remote setting have been well defined and are generally applicable:

1. Glasgow Coma Score (GCS) < 9 after resuscitation.
2. Neurological deterioration of 2 or more points on GCS or development of neurological deficit.
3. Drowsiness or confusion (GCS 9–13 persisting > 2 hours).
4. Persistent headache, vomiting.
5. Focal neurological signs.
6. Fracture: known or suspected.
7. Penetrating injury: known or suspected.
8. Age: over 50.
9. Postoperative assessment.

Box 4.2 outlines the signs to look for in the trauma head CT.

Surface collections

Surface collections following trauma are primarily due to:

- acute subdural haemorrhage
- chronic subdural haemorrhage
- extradural haemorrhage.

Acute blood is hyperdense (bright) on CT and the density decreases with the interval from the bleed. At approximately 2 weeks the haemorrhage is isodense to brain parenchyma and can be difficult to see. After this it becomes gradually darker and chronic haemorrhage is hypodense. In patients with severe anaemia the acute haemorrhage may not be hyperdense due to the low haemoglobin content of the blood.

WHAT TO LOOK FOR   Box 4.2

on the head-trauma CT scan

- Scalp swelling
- Fracture (linear or depressed)
- Midline shift
- Ventricular size and shape
- Contusions
- Intracerebral haematoma
- Subarachnoid or intraventricular haemorrhage
- Surface collections (extradural, subdural)

Acute subdural haematoma

Acute subdural haematoma is usually associated with severe injury (e.g. motor vehicle crash) or anticoagulants (Fig. 4.1). It carries a poor prognosis and requires craniotomy. Typical features on the CT scan include:

- a crescentic collection
- high density (i.e. white)
- swelling of the underlying hemisphere.

Chronic subdural haematoma

Chronic subdural haematoma often occurs in elderly or alcoholic patients following a trauma that might be trivial or forgotten. The collection can be large with a major mass effect and yet little neurological deficit because these lesions accumulate slowly (Fig. 4.2). They can usually be drained easily through burrholes. Typical features on the CT scan include:

- characteristic appearance of a low density (i.e. black) collection
- possibly some elements of recent haemorrhage (white)
- a crescentic appearance (i.e. parallel to the skull)
- posterior layering (with a fluid level) in more recent haemorrhage.

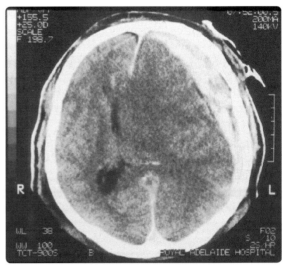

Fig. 4.1 Acute subdural haematoma showing bilateral scalp swelling, a high density, crescentic surface collection and massive swelling of underlying hemisphere with midline shift.

Extradural haematoma

Extradural haematomas are often associated with sporting injuries or falls in children. They tend to occur in younger patients (Fig. 4.3). An extradural haematoma requires craniotomy but generally there is a good prognosis as long as it is treated early. Typical features on the CT include:

- biconvex (i.e. lens shaped) collection
- high density (i.e. white)
- a fracture (although this may not be visible on the CT.

Subarachnoid haemorrhage

Subarachnoid haemorrhage can be secondary to trauma or spontaneous rupture of a berry aneurysm (Fig. 4.4). If there is no convincing history of trauma, further investigation will be required. A CT angiogram is often used as a screening test and will usually show the causative aneurysm, but most units still require cerebral angiography before proceeding to surgery or endovascular coiling. Interpretation of scans can be difficult if the patient has had a previous high dose of contrast. Changes on a CT scan may include:

- high density following the contour of the brain, extending into sulci
- high density around the brainstem in the basal cisterns
- blood in the ventricles
- intracerebral haematomas, particularly in the medial frontal lobe with anterior communicating artery aneurysms and in the temporal lobe with middle cerebral artery aneurysms.

MASS LESIONS

The most common intracranial mass lesions seen in general surgical practice are metastases. Although this may seem an obvious diagnosis in the clinical context of a patient with a known malignancy, there are other possibilities that need to be considered. These include glioma, meningioma and abscess. There are some radiological features that can help differentiate these (see Box 4.3) but sometimes biopsy will be required.

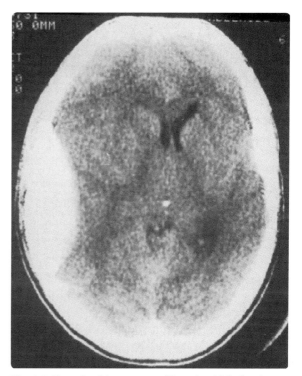

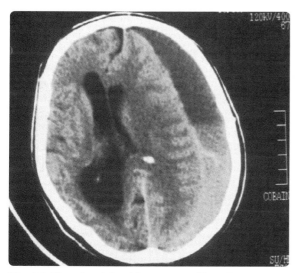

Fig. 4.2 Chronic subdural haematoma. There is a crescentic surface collection. The low density (black) blood lies anteriorly with higher density blood layering posteriorly. There is marked midline shift.

Fig. 4.3 Extradural haematoma. There is a high density biconvex (lens shaped) collection. The midline shift and brain swelling is not as severe as in acute subdural haematoma.

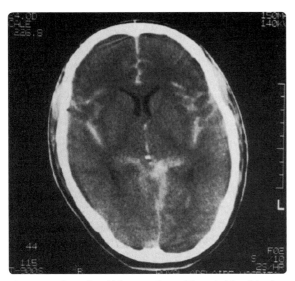

Fig. 4.4 Subarachnoid haemorrhage. There is blood in the subarachnoid space outlining the anterior interhemispheric fissure, both Sylvian fissures and the basal cisterns. There is also blood in the third ventricle and the occipital horn of the left lateral ventricle.

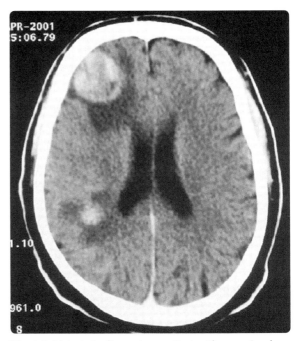

Fig. 4.5 Metastatic disease in a patient with a previously treated adenocarcinoma of the oesophagus.

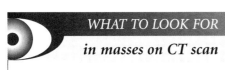
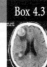

WHAT TO LOOK FOR — Box 4.3
in masses on CT scan

- Site of the lesion
- Single or multiple
- Associated mass effect
- Calcification
- Haemorrhage
- Contrast enhancement

Metastases

Cerebral metastases are most commonly seen in patients with primary sites in the lung, breast, gastrointestinal tract, kidney or melanoma (Fig. 4.5). Most are multiple and they are most commonly situated at the grey–white junction. They are usually iso-dense to brain parenchyma on plain scans and enhance after contrast. Melanoma is frequently hyperdense on plain scans. The centre may be necrotic (low density), but truly cystic metastases are quite uncommon.

Haemorrhage (high density on non-contrast scans) may occur, especially with melanoma and choriocarcinoma. Lymphoma often spreads diffusely along the ependyma of the ventricles. Malignant meningitis produces diffuse enhancement over the surface of the brain and often along the ependyma.

MRI is often used as a more sensitive screening test for cerebral metastases. Most will appear slightly hypointense but melanoma is typically hyperintense on T1-weighted scans due to the melanin content. T2-weighted scans usually show the tumour as hyperintense and highlight the surrounding oedema. Most metastases will enhance with gadolinium.

Primary intracerebral tumours

Glioma

Most primary brain tumours are gliomas and most of these are astrocytomas. The other types of gliomas are oligodendrogliomas and ependymomas. In adults, the majority of gliomas are malignant (glioblastoma multiforme). Most are solitary lesions but 5% of malignant gliomas are multicentric.

Low-grade gliomas appear as poorly defined hypodense areas on CT, just like cerebral oedema, and do not enhance (Fig. 4.6). They may produce large cysts and calcification is common in oligodendrogliomas, as is spontaneous haemorrhage. The more malignant tumours often have necrotic centres with irregular peripheral enhancement and considerable surrounding oedema and mass effect. There may be areas of haemorrhage or calcification if the tumour has evolved from a lower grade glioma.

MRI shows similar appearances with the low grade tumours looking very much like areas of oedema and the higher grade tumours showing considerable heterogeneity in keeping with the descriptive term glioblastoma multiforme. Higher grade gliomas usually enhance after gadolinium whereas lower grade tumours do not.

Meningioma

Meningiomas are the most common benign primary brain tumour. They can occur anywhere there is dura and also within the orbit and the ventricles. They are more common in females, often possess hormone receptors and have an association with breast cancer. Meningiomas may be multiple, especially when associated with type 2 neurofibromatosis.

Plain CT shows a well defined, hyperdense extra-axial lesion (Fig. 4.7). There may be tumour calcifica-tion and adjacent bone may be hyperostotic. Oedema in the adjacent brain is a common finding (Fig. 4.8). Most meningiomas enhance fairly uniformly after contrast. Rarer variations include cystic meningiomas and rim-enhancement mimicking abscess or glioma.

MRI can be helpful in confirming the extra-axial nature of these tumours as it will show the brain tumour interface more clearly (Fig. 4.9). The most common appearance is an isointense lesion on T1 images with strong, uniform enhancement after contrast. There is often high T2 signal in the adjacent white matter due to oedema.

Cerebral abscess

Pyogenic cerebral abscess can be very difficult to distinguish from malignant glioma or metastasis on CT and it is usually the clinical history that is most important. Important factors include previous intracranial surgery or trauma, long term steroid therapy and other causes of immunosuppression, middle ear infection, frontal sinusitis and bacterial endocarditis. Patients with AIDS are particularly prone to developing multiple cerebral abscesses due to *Toxoplasma*

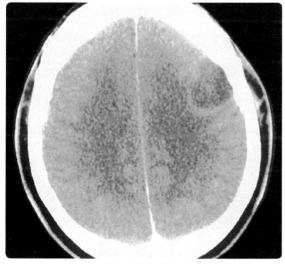

Fig. 4.6 A low grade glioma.

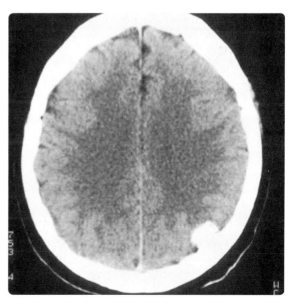

Fig. 4.7 Meningioma. This scan shows a small convexity meningioma, often seen as an incidental finding. The scan is non-contrast so the white colour is due to calcification. There is no surrounding oedema.

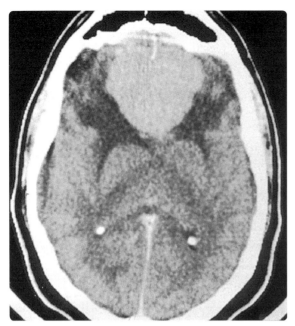

Fig. 4.8 Meningioma. This contrast CT scan shows a large subfrontal meningioma. There is bifrontal oedema and considerable mass effect. Because the frontal lobes are a relatively 'silent area' of the brain and meningiomas grow very slowly, they can often reach a large size before producing symptoms (often personality change, poor memory and headaches). Anosmia will almost always be present with tumours in this location but it is unusual for a patient to complain of this (and also unusual for a doctor to test for it!).

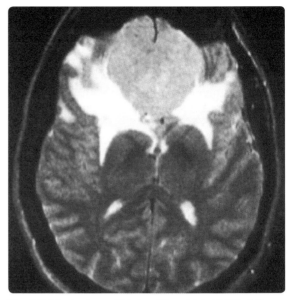

Fig. 4.9 Meningioma. This is a T2-weighted MRI of the same patient as Fig. 4.8. It shows the tumour as a hyperintense mass surrounded by oedema. The extra-axial nature of the tumour is clearly shown.

gondii. The possibility of missing a treatable abscess is a major underlying reason for biopsy of cerebral mass lesions.

In the early stages of cerebritis, CT may show only diffuse low density. As the abscess matures there will usually be a well-defined ring of contrast-enhancement, surrounded by oedema (Fig. 4.10). MRI reveals similar findings with the rim appearing hyper-intense on T1- and hypointense on T2-weighted images. There is intense enhancement with gadolin-ium. Magnetic resonance spectroscopy collects data over a range of frequencies (unlike MRI) and can provide information on the chemical composition of a lesion. This can be very helpful in determining whether a ring-enhancing lesion is more likely to be a tumour or an abscess.

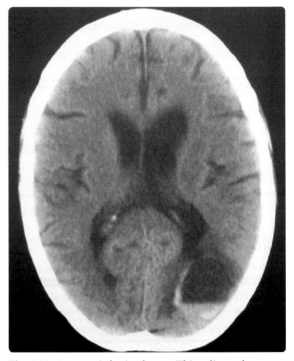

Fig. 4.10 A pyogenic brain abscess. This solitary abscess has an enhancing rim with a low density centre. A fluid level is present.

COMPUTED TOMOGRAPHY OF THE CHEST

A. Chew

Background

Computed tomography (CT) has largely replaced the plain chest radiograph as the definitive imaging investigation of the chest. This is particularly so in the assessment of many surgically related problems such as trauma and malignancy (Chapter 25).

The sensitivity of CT imaging of the chest owes much to the speed of current machines, which allow the whole chest cavity to be scanned within a single breath hold, thus minimizing motion artefact. CT angiography is now a mainstream investigation in the detection of pulmonary emboli and significant developments in coronary artery imaging are promising to challenge conventional coronary angiography.

ANATOMY AND INTERPRETATION OF THE CHEST COMPUTED TOMOGRAPHY SCAN

Assessment of a chest CT involves looking at both lung and mediastinal window settings to ensure adequate visualisation of all structures. In addition it may be useful to look at bone windows to determine the extent of any bone erosion from an underlying lesion or metastasis. Three of the key anatomical sections are illustrated below (Figs 4.11, 4.12 and 4.13).

On lung windows the pulmonary parenchyma is optimally visualised and any focal masses, consolidation or cavities will be easily seen. Pneumothoraces will only be visualised on lung windows, but the mediastinum will be too bright for assessment. On mediastinal windows the heart, great vessels, trachea and oesophagus are well defined and are surrounded by low-density mediastinal fat (Fig. 4.13). Any increased density within this fat may be due to lymph

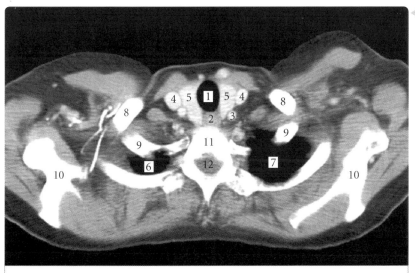

◀ **Fig. 4.11** CT of thoracic inlet.

KEY

1 Trachea	8 Clavicle
2 Oesophagus	9 First rib
3 Left common carotid artery	10 Scapula
4 Internal jugular vein	11 Vertebral body
5 Thyroid gland	12 Spinal cord
6 Right lung	
7 Left lung	

Fig. 4.12 CT chest at the level of the great vessels.

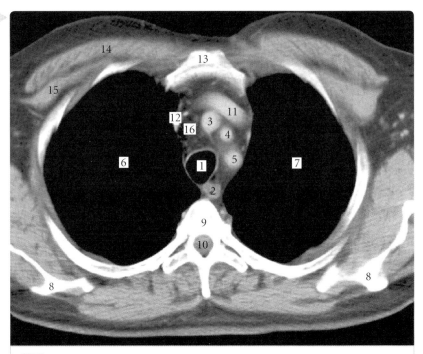

KEY

1	Trachea	9	Vertebral body
2	Oesophagus	10	Spinal canal
3	Brachiocephalic trunk	11	Left brachiocephalic vein
4	Left common carotid artery	12	Right brachiocephalic vein
5	Left subclavian artery	13	Sternum
6	Right lung	14	Pectoralis major
7	Left lung	15	Pectoralis minor
8	Scapula	16	Mediastinal fat

nodes, tumour or mediastinal haematoma. Pleural effusions can be distinguished from collapsed lung and pleural thickening on mediastinal windows as they are of lower density consistent with fluid.

CLINICAL APPLICATIONS OF THE CHEST COMPUTED TOMOGRAPHPY SCAN

Diagnosis and staging of lung cancer

Small-cell lung cancer usually presents at a relatively late stage and remains, on the whole, a non-surgical disease with chemotherapy and radiation therapy the mainstay of treatment.

Non-small-cell lung cancer (NSCLC), constitutes 80% of newly diagnosed lung cancer. The overall 5-year survival for NSCLC is approximately 10% with over half harbouring extrapulmonary spread at diagnosis. Only 20% of cases are surgically curable and accurate staging of this aggressive disease decreases the proportion of non-curative resections. Stage is determined by tumour characteristics, nodal status and the presence or absence of metastases. The role of CT is to assess the primary tumour, to determine local invasion and the presence or absence of lymph node involvement and distant metastases. Invasion of proximal airways, aorta, pulmonary vessels, SVC, heart, oesophagus or vertebral bodies indicate unresectability (Fig. 4.14).

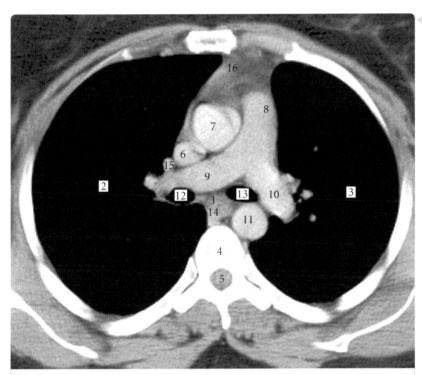

Fig. 4.13 CT chest at the level of the pulmonary bifurcation.

KEY

1	Oesophagus	9	Right pulmonary artery
2	Right lung	10	Left pulmonary artery
3	Left lung	11	Descending thoracic aorta
4	Vertebral body	12	Right main bronchus
5	Spinal canal	13	Left main bronchus
6	Superior vena cava	14	Azygos vein
7	Ascending aorta	15	Right superior pulmonary vein
8	Pulmonary trunk	16	Mediastinal fat

With clinically apparent localised disease, evaluation of nodal status is critical as it discriminates between disease stages and thus suitability for surgical resection. However, CT alone is inadequate in assessing mediastinal nodal status (sensitivity 57%, specificity 75%) as enlarged nodes are often benign and subcentimetre nodes may contain metastatic disease. PET scans have an overall accuracy of 79% in this setting and when combined with CT images, improves the overall accuracy to 88%. PET scanning has the added advantage of imaging the whole body for occult metastasis. Combining CT with PET scanning allows targeted biopsies of suspicious nodes resulting in more accurate preoperative staging.

Staging of non-bronchogenic malignancies

CT scans of the chest are often performed to stage non-bronchogenic malignancies. Its role is to:

- detect the presence of pulmonary metastases
- assess loco-regional spread (e.g. from carcinoma of the oesophagus).

The presence of multiple pulmonary lesions is usually diagnostic of metastatic disease but biopsy may be required for confirmation if there is doubt in the clinical setting (Fig. 4.15). CT is often used to monitor response to treatment and assess disease progression, allowing some prediction of prognosis.

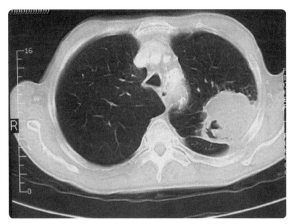

Fig. 4.14 A non-small-cell carcinoma in the left upper lobe. This CT slice shows that the tumour has invaded the pleura.

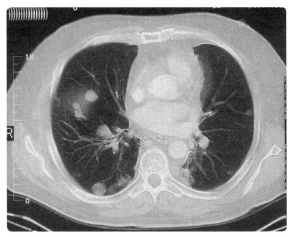

Fig. 4.15 Metastatic pulmonary disease in a patient with a carcinoma of the oesophagus. The patient was being staged prior to treatment. The CT scan shows numerous deposits in both lungs.

Solitary pulmonary nodules

Solitary pulmonary nodules (SPN), defined as focal areas of increased density in the lung measuring <3 cm, are a common radiological abnormality. Whereas the majority have benign causes, 30–40% are malignant and may represent curable, early-stage lung cancer. Specific morphological features of size, contour, margins, pattern of calcification and presence of fat can help differentiate benign from malignant lesions in conjunction with the clinical features (patient age, smoking history, prior malignancy, presenting symptoms). Morphological criteria, however, are not specific allowing up to 40% of malignant nodules to be incorrectly classified as benign.

The morphologic criteria used in evaluating SPN are:

- Size:
  - 80% benign nodules <2 cm
  - 40% malignant nodules <2 cm
- Margins/contour:
  - spiculated, irregular margin indicates malignant process
  - smooth, well-defined usually benign (20% malignant nodules well defined)
  - lobulation (uneven growth) usually malignant (25% benign nodules lobulated)

- Pattern of calcification:
  - benign: central, diffuse solid, laminated, 'popcorn' like
  - malignant: diffuse, amorphous, punctate
- Intranodular fat: hamartoma.

Subcentimetre lesions are difficult to assess as they are below the resolution of CT scans and biopsy is difficult. Tumour doubling time is a useful predictor as malignant nodules double in volume in 30–400 days; nodules doubling more slowly or quickly are usually benign. However, this is also a difficult generalisation for small nodules as a 1 cm nodule increases its diameter by less than 3 mm when it doubles in volume, which is at the limits of accuracy for measurement.

Pulmonary embolism

The mortality of untreated PE is high and prompt diagnosis with early treatment is vital. As there are no specific symptoms or signs associated with pulmonary embolism, the diagnosis is often missed. Conversely, many patients suspected of PE eventually prove to have an alternative explanation for their illness. In one study an antemortem diagnosis of PE was made in only 18% of cases. Findings from a large multi-institutional trial showed that a high-probability ventilation–perfusion scan was diagnostic of pulmonary embolism and a normal scan virtually excluded it. However, only a quarter of patients had diagnostic scans and the majority required further imaging, of whom one-fifth proved to have the disease. Indeterminate scans were typical of patients with cardiopulmonary disease, and only 10% of scans were diagnostic in patients with chronic obstructive pulmonary disease. The advent of multislice CT with its faster acquisition times and higher spatial resolution has resulted in decreased motion artifact, facilitating diagnosis of central, segmental and subsegmental pulmonary emboli, making it preferable to conventional angiography (Fig. 4.16). The added advantage of a CT pulmonary angiogram (CTPA) is that it may demonstrate other pleural or pulmonary parenchymal conditions.

As a general rule, if the patient with a low clinical probability of a PE has a normal chest radiograph, a V/Q scan, with its high negative predictive value may be more appropriate than a CTPA (see Chapter 7). If the patient has an intermediate to high probability of PE and an abnormal chest radiograph, a CTPA is likely to have a greater diagnostic yield (see Box 4.4). The main limiting factor for CTPA is the requirement of a large bolus of intravenous contrast (contra-indicated in patients with renal failure). It is also necessary to perform the examination as soon as possible after the

acute event as after 48 hours thrombus may fragment and progress into smaller vessels beyond the resolution of the CTPA.

INTERVENTIONAL RADIOLOGY IN THE CHEST

Computed-tomography-guided intervention

CT scans are used to guide the following interventional procedures:

- fine needle aspiration cytology
- core biopsy
- aspiration of fluid collections
- insertion of drains into cavities and collections (see Chapter 9).

Advances in cytopathological techniques have allowed needle biopsy to become the procedure of choice in evaluating thoracic masses as it has high diagnostic accuracy and a relatively low morbidity. Its roles in the chest include:

- staging lung cancer
- evaluation of pulmonary nodules (avoiding thoracoscopic biopsies)
- diagnosis of mediastinal masses
- diagnosis of pleural disease
- sampling of suspected focal infectious lung lesions.

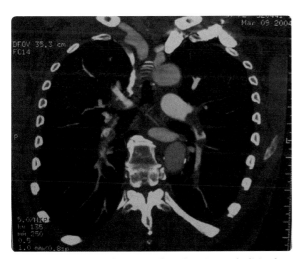

Fig. 4.16 An axial oblique CT slice showing emboli in the right and left pulmonary arteries.

WHAT TO LOOK FOR   Box 4.4

in suspected acute PE

- Direct sign: partial/complete filling defects within contrast enhanced lumen of pulmonary arteries – direct visualisation of thrombus
- Indirect signs:
  - wedge-shaped, pleurally based consolidation
  - dilated central/segmental pulmonary arteries

Advantages of CT guided transthoracic biopsies are the:

- ability to accurately localise the lesion and plan a direct path to avoid important chest wall and mediastinal structures.
- relative low morbidity and high cost effectiveness.

Assessment of response to treatment

Uncomplicated pleural effusions usually resolve with appropriate conservative management (e.g. timely treatment of pneumonia, cardiac failure) and are generally transudative in nature. However, complicated effusions may not resolve without drainage and these are likely to include:

- late-stage parapneumonic effusions
- empyema
- haemothoraces
- malignant effusions.

Drainage allows:

- control of sepsis
- re-expansion of lung, preventing subsequent lung trapping from pleural fibrosis.

The advent of CT has allowed a more precise definition of many of these collections and at the same time, access into the cavity with various forms of self-retaining catheters. It must be remembered that these catheters usually have a small lumen and the contents of a cavity may be loculated, viscous, of high fibrin content or contain necrotic debris. To maximize the chances of a CT-guided drain achieving success, addition of fibrinolytic agents (principally recombinant tissue plasminogen activator) should be considered. In many cases it is also practical to insert drains under ultrasound guidance with the same considerations.

Failure of image-guided drainage may necessitate closed tube thoracostomy, video-assisted thoracostomy or thoracotomy. Closed tube drainage has a lower morbidity but may be limited by the presence of fluid loculations or high fibrin content of the collection causing tube occlusion. Surgery is indicated when tube drainage fails or when the lung is trapped by fibrin peel.

COMPUTED TOMOGRAPHY OF THE ABDOMEN

P. Gallagher, G. Maddern

Background

As with any other investigation, CT of the abdomen is an adjunct to clinical history and examination. With greater availability, its place in the diagnostic pathway has risen to being the first choice investigation in some conditions, such as the stable trauma patient, whereas in other disorders it has a complementary role. A CT of the abdomen must be requested to confirm or refute specific clinical questions, and not seen as an infallible solution in the patient who is critically ill or in whom there is a diagnostic dilemma.

INTERPRETATION AND ABDOMINAL COMPUTED TOMOGRAPHY ANATOMY

As with any imaging investigation, a methodical routine is required to fully examine a CT scan. The major solid organs are easily identified and provide landmarks by which to orientate other structures. Key anatomical sections are illustrated in Figs 4.17–4.21. The liver, spleen and kidneys should be readily distinguishable in the upper abdomen, and the aorta and inferior vena cava identified in the retroperitoneum. The rectum, bladder and uterus will usually be identifiable in the pelvis (see Box 4.5). The most useful information is then gained by reviewing individual organ systems in the light of clinical suspicions.

Scans are usually obtained with intravenous contrast and it is important to note if a patient has an iodine allergy, renal dysfunction or is on metformin (see above). The interpretation of the different timings of postcontrast scans is discussed below.

Phases of intravascular contrast enhancement

More than anywhere else in the body, in a CT abdomen the timing of scanning following the injection of intravenous contrast will alter the appearance and diagnostic usefulness of the images. Familiarity with the different timings and their uses will be of great use in interpreting the scan.

Unenhanced scans are obtained before an injection of intravenous contrast, although the patient has usually been given oral contrast. These unenhanced images are particularly useful for detecting calcification, which will appear as high density (white), for example in the pancreas, the wall of a renal cyst or a liver lesion (Fig. 4.22). Assessment of an adrenal lesion is also best performed on unenhanced images, as if the lesion has an attenuation <10 HU it is most likely an adrenal adenoma (see Chapter 22).

Arterial-phase scans are acquired immediately after the injection of contrast. The exact timing will vary with the speed of the injection and of the scanner, and ranges from 10 to 35 seconds. Early arterial scans are used for angiograms (e.g. aortic aneurysms) as the majority of the contrast is within the arteries, providing good definition. The arterial phase is good for hypervascular lesions within the liver or pancreas such as neuroendocrine tumours and hepatocellular carcinomas (Fig. 4.23). In this phase the hypervascular lesions usually appear denser than the surrounding normal parenchyma, and the lesions are well seen. In

the arterial phase the spleen demonstrates patchy enhancement, which can be mistaken for diffuse disease or traumatic injury if the timing of the scan is not appreciated.

Venous phase scans can also be acquired at different timings, which will vary with the reason for the scan. The typical venous phase scan is termed the 'portal-venous' phase and is acquired when the portal vein is opacified and there is maximal splenic and hepatic parenchymal enhancement (approximately 50–70 s). At this time hypovascular lesions will be of lower density than the surrounding parenchyma, but hypervascular lesions seen well on the arterial phase may be isodense and thus 'invisible'.

The standard 'triple phase' scan of the liver usually refers to unenhanced, arterial and portal-venous phase images. Other timings will be used for specific situations, for example a delayed scan to show the characteristic 'filling-in' of a haemangioma or drainage from the kidneys, a later venous phase scan to view thrombus in the IVC, or an intermediate phase to view the pancreatic parenchyma.

To determine the timing of the scan it is necessary to look at the large vessels and kidneys. In the arterial phase scans the aorta will appear denser (brighter) than the IVC, whereas on venous phase scans these two vessels will be of similar density. Contrast flowing back from the leg veins takes longer than contrast returning from the renal veins, and there is mixing of blood within the IVC at the level of the renal veins. On early venous phase scans the mixing of blood with and without contrast will appear irregular and should not be mistaken for thrombus within the IVC. The kidneys rapidly excrete contrast and display appearances identical to an IVU. Initial cortical enhancement is followed by enhancement of the cortex and medulla, then by excretion of contrast into the renal pelvis and ureters. Often the timing of the scan following injection will be labelled in seconds on the film, however it is preferable to use the above information as a true indicator of timing, as there is significant variability in cardiac output between patients, and what may be venous phase for one patient may still be arterial phase for another.

Oral contrast

Oral contrast is given to opacify the bowel, and aids differentiation between an abdomino-pelvic mass and

Fig. 4.17 Normal abdominal CT at the level of the oesophagogastric junction. The superior liver segments are well visualised at this level.

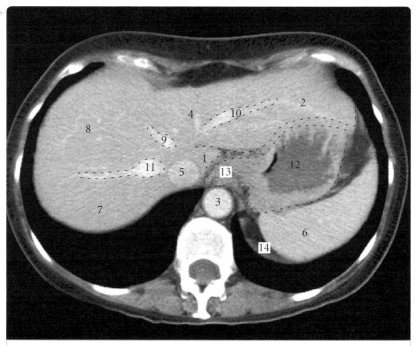

KEY

1	Liver segment 1	8	Liver segment 8
2	Liver segment 2	9	Middle hepatic vein
3	Aorta	10	Left hepatic vein
4	Liver segment 4a	11	Right hepatic vein
5	Inferior vena cava	12	Stomach
6	Spleen	13	Oesophagogastric junction
7	Liver segment 7	14	Left hemidiaphragm

bowel loops. It may also be useful in the assessment of fistulae. For studies of the pancreas and upper abdomen contrast can be administered 15–30 minutes before the scan, whereas studies of the pelvis require at least 1 hour of oral preparation. Traditionally, a dilute barium or iodine based contrast agent is used (which will appear white), however many centres are now using water instead. Occasionally rectal contrast is administered if there is a pelvic mass or collection.

CLINICAL APPLICATIONS OF ABDOMINAL COMPUTED TOMOGRAPHY

- Abdominal trauma (see Chapter 25)
- Staging of malignancy (see Chapter 23)
- Investigation of abdominal sepsis
- Investigation of the acute abdomen (see Chapter 10)
- Ureteric colic (see Chapter 18)
- Assessing cause and level of intestinal obstruction (see Chapter 10)
- Assessment of disease progression, response or recurrence
- Preoperative planning
- Aortic aneurysms/vascular (see Chapter 21).

Most of the above applications are covered in the relevant chapters. This chapter will discuss the use of abdominal CT for assessment of:

- peritoneal disorders
- mesenteric disorders

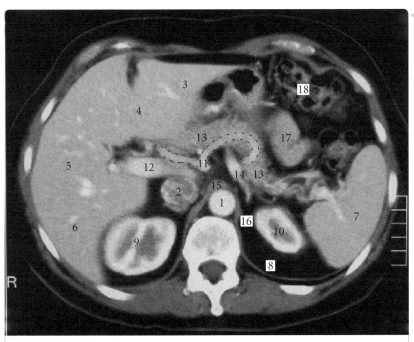

Fig. 4.18 Normal CT taken at the level of the coeliac axis.

KEY

1	Aorta	10	Left kidney
2	Inferior vena cava	11	Coeliac axis
3	Liver segment 3	12	Portal vein
4	Liver segment 4b	13	Pancreas
5	Liver segment 5	14	Left adrenal
6	Liver segment 6	15	Right diaphragmatic crus
7	Spleen	16	Left diaphragmatic crus
8	Left hemidiaphragm	17	Small bowel
9	Right kidney	18	Transverse colon

- spleen
- lymph nodes
- retroperitoneum
- abdominal wall lesions
- sepsis
- postoperative patients
- intervention.

Peritoneal disorders

The peritoneum may be involved in inflammatory or malignant processes, with metastatic disease being the most common form of malignancy. Fluid within the peritoneal cavity is most frequently ascites or blood.

Peritoneal carcinomatosis

This refers to the presence of carcinoma cells within the peritoneum and is often due to metastatic spread from primary tumours such as ovarian and gastric carcinoma. On CT the disease may appear as plaque like 'omental cake' or as focal nodular deposits. Lesions are best seen over the surface of the liver, deep to the anterior abdominal wall and in the right para-colic gutter (Fig. 4.24). The mesentery may appear diffusely thickened and coating of the serosal surfaces of the bowel often appears as ill-defined enhancing bowel wall thickening. Focal lesions may calcify. Peritoneal carcinomatosis is often associated with large volumes of ascites, and plaques of disease are frequently better

Fig. 4.19 Normal abdominal CT taken at the level of the superior mesenteric artery.

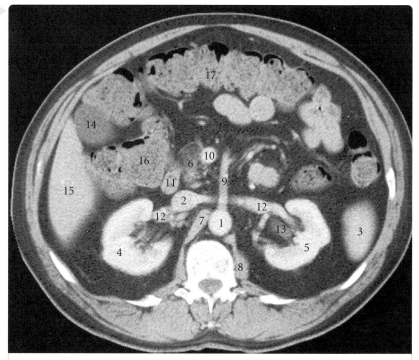

KEY

1	Aorta	10	Superior mesenteric vein
2	Inferior vena cava	11	Second part of duodenum
3	Spleen	12	Renal veins
4	Right kidney	13	Left renal pelvis
5	Left kidney	14	Gall bladder
6	Pancreas	15	Liver
7	Right diaphragmatic crus	16	Ascending colon
8	Left diaphragmatic crus	17	Transverse colon
9	Superior mesenteric artery		

appreciated if the scan is performed prior to ascitic drainage.

Due to the diffuse nature of the disease process, CT has a lower sensitivity for detecting peritoneal deposits than laparoscopy.

Pseudomyxoma peritonei

This condition is characterised by the presence of large amounts of gelatinous material within the peritoneal cavity and is thought to be due to rupture of a mucinous cystadenoma or cystadenocarcinoma of the appendix or ovary.

On CT the gelatinous material is of relatively low attenuation, and may not appear much denser than ascitic fluid. However, it can be differentiated from ascites by the presence of mass effect, which produces the classic 'scalloped' edges of the liver and spleen and displaces the bowel loops posteriorly (Fig. 4.25).

Mesothelioma

This is a primary tumour of the peritoneum arising from the mesothelial cells, and is associated with previous asbestos exposure. On CT it may appear as nodular masses or diffuse thickening of the mesentery,

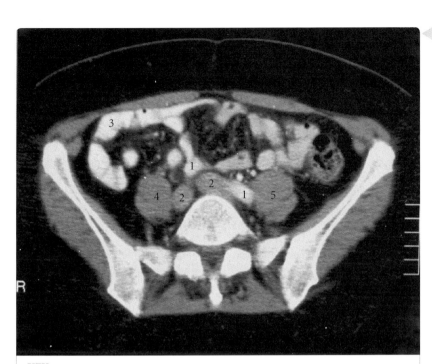

R

KEY

1 Common iliac artery
2 Common iliac vein
3 Small bowel
4 Right psoas
5 Left psoas

omentum, peritoneum and bowel wall. These masses may calcify, and if ascites is present it is usually of small volume. Patients usually present late, and direct invasion of the viscera may be identified.

Peritoneal fluid

Free fluid within the peritoneal cavity is usually ascites or blood. Small volumes of fluid are seen in either the pelvis or right paracolic gutter. As the volume increases, fluid will be seen to fill the pelvis, extend into the upper abdomen and in severe cases cause significant distension of the abdominal wall. In ascites the loops of small bowel tend to float anteriorly, which helps differentiate it from pseudomyxoma peritonei. Often the attenuation of the fluid is near 0HU and it is not possible to differentiate the cause of the fluid on CT. In cases of severe acute haemorrhage the fluid may appear dense, but a haemoperitoneum is usually assumed by the history rather than the imaging appear-

ances. Other signs such as a cirrhotic liver, pelvic mass or dilated right heart may provide clues to the cause.

In cases of peritoneal tuberculosis peritoneal fluid is often of increased density and irregular soft tissue masses may be seen in the omentum or mesentery. Retroperitoneal lymphadenopathy may also be a feature.

Mesenteric disorders

The mesentery is identified by the mesenteric vessels, surrounded by an area of low attenuation fat. It is occasionally the site of primary intra-abdominal lesions, and is often involved by metastatic disease or lymphoma. The mesenteric vessels may become congested (enlarged) with fluid overload, venous obstruction or tumour. 'Stranding' of the mesentery refers to increased density within the mesenteric fat, and may be a sign of oedema, inflammation, fibrosis, haemorrhage or tumour.

Fig. 4.21 Normal CT of the female pelvis.

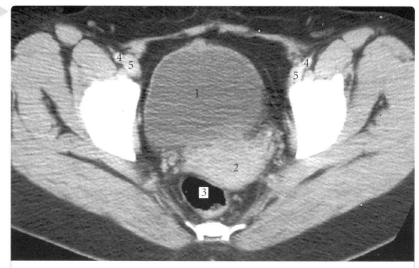

KEY

1. Bladder
2. Uterus
3. Rectum
4. External iliac artery
5. External iliac vein

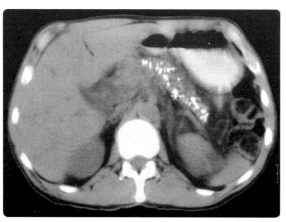

Fig. 4.22 An unenhanced CT scan showing calcification in the body and tail of the pancreas. Note that the patient has already been given oral contrast.

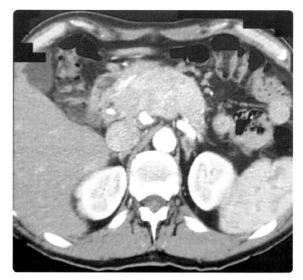

Fig. 4.23 An arterial phase scan showing a large neuroendocrine tumour in the body of the pancreas.

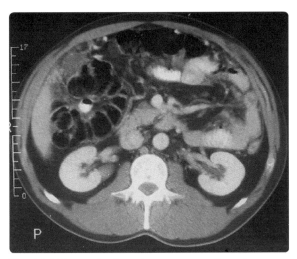

Fig. 4.24 Metastatic phaeochromocytoma. Several tumour deposits can be seen immediately under the anterior abdominal wall.

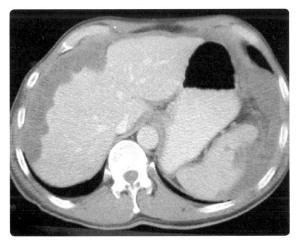

Fig. 4.25 Pseudomyxoma peritonei. The scalloped indentations can clearly be seen on the lateral aspects of the liver and spleen.

Trauma

Mesenteric haematoma may be a feature following blunt abdominal trauma and is discussed in Chapter 25.

Mesenteric ischaemia

Acute occlusion of the superior mesenteric artery may be due to either thrombosis or embolisation and is the cause of acute bowel ischaemia in 60–70% of cases. It is commonly associated with left atrial thrombus in a patient with atrial fibrillation. Bowel ischaemia is discussed in Chapter 10.

Sclerosing mesenteritis

Also termed retractile mesenteritis, mesenteric panniculitis and mesenteric lipodystrophy, this is a condition characterised by chronic inflammation of the mesentery. Depending upon whether the dominant histological finding is inflammation, fat necrosis or fibrosis, the appearance on CT will range from a diffuse increase in the density of the mesentery (misty mesentery) to a focal mass. In the latter case it can be difficult to differentiate from other causes of a mesenteric mass such as carcinoid, desmoid tumour and lymphoma.

Desmoid tumours/cysts

Desmoid tumours are uncommon locally invasive connective tissue lesions. They may arise from the abdominal wall or mesentery. Abdominal wall desmoids usually involve the rectus abdominus muscle and most commonly occur in young women of childbearing age, often within 2 years of a pregnancy (Fig. 4.26). Intraabdominal desmoids may occur in association with familial adenomatous polyposis and are often ill defined. The differential diagnosis on imaging is of any other cause of a mesenteric mass as listed above. Mesenteric cysts may be found incidentally on imaging and can be up to several centimetres in size. They should be well defined, but can be of varying attenuation.

Spleen

The spleen is easily seen in the left upper quadrant, and is a guide to the position of the tail of the pancreas. Care should be taken in assessing the spleen as it has normal patchy enhancement on arterial phase scans which may be mistaken for disease. Ideally the spleen should be assessed on venous phase images, when it should demonstrate homogeneous contrast enhancement. Haematological conditions may cause splenomegaly, as may a variety of other conditions such as cirrhosis and viral infections. There may be other features of disease seen on the CT, which may suggest a diagnosis, such as portal hypertension or lymphadenopathy from lymphoma. Focal lesions

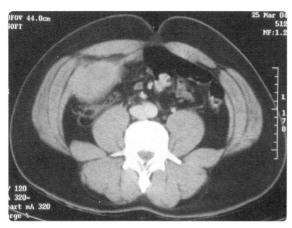

Fig. 4.26 A desmoid tumour arising from the anterior abdominal wall.

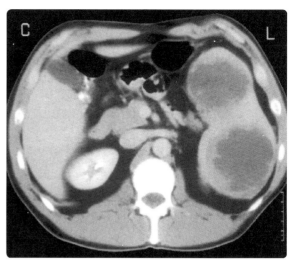

Fig. 4.27 An abdominal CT slice taken from a patient with metastatic melanoma. There are two deposits within the spleen.

in the spleen may be due to a variety of causes including:

- simple cysts
- hydatid disease
- metastatic deposits (e.g. malignant melanoma) (Fig. 4.27)
- infarcts.

The CT grading of splenic trauma may decide whether a conservative or operative approach is adopted (see Chapter 25).

Lymph nodes

Lymph nodes may be identified throughout the abdomen and pelvis, including in the coeliac axis, retroperitoneum, mesentery and pelvis. The CT assessment of nodes is based on size and morphology. Generally a maximum short axis diameter of >1 cm is taken to indicate a suspicious node in malignancy, (smaller in the retrocrural, gastrohepatic ligament and porta hepatis regions) although the specificity of this is relatively low, including many reactive nodes. Sometimes nodes will have a low attenuation centre suggestive of tuberculosis, pyogenic infection or lymphoma (see Chapter 16).

Other retroperitoneal structures

The large retroperitoneal vessels are well defined on post contrast images and CT angiograms can be per-

formed for the assessment of aortic aneurysms and other vessels (see Chapter 16). Retroperitoneal masses include renal, adrenal, and pancreatic tumours and soft tissue sarcomas (see Chapter 16).

Abdominal wall

CT may be of use in the diagnosis of abdominal wall hernia (see Chapter 17) or characterising masses such as tumours of the abdominal wall (Figs 4.28 and 4.29). Foreign bodies are usually well seen. This may be of particular use in the stable trauma patient with bullet wounds to determine if a tangential course outside of the peritoneal cavity has occurred and so allowing a non-operative approach.

Role of computed tomography abdomen scan in abdominal sepsis

Abdominal sepsis can be a difficult management problem, for example in the ICU setting or in a neutropaenic patient unfit for laparotomy. CT is becoming the main investigation for detecting intra-abdominal collections, particularly if they are deep and covered by bowel gas, making them unlikely to be defined on ultrasound. If an abscess is present it should be well seen as a focal fluid collection, often containing locules of gas (Fig. 4.30). In this case, CT may be used for image guided drain insertion. Often there are non-specific features such as increased density of the mesenteric or omental fat, and the presumed diagnosis of local infection is inferred from the clinical findings.

Relatively little has been published on the effectiveness of CT as a diagnostic tool in the management of

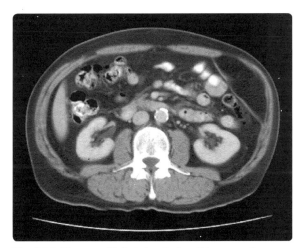

Fig. 4.28 Lipoma of left abdominal wall between the internal oblique and transversus abdominis layers

suspected intra-abdominal sepsis. In cases of severe trauma where there has been a penetrating abdominal injury or an emergency laparotomy, the sensitivity of CT in the diagnosis of an intra-abdominal focus of infection can approach 95%, with a specificity of about 60%. Even with a substantial false positive rate, it might be argued that the percutaneous aspiration of a sterile collection is less invasive than a negative laparotomy.

Effective control of intra-abdominal abscesses by CT-guided percutaneous drainage can be obtained in up to 70% of cases, particularly if the collection is a postoperative one, is unilocular and not related to a pancreatic problem. The role of CT guided drainage of peri-diverticular collections is discussed in Chapter 13.

The postoperative computed tomography scan

Following laparotomy the CT will often reveal small volumes of free fluid and increased density ('stranding') within the mesentery and peritoneum, consistent with oedema. The degree of change will gradually decrease as the time interval between surgery and the CT increases. A CT scan may be useful to assess the position of drains or to confirm the resolution of a collection when drainage has ceased. A scan is often

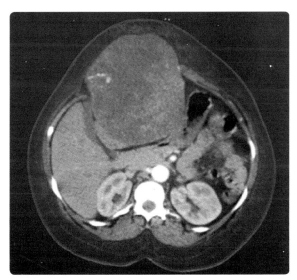

Fig. 4.29 Soft tissue tumour (chondrosarcoma) of the anterior abdominal wall.

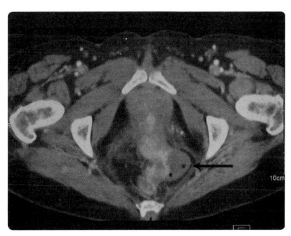

Fig. 4.30 A small pararectal abscess in a patient who presented with chills and rigors one month after an episode of acute diverticulitis. The abscess cavity (arrow) contains two locules of gas.

requested to look for evidence of an anastomotic leak or focal collection, and CT will provide information on both the size and location of any such collection, as well as being able to guide drainage if necessary.

Intervention

CT can be used to guide interventional procedures in the abdomen and pelvis, including biopsies and drain insertion (see Chapter 9).

Further reading

Bearcroft PW, Miles KA. Leucocyte scintigraphy or computed tomography for the febrile post-operative patient? Eur J Radiol 1996; 23:126–9

Boiselle PM. Multislice helical CT of the central airways. Radiol Clin N Am 2003; 41:561–74

Cho K, Morehouse H, Alterman D, Thornhill B. Sigmoid diverticulitis: diagnostic role of CT – comparison with barium enema studies. Radiology 1990; 176:111–15

Cinat ME, Wilson SE, Din AM. Determinants for successful percutaneous image-guided drainage of intra-abdominal abscess. Arch Surg 2002; 137:845–9

Dodds WJ, Taylor AJ, Erickson SJ et al. Radiological imaging of splenic anomalies. AJR 1990; 155:805–10

Erasmus JJ, Connolly JE, McAdams HP, Roggli VL. Solitary pulmonary nodules: part 1. Morphologic evaluation for differentiation of benign and malignant lesions. RadioGraphics 2000; 20:43–58

Erasmus JJ, McAdams HP, Connolly JE. Solitary pulmonary nodules: part 2. Evaluation of the indeterminate nodule. RadioGraphics 2000; 20:59–66

Farr RF, Allisy-Roberts PJ. Physics for medical imaging. WB Saunders, London, 1998

Fletcher JG, Wiersema MJ, Farrell MA et al. Pancreatic malignancy: value of arterial, pancreatic, and hepatic phase imaging with multi-detector row CT. Radiology 2003; 229:81–90

Fritscher-Ravens A, Bohuslavizki KH, Brandt L et al. Mediastinal lymph node involvement in potentially resectable lung cancer: comparison of CT, positron emission tomography, and endoscopic ultrasonography with and without fine-needle aspiration. Chest 2003; 123:442–51

Goldsmith SJ, Kostakoglu L. Nuclear medicine imaging of lung cancer. Radiol Clin N Am 2000; 38:511–23

Grainger RG, Allison DJ. Grainger and Allison's Diagnostic radiology. A textbook of medical imaging, vol 1, 4th edn. Churchill Livingstone, New York, 2001

Horton K, Lawler LP, Fishman EK. CT findings in sclerosing mesenteritis (panniculitis): spectrum of disease. Radiographics 2003; 23:1561–7

Husband JES, Reznek RK. Imaging in oncology, vol. 2, chapter 41. ISIS Medical Media, Oxford, 1998

Karwinski B, Svendsen E. Comparison of clinical and postmortem diagnosis of pulmonary embolism. J Clin Pathol 1989; 42:135–9

Kaye A, Laws E. Brain tumours – an encyclopedic approach, 2nd edn. Churchill Livingstone, Edinburgh, 2001

Kim EA, Lee KS, Shim YM et al. Radiographic and CT findings in complications following pulmonary resection. RadioGraphics 2002; 22:67–86

Klein JS, Zarka MA. Transthoracic needle biopsy. Radiol Clin N Am 2000; 38:235–66

Lee MJ. Non-traumatic abdominal emergencies: imaging and intervention in sepsis. Eur Radiol 2002; 12:2172–9

McLaughlin JS, Krasna MJ. Parapneumonic empyema. In: Shields TW (ed) General thoracic surgery, 5th edn. Lippincott, Williams & Wilkins, Baltimore, 2000

Moulton JS. Image guided management of complicated pleural fluid collections. Radiol Clin N Am 2000; 38:345–74

Mueller P, Saini S, Wittenburg J et al. Sigmoid diverticular abscesses: percutaneous drainage as adjunct to surgical resection in 24 cases. Radiology 1987; 164:321–5

Pannu HK, Bristow RE, Montz FJ, Fishman EK. Multidetector CT of peritoneal carinomatosis from ovarian cancer. Radiographics 2003; 23:687–701

Park B, Louie O, Altorki N. Staging and the surgical management of lung cancer. Radiol Clin N Am 2000; 38:545–61

Reilly PL, Bullock R. Head injury. Pathophysiology and management of severe closed injury. Chapman and Hall, London, 1997

Rivas LA, Fishman JE, Munera F, Bajayo DE. Multisclice CT in thoracic trauma. Radiol Clin N Am 2003; 41:599–616

Rydberg J, Liang Y, Teague SD. Fundamentals of multichannel CT. Radiol Clin N Am 2003; 41:465–74

Schoepf UJ, Becker CR, Hofmann LK, Yucel EK. Multidetector-row CT of the heart. Radiol Clin N Am 2003; 41:491–506

Sheth S, Horton KM. Garland MR, Fishman EK. Mesenteric neoplasms: CT appearances of primary and secondary tumours and differential diagnosis. Radiographics 2003; 23:457–73

Siewert B, Raptopoulos V. CT of the acute abdomen: findings and impact on diagnosis and treatment. AJR 1994; 163:1317–24

Stojadinovic A, Hoos A, Karpoff HM et al. Soft tissue tumours of the abdominal wall: analysis of disease patterns and treatment. Arch Surg 2001; 136:70–9

The PIOPED Investigators. Value of the ventilation/perfusion scan in acute pulmonary embolism: results of the Prospective Investigation of Pulmonary Embolism Diagnosis (PIOPED). JAMA 1990; 263:2753–9

Thomsen HS, Morcos SK. Contrast media and the kidney: European Society of Urogenital Radiology (ESUR) Guidelines. BJR 2003; 76:513–18

Urban BA, Fishman EK. Tailored helical CT evaluation of acute abdomen. Radiographics 2000; 20:725–49

Velmahos GC, Kamel E, Berne TV et al. Abdominal computed tomography for the diagnosis of intra-abdominal sepsis in critically injured patients: fishing in murky waters. Arch Surg 1999; 134: 831–6

Washington L, Miller WT Jr. Computed tomography of the lungs, pleura and chest wall. In: Shields TW (ed) General thoracic surgery, 5th edn. Lippincott, Williams & Wilkins, Baltimore, 2000

Wiesner W, Khurana B, Ji H, Ros PR. CT of acute bowel ischemia. Radiology 2003; 226:635–50

Yankelevitz DF, Henschke CI. Small pulmonary nodules. Radiol Clin N Am 2000; 38:471–8

Ultrasound 5

K.L. Gormly, D. Walters, J.R. Bessell, N.A. Rieger, I. Martin

INTRODUCTION

K.L. Gormly

Background

Ultrasound is one of the most widely used modalities of imaging as it is a versatile examination that can be used for many areas of the body. It has the advantage of being mobile, enabling the investigation to be used at the bedside in intensive care units, the trauma room, and the operating theatre. The development of small portable hand held units has allowed ultrasound to be used further afield, for example in rural settings.

The lack of ionizing radiation provides significant advantages, particularly in the imaging of children and women of reproductive age. Ultrasound is a dynamic procedure and there is no substitute for being present at the actual examination or performing it yourself. This is why a number of surgeons are choosing to become qualified in ultrasound and performing pre-operative scans to allow a better appreciation of the anatomy and relations of a mass before going to surgery.

Interventional procedures are frequently performed under ultrasound guidance, particularly biopsies and drainages. Other procedures include thrombin embolisation of false aneurysms, central venous catheter insertion and radiofrequency ablation.

Advantages of ultrasound as an imaging modality

- No ionizing radiation
- Relatively inexpensive
- Portable
- Real-time imaging
- Guidance of intervention
- Good tissue resolution of many structures (thyroid, muscles, ovaries)

BASIC PRINCIPLES OF ULTRASOUND

Ultrasound (US) uses high-frequency sound waves transmitted into the body, which when reflected by interfaces provide information about the sampled tissue. Piezoelectric crystals are used to generate ultrasound waves with frequencies in the range of 1–20 MHz. These crystals are embedded in the ultrasound probe and each crystal has a specific frequency. A pulse is initiated from the probe and a longitudinal sound wave propagates through the body. Some of the energy is absorbed by the soft tissue and some is reflected at interfaces between tissues of different densities. This reflected energy is received by the probe, which calculates the depth of the interface by measuring the time taken to return. Soft tissue interfaces only reflect part of the energy and the residual energy continues and is able to provide information about deeper structures. At soft tissue-gas and soft tissue-bone interfaces almost all of the energy is reflected and therefore it is not possible to gain information about deeper tissues.

Higher ultrasound frequencies (7–15 MHz) have higher resolution, but are strongly absorbed by soft tissue and are therefore used to assess superficial structures such as the thyroid gland, breast, testis and tendons. The highest frequencies (15–20 MHz) will travel for only a few millimetres within tissue and so are limited to intravascular and ocular studies. Lower frequencies (3–7 MHz) are of lower resolution, but are less strongly absorbed and so can be used to assess deeper structures such as the abdominal and pelvic organs.

With the trade-off between resolution and depth, obesity is a limiting factor in transabdominal scanning. In obese patients with many centimetres of subcutaneous fat, much of the ultrasound wave is absorbed before it reaches the area of interest and therefore the images are suboptimal. The structure to be assessed also has to be accessible to the ultrasound wave and not covered by gas or bone.

Many different probes have been developed for a variety of clinical uses, with the main differences being the frequency and the shape/size of the probe and 'footprint'. As described above, higher frequencies are good for assessing superficial structures and these probes usually have a small footprint (i.e. the part in contact with the patient's skin). This enables the majority of the footprint to be in contact with the area of interest, for example the thyroid gland. Abdominal probes are of lower frequencies, and are usually curved, producing a sector image like a fan. Endoluminal probes are shaped to allow them to be inserted into the vagina or rectum, and use medium frequencies.

The use of a 'coupling gel' is important to remove any air between the probe and the skin surface. If this is not done the air will reflect the ultrasound wave and no picture will be obtained. If necessary sterile gel can be used over wounds and for internal or intra-operative scans.

MODALITIES OF ULTRASOUND

There are different modes of displaying the amplitude of the reflected sound waves. These different modalities of ultrasound are:

- A mode
- M mode
- B mode
- Doppler:
  - colour Doppler
  - spectral Doppler
  - power Doppler.

A and M mode ultrasound

A mode (amplitude) ultrasound calculates only the depth of the interface and is mostly of historical interest. M mode (movement) uses the transmitted pulse repeated rapidly, enabling a trace of depth versus time to be obtained for different interfaces. This is used in cardiac ultrasound.

B mode ultrasound

B mode (brightness) is the routine ultrasound image for most general surgical applications. It is the production of a 2D grey-scale image by a beam sweeping through a slice of tissue while multiple pulses are sent out and received.

Doppler ultrasound

Doppler ultrasound uses the Doppler effect, whereby when ultrasound is reflected from a moving structure (i.e. blood) the frequencies of the incident and reflected waves are different. The amount of frequency change is determined by the speed and direction of blood flow, enabling the calculation of these two parameters.

Colour Doppler refers to the overlay of a colour image on the grey scale image. This provides information on the direction of flow and an indica-tion of velocity given by a colour scale, the sensitivity and direction of which can be altered by the operator.

Spectral Doppler is the interrogation of a single vessel to provide quantitative measurements of velocity. This information is displayed graphically as a spectral trace (velocity versus time). The angle of incidence of the beam to the vessel and the size of the 'gate' affect the accuracy of the measurement and need to be optimised by a skilled operator.

Power Doppler gives no information on direction of flow or velocity. It is useful for detecting blood flow in low flow states and provides an overview of the extent of vascularity e.g. perfusion assessment in a transplanted kidney.

Characteristics of blood flow have an obvious role in vascular investigation (see Chapter 21) but are also pivotal to all areas of diagnostic ultrasound. This extra information can assist in differentiating pathologies. Increased vascularity throughout an organ can suggest inflammation (e.g. epididymo-orchitis), whereas the absence of flow suggests ischaemia (e.g. testicular torsion). The pattern of vessels may also be useful, for example in lymph nodes, where normal or reactive nodes have a dominant hilar blood vessel, and malignant nodes usually have vessels growing in from the periphery.

APPEARANCE OF ULTRASOUND IMAGES

Grey-scale pictures are exactly that – a mixture of shades of grey ranging from white to black. Each pixel in the image is assigned a brightness based on the relative amplitude of the reflected sound wave. Structures that reflect almost all the ultrasound beam will appear white and are termed 'hyperechoic' (e.g. fat, calcification). Structures that absorb, refract or scatter the ultrasound appear dark grey and are termed 'hypoechoic' (e.g. fluid in cysts, vessels, oedema). A structure containing no internal echoes appears black and is termed 'anechoic' (Fig. 5.1).

It is important to be aware that the physical properties of sound can affect the image appearance. Features such as acoustic shadowing and enhancement may provide useful diagnostic information

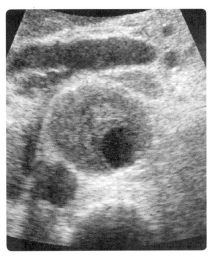

Fig. 5.1 This ultrasound image of an abdominal aortic aneurysm shows a small anechoic segment of vessel, which is the patent lumen, and a larger hypochoic area which is the mural thrombus.

while artefacts can degrade the image and prove misleading.

Acoustic shadowing and enhancement

Acoustic shadowing refers to decreased echogenicity deep to a structure and can be due to reflection or increased absorption of US by a tissue. This can be useful in identifying calcified structures such as gallstones, as the eye is drawn to the area of shadowing. Edge shadows are seen beyond the edges of curved structures and again may make them more noticeable.

Acoustic enhancement refers to increased echogenicity deep to a structure. This is caused by decreased absorption of ultrasound by a tissue, with the area deep to that tissue appearing brighter due to over compensation during processing. Prominent acoustic enhancement helps confirm the fluid nature of a lesion with low echogenicity, for example a breast cyst versus a mass (Fig. 5.2).

Ultrasound contrast agents

One of the recent advances in ultrasound has been the development of intravascular contrast agents that are

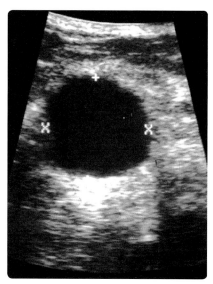

Fig. 5.2 The decreased echogenicity of this breast cyst has produced an areas of brightness beyond the cyst.

visible on ultrasound. These agents consist of 'microbubbles' injected intravenously and act as vascular echo enhancers. Microbubbles comprise gas (air or perflurocarbon) stabilized by a shell of albumin or surfactant. Newer microbubble agents are less than 10 μm in diameter and can cross capillary beds and they can be visualized spreading throughout tissues in real time. In addition to providing improved images they can also be used to provide functional information about microcirculations and have potential to be used for targeted therapeutic agents. Liver specific microbubbles have been developed and are effective in the assessment of liver lesions, by using enhancement characteristics similar to those seen on CT, for example to differentiate between a metastasis and a haemangioma.

PREPARATION AND PRECAUTIONS

Preparation for ultrasound

For abdominal ultrasound the patient should be fasted for 6 hours to minimise bowel gas and promote gall bladder distension. Bowel gas degrades the images and impairs visualisation of deeper structures, e.g. pancreas. A collapsed gall bladder can appear pathologically thickened and small stones may go undetected.

If patients are being sent for a renal scan to include assessment of the urinary bladder, an indwelling urinary catheter should be clamped before the procedure to ensure adequate bladder distension.

Pelvic transabdominal imaging is facilitated by a full bladder which acts as an 'acoustic window.' This produces superior images of deeper structures and reduces the chances of intervening bowel loops. The bladder is emptied for transvaginal scanning, or occasionally to assess a large pelvic cystic mass.

Precautions/contraindications

Ultrasound does not expose the patient to ionising radiation but there are potential thermal and mechanical bioeffects. These effects are still under investigation, particularly in pregnancy, but have not been reported using diagnostic modalities. They are more likely in lengthy focused Doppler applications using high frequency transducers, contrast agents or at soft tissue-bone interfaces. Heat is also produced at the transducer point of contact e.g. endocavity scanning. As with any procedure the scan should only be performed if clinically justified.

While there are no contraindications to ultrasound, patient cooperation, body habitus and any skin wounds (which may prevent access) should be considered before ordering an examination.

NEW DEVELOPMENTS IN ULTRASOUND

There have been a number of major recent developments in ultrasound. These include the development of 3D ultrasound using multiplanar image reconstruction and new imaging modalities such as tissue harmonic imaging. Tissue harmonic imaging is a new modality of ultrasound which differs from conventional ultrasound. It is particularly useful for imaging 'difficult' areas such as the retroperitoneum and may have application in obese patients. Other new modalities are beyond the scope of this text but include elastography and vibro-acoustography which utilize the physical behaviour of tissue and are likely to come into clinical practice in the next few years. Recent advances have also seen the development of therapeutic ultrasound.

ABDOMINOPELVIC ULTRASOUND

D. Walters, K. Gormly

Background

Ultrasound of the abdomen is one of the most frequently performed radiological investigations in general surgery. This chapter deals with the interpretation of abdomino-pelvic ultrasound images and the application of this imaging modality in the management of patients with suspected appendicitis. Ultrasound has many other uses within the abdomen and these are dealt with in the appropriate chapters:

- Gallstones/biliary obstruction (see Chapter 12)
- Liver lesions (see Chapter 12)
- Renal obstruction/focal lesions (see Chapter 18)
- Abdominal aortic aneurysms (see Chapter 21)
- Appendicitis (see Chapter 10)

ABDOMINAL ULTRASOUND

Image interpretation

Abdominal scans tend to be performed by sonographers and reported by radiologists. This means a relatively standard format of images is obtained on hard copy to ensure adequate representation of the organs assessed. Images are obtained in sagittal ('sag' or 'LS' for longitudinal section) and axial/transverse planes ('trans' or 'TS'). On axial images the right of the patient usually appears on the left side of the image as in CT, and on sagittal images superior is often on the left, although this may be variable. The plane should be indicated on the film by an annotation or body diagram, and the main structure assessed is usually annotated. Callipers are used for measurements and a colour Doppler box may be seen on the black and white image (e.g. indicating flow in the portal vein).

Key images are:

- liver in transverse and sagittal sections
- gall bladder
- pancreas lying anterior to the splenic vein and portal confluence
- CBD lying anterior to the portal vein (with CBD diameter measurement)
- kidneys in maximal length
- spleen in maximal craniocaudal length
- aorta in transverse plane.

It is important to remember that ultrasound is a dynamic test and best appreciated by performing, or watching, the procedure. The hard copy images provide only representative images and lesions may be missed, or normal structures made to look abnormal, in the image acquisition. Confidence in the person performing the scan is of utmost importance and if there are difficult clinical questions, particularly regarding anatomy or the location of a lesion, there is no substitute for attending the scan in person. In certain situations a limited targeted ultrasound will be performed to answer a particular clinical question.

Appendicitis

Despite advances in imaging and laboratory testing, early surgical consultation remains pre-eminent in the evaluation of patients suspected of having appendicitis. Recently, ultrasonography (± saline enema), limited pelvic CT (± rectal contrast) and early diagnostic laparoscopy have each been advocated to limit the duration of hospital stay, prevent inappropriate discharge, screen for alternate pathology and reduce negative laparotomy and perforation rates (1–3%).

Ultrasound may be used in the assessment of patients with possible appendicitis, but the role of routine imaging is controversial. The rate of non-therapeutic interventions range from 7% to 40% in reproductive age females. It is in this subgroup where evidence supports imaging as a cost-effective adjunct to clinical examination (see Chapter 10). However, ultrasound offers little benefit in the clinically unequivocal patient and may delay definitive management.

The use of graded compression ultrasound (i.e. gradually increasing the pressure of the ultrasound probe over the right iliac fossa to displace the bowel gas) has a sensitivity ranging from 75 to 90% and a specificity of 78–100% in the diagnosis of appendicitis. The diagnostic accuracy of transabdominal US depends on the habitus of the patient as well as the experience and enthusiasm of the sonologist. Visualisation of an enlarged (>6 mm) appendix at the point of tenderness has a positive predictive value of >85%, however the appendix can be difficult to visualize especially if retrocaecal. If the examination is performed by an experienced operator, the benefit to the surgeon will be increased and this will probably become more widely accepted with time.

If the appendix can be visualised it will appear as a blind ending tubular structure. An inflamed appendix will have a transverse diameter of greater than 6 mm and be non-compressible. Sometimes a target appearance is seen due to hypoechoic fluid within the lumen, a hyperechoic inflamed submucosa and hypoechoic outer muscle. Supporting findings for a diagnosis of appendicitis are the presence of an appendicolith, which will appear as an echogenic structure with distal acoustic shadowing, and the presence of an adjacent fluid collection (Fig. 5.3) (Box 5.1).

WHAT TO LOOK FOR — Box 5.1

on ultrasound in suspected appendicitis

- Appendix > 6 mm diameter
- Appendicolith
- Periappendiceal fluid collection or mass
- Enlarged mesenteric nodes

FEMALE PELVIC ULTRASOUND

Image interpretation

Transabdominal and transvaginal ultrasound are valuable investigations of the female pelvis and provide better visualisation of the uterus and ovaries than CT. The lack of ionising radiation is an important factor in assessing the reproductive organs. Transabdominal (TA) scanning is performed with a full bladder, which is used as an 'acoustic window', pushing bowel out of the way and allowing the ultrasound beam to reach the uterus and ovaries. It is useful in assessing large pelvic masses, free fluid in the pouch of Douglas, intrauterine and ectopic pregnancies. The hypoechoic, fluid-filled bladder is seen anteriorly, with the uterus imaged in sagittal and transverse planes (Fig. 5.4). The uterus and ovaries are often magnified, with only a small portion of the bladder being visible.

Transvaginal (TV) scanning is performed with the bladder empty and uses an intra-cavity probe. These images may appear different to look at, with the probe seen at the superior or inferior aspect of the image. Normally, the uterus is much better visualised with TV scans (Box 5.2), providing an accurate measurement of endometrial thickness, assessment of the myometrium and reliable visualisation of an intrauterine pregnancy from six weeks onwards. Occasionally large calcified fibroids make the examination very difficult and visualisation is suboptimal. If the ovaries can be

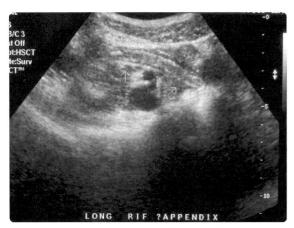

Fig. 5.3 A mildly inflamed appendix. The ultrasound examination was performed because of doubt over the clinical diagnosis.

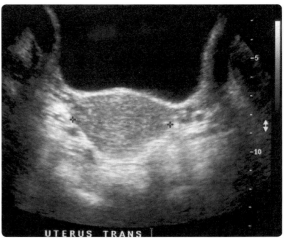

Fig. 5.4 Normal uterus and bladder in the transverse plane.

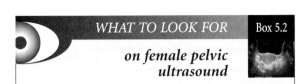

WHAT TO LOOK FOR — Box 5.2

on female pelvic ultrasound

- Uterus:
  - size and shape
  - endometrial thickness
  - homogeneity of myometrium
  - intrauterine gestational sac, yolk sac, fetal pole
- Ovaries:
  - size
  - presence and distribution of follicles
  - cysts (size, internal echogenicity, septations, mural nodules)
- Free fluid: anechoic or containing echoes suggestive of haemorrhage or pus
- Adnexal mass:
  - size and shape
  - echogenicity
  - vascularity

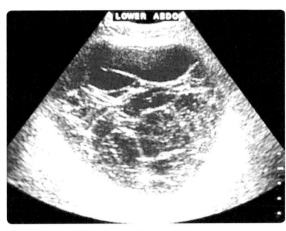

Fig. 5.5 A multilocular ovarian cyst.

identified on TV scanning the internal architecture is much better defined than on TA scans.

Adnexal masses

Adnexal masses are common in reproductive age women. Most adnexal masses in this group are non-neoplastic and include functional ovarian cysts, para-ovarian cysts (10% arising from broad ligament), peritoneal inclusion cysts (postsurgery or inflammation) and complications of ovarian torsion, endometriosis and pelvic inflammatory disease. Neoplastic masses become more common with increasing age, but do not usually present until they are large with associated peritoneal disease. Complex cystic lesions, solid ovarian tumours, rapidly growing masses and any lesion over 5 cm are significant (Fig. 5.5). Small ovarian masses and cysts are best assessed by transvaginal scanning, which will detect any cyst septations or wall thickening. Even completely simple cystic structures >5 cm warrant follow-up to resolution.

Gastrointestinal causes of 'adnexal' masses should also be considered, including primary and secondary malignancy and inflammatory masses. Faecal material in the rectum can masquerade as a pseudo-mass and a follow-up scan after saline enema or evacuation may be helpful.

Ectopic pregnancy

The purpose of imaging in the suspected ectopic pregnancy is to confirm an intrauterine pregnancy, as this greatly reduces the chances of an ectopic (1 in 30 000). The classic triad of an empty uterus, adnexal mass and free fluid appears in only 20%.

A TA scan should be performed initially while the patient's bladder is full. This will detect an adnexal mass which may be distant from the uterus and not appreciated if only TV scanning is performed. If there is no abnormality, or further assessment is required, the patient can then empty their bladder and a TV scan performed. On TV scanning a yolk sac should be visible within the gestational sac at 5 weeks, and a fetal pole with cardiac activity visible at 6 weeks gestation.

Pelvic pain

Other gynaecological conditions which may cause acute pelvic pain and can be assessed on ultrasound include torsion or rupture of an ovarian cyst, endometriosis and pelvic inflammatory disease, although US is often normal in the latter two conditions.

In ovarian torsion the US appearances are variable, but the ovary is usually enlarged and may demonstrate absence of flow on Doppler imaging. There is often free fluid in the pouch of Douglas, which is usually the only finding in the case of a ruptured ovarian cyst. Endometrial implants may occur anywhere in the peritoneal cavity and are often sonographically occult. Large cystic masses (chocolate cysts) may be visible and appear as a cyst containing homogeneous mid/low level echoes, possibly with a fluid level. Acute rupture of an endometrioma can cause acute pain and also produce free fluid. In acute pelvic inflammatory disease free fluid may be present containing low-level echoes due to pus. Enlargement of the fallopian tubes suggests a hydro/pyosalpinx or progression to tuboovarian abscess.

ENDOLUMINAL AND INTRAOPERATIVE ULTRASOUND

J.R. Bessell, N.A. Rieger, I. Martin

Background

Endoscopic ultrasound (EUS) refers to the integration of two imaging techniques – endoscopy and ultrasound. EUS does not differentiate malignancy from benign inflammation as both processes cause similar changes in the gastrointestinal wall. EUS provides information about the layer of origin of a lesion, the echotexture, and margins. With developments in endoscopic resection of mucosal neoplasms of the oesophagus and stomach and wider use of neo-adjuvant chemotherapy, there is a real need for accurate staging pre- and post-treatment. EUS is most useful when the histology is already known, to provide more detailed investigative information that may change management.

The learning curve for EUS can be long, with approximately 100 examinations required to reach an acceptable T-stage accuracy. The accuracy of EUS varies with the expertise of the user and the sophistication of the equipment.

Recently, 3D EUS has become available using a high-resolution mini-probe. It can measure tumour volume, which may be a better discriminator of prognosis than the level of invasion or tumour thickness and expand the applications of EUS.

THE UPPER DIGESTIVE TRACT

Equipment

There are two main EUS probes:
- dedicated echoendoscopes
- blind mini-probes.

The most common echoendoscope is a rotating sector scanner (Fig. 5.6). This is a side-viewing endoscope with a transducer on the tip giving a 360 degree image. Many scopes use both 5 and 20 MHz. The higher frequency increases image resolution but decreases the penetration depth.

A second type of dedicated echoendoscope has an oblique-viewing endoscope with a linear array scanner at the tip. This provides a 100 to 270 degree image and allows FNA and colour Doppler to be performed.

Blind mini-probes are inserted through the instrument channel of a standard gastro/duodenoscope. They can be used to examine obstructing oesophageal tumours, or be passed intra-ductally into the common bile duct or pancreatic duct (see Box 5.3).

Clinical uses
- Locoregional staging of malignancy, e.g. oesophageal, gastric, duodenal and periampullary carcinomas.

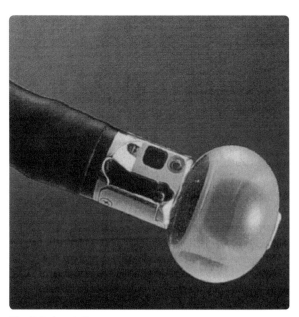

Fig. 5.6 A rotating sector scanner.

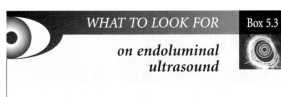

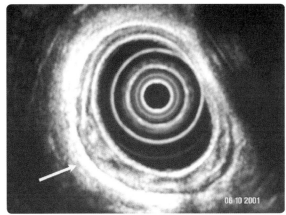

Fig. 5.8 A T1/2 tumour of the oesophagus. The (bright) adventitial layer (arrow) is not involved.

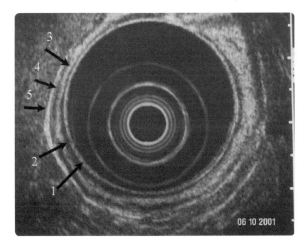

Fig. 5.7 An assessment of the normal oesophagus by endoscopic ultrasonography. From the outermost ring, the five layers of the digestive tract are: 5, adventitia/serosa (bright); 4, muscularis propria (dark); 3, submucosa (bright); 2, muscularis mucosae (dark); 1, mucosal surface (bright).

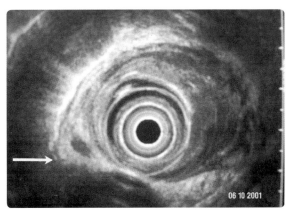

Fig. 5.9 A T3/4 carcinoma of the oesophagus. The bright adventitial layer (arrow) has been lost by tumour invasion.

- Assessment of lesions in the gastrointestinal wall, e.g. stromal tumours, gastric lymphoma.
- Assessment of mediastinal lymphadenopathy.
- Biopsy of potentially malignant nodes from the lung, oesophagus, liver.
- Investigation of jaundice.
- Diagnosis of chronic pancreatitis and pancreatic ductal calculi.
- Assessment of pancreatic tumours (including islet cell tumours) (see Chapter 12).
- Therapeutic alcohol injection into coeliac plexus.

Oesophagus

At a scanning frequency of 7.5 MHz the normal oesophageal wall is a five layered structure of alternating bright and dark bands (Fig. 5.7).

EUS staging of oesophageal carcinoma is more accurate than CT for detection of local tumour, with up to 92% correct T stage prediction. It is particularly effective in differentiating between T1/2 and T3/4 tumours (Figs 5.8 and 5.9). This has important implications in management (see Chapter 11). It is important to emphasize that loss of the fifth layer represents local organ invasion, and this usually renders tumours irresectable.

Malignant oesophageal strictures precluding passage of the EUS scope are a common problem, and

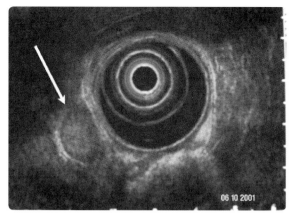

Fig. 5.10 A benign, enlarged lymph node (arrow). It is elongated, hyperechoic, heterogenous, and has an echogenic hilum with instinct borders.

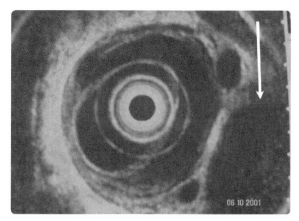

Fig. 5.11 The ultrasonographic appearances of a malignant lymph node (arrow). It is round, sharply demarcated, hypoechoic, homogenous, and there is no echogenic hilum.

attempts to dilate the tumour prior to EUS can be associated with a high perforation rate. However, EUS is still worthwhile because stenotic tumours are virtually always full-thickness, and excellent staging can be achieved by scanning proximal to the tumour.

Pancreas

EUS has been widely used as a diagnostic and staging tool for pancreatic cancer. With new development in 3D CT and MRCP, the place of EUS is less clear. However it is a reliable investigation with a diagnostic accuracy of over 90%. EUS and FNA is particularly useful in patients who have a small pancreatic cancer which may not be visible as a mass lesion on CT. Absence of a visible lesion on EUS can effectively exclude the presence of a pancreatic cancer.

Lymph nodes

When examining lymph nodes, EUS provides information regarding shape, border demarcation, echo intensity and echo texture (Figs 5.10 and 5.11).

Features suggesting malignancy are:

- roundness and absence of an echogenic hilum
- sharply demarcated, homogenous, hypoechoic features.

There is good agreement between the number of mediastinal nodes detected by EUS and the number recovered by pathology. Overall EUS yields 86% correct

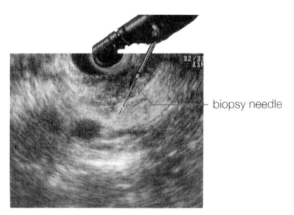

Fig. 5.12 EUS-guided needle biopsy for FNA of a peri-oesophageal lymph node. The needle is in the lymph node.

N-stage prediction. Limitations of lymph node evaluation are:

- overestimation of malignant involvement
- failure to detect regional nodes in the abdominal cavity.

EUS-guided FNA lymph node staging The accuracy of nodal staging can be improved by using a linear array probe. A needle is passed down the biopsy channel of the sonoscope, through the wall of the oesophagus and into adjacent structures such as lymph nodes (Fig. 5.12). The orientation of the ultrasound beam allows continuous monitoring of the needle tip.

Mediastinal tumours, liver metastases, and upper abdominal lymph nodes can also be biopsied this way. The addition of FNA to EUS nodal (N) staging can improve sensitivity and accuracy from 86 to 93%, and specificity to 100%, with minimal complications.

LOWER DIGESTIVE TRACT

Endoanal ultrasound

Clinical applications of EAUS

Endoanal ultrasound (EAUS) is used principally as an investigative tool in the management of faecal incontinence. It has an adjunctive role in the management of perianal abscess and anal fistula. Patients with other disorders such as ill-defined anal pain, constipation, anal canal tumours and congenital anorectal malformations may benefit to a lesser degree from the use of this investigation.

EAUS involves inserting a specially designed ultrasound probe into the anal canal. EAUS is safe and easy to perform with little patient discomfort. It has surpassed electromyelography (EMG) in the evaluation of the integrity of the anal sphincters. It allows accurate anatomical delineation of the anal sphincters (Fig. 5.13). A defect in the anal sphincter, if present may be amenable to direct repair (sphincteroplasty). Defects seen on EAUS have been correlated with histological examination and operative findings and found to be accurate (Fig. 5.14).

Endorectal ultrasound

Endorectal ultrasound (ERUS) is an accurate investigation for local staging of rectal tumours. It can assess the depth of tumour invasion through the rectal wall and the involvement of mesorectal lymph nodes (Fig. 5.15). With this knowledge, tumours deemed at high risk of local recurrence (T3, T4 or N1) may be offered preoperative radiotherapy or chemo-radiation. Early tumours (T0, T1) in appropriate circumstances may be more confidently treated by local excision. Each of the anatomical layers of the rectum can be seen clearly with ERUS. Imaging however may be hampered by retained faeces, large and stenosing tumours.

The accuracy of ERUS for evaluating the depth of local tumour invasion ranges from 63 to 95% and for assessing nodal metastases the accuracy ranges from 61 to 86%.

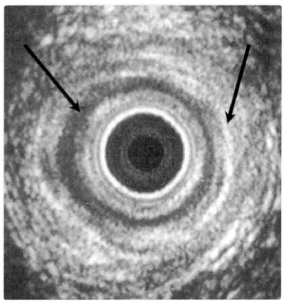

Fig. 5.13 Normal anal ultrasound at the middle of the anal canal. The internal anal sphincter is easily seen as a hypoechoic (black) ring within the anal canal. The external anal sphincter is seen as a less well defined hyperechoic (white) ring outside the internal anal sphincter.

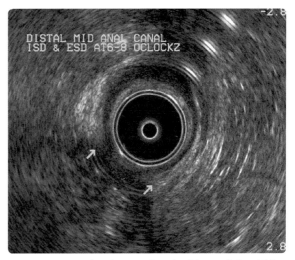

Fig. 5.14 External and internal anal sphincter defect. This defect to both the external and internal anal sphincters are due to trauma. The normal rings of muscle are disrupted between 6 and 8 o'clock.

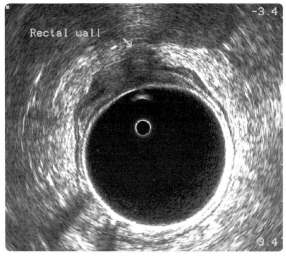

Fig. 5.15 Rectal ultrasound of a T3 tumour with spread of tumour into the perirectal fat (arrow).

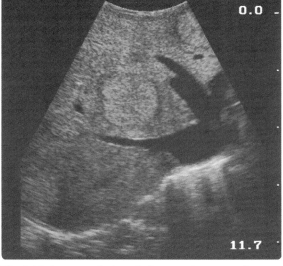

Fig. 5.16 A metastatic deposit from a colon cancer in segment VIII liver (between right and middle hepatic veins).

INTRAOPERATIVE ULTRASOUND

Intraoperative ultrasound (IOUS) is used to characterise and accurately localise pathology in various organs and at times to assess operability. The use of laparoscopic ultrasound probes may avoid open surgery in patients who are deemed non-resectable.

Clinical uses of IOUS are principally:

- liver
- pancreas.

Liver

Intraoperative ultrasound has a well-defined role in liver surgery. It can be used to:

- identify subcentimetre metastases (often missed with CT or MRI)
- characterise liver lesions and their relationship to hepatic vasculature (Fig. 5.16)
- target treatment of tumours with positional probes, e.g. thermal ablation
- identify gallstones and stones in the common bile duct.

Pancreas

Although invasive, laparoscopic ultrasound is as accurate as spiral CT in the assessment of resectability of tumours. The procedure may be used to detect small volume peritoneal or liver metastases. IOUS can:

- define the limit of a tumour
- define portal or mesenteric vein involvement with tumour
- assess lymph node involvement
- locate small functioning endocrine tumours.

Further reading

Agargwal B, Abu-Hamda E, Molke KL et al. Endoscopic ultrasound-guided fine needle aspiration and multidetector spiral CT in the diagnosis of pancreatic cancer. Am Gastroenterol 2004; 99;844–50

Bergman JGHM, Fockens P. Endoscopic ultrasonography in patients with gastro-esophageal cancer. Eur J Ultrasound 1999; 10:127–38

Beynon J, Mortensen NJ, Foy DM et al. Pre-operative assessment of local invasion in rectal cancer: digital examination, endoluminal sonography or computed tomography? Br J Surg 1986; 73:1015–17

Branda H, Vlad L, Sparchez Z et al. In situ thermal ablation of focal liver neoplasms, with a special emphasis on the intraoperative ultrasound-guided radio frequency ablation method. Rom J Gastroenterol 2003; 12:57–64

Calculli L, Casadei R, Amore B et al. The usefulness of spiral computed tomography and colour-Doppler ultrasonography to predict portal-mesenteric trunk involvement in pancreatic cancer. Radiol Med (Torino) 2002; 104:307–15

Caletti G, Fusaroli P, Bocus P. Endoscopic ultrasonography. Digestion 1998; 59:509–29

Conlon R, Jacobs M, Dasgupta D, Lodge JP. The value of intraoperative ultrasound during hepatic resection compared with improved preoperative magnetic resonance imaging. Eur J Ultrasound 2003; 16:211–16

Deen KI, Kumar D, Williams JG et al. Anal sphincter defects: correlation between endoanal ultrasound and surgery. Ann Surg 1993; 218:201–5

Edwards MJ. Office-based and intraoperative ultrasound enhance surgeon's care of breast disease patients. Ann Surg Oncol 2003; 10:201

Grainger RG, Allison DJ. Grainger and Allison's Diagnostic radiology. A textbook of medical imaging, vol 1, 4th edn. Churchill Livingstone, New York, 2001

Harness JK, Wisher DB. Ultrasound in surgical practice, basic principles and clinical applications. Wiley-Liss, New York, 1999

Hofer M. Ultrasound teaching manual, the basics of performing and interpreting ultrasound scans. Thieme, New York, 1999

Hohmann J, Albrecht T, Hoffmann CW, Wolf KJ. Ultrasonographic detection of focal liver lesions: increased sensitivity and specificity with microbubble contrast agents. Eur J Radiol 2003; 46:147–59

Holdsworth PJ, Johnston D, Chalmers AG et al. Endoluminal ultrasound and computed tomography in the staging of rectal cancer. Br J Surg 1988; 75:1019–22

Hunerbein M, Ghadimi BM, Gretschel S, Schlag PM. Three-dimensional endoluminal ultrasound: a new method for the evaluation of gastrointestinal tumors. Abdom Imaging 1999; 24:445–8

Isozaki T, Numata K, Kiba T et al. Differential diagnosis of hepatic tumors by using contrast enhancement patterns at US. Radiology 2003; 229:798–805

Kelly S, Harris KM, Berry E et al. A systematic review of the staging performance of endoscopic ultrasound in gastro-oesophageal carcinoma. Gut 2001; 49:534–9

Kim LS, Koch J. Do we practice what we preach? Clinical decision making and utilization of endoscopic ultrasound for staging esophageal carcinoma. Am J Gastroenterol 1999; 94:1847–52

Kumar A, Scholefield JH. Endosonography of the anal canal and rectum. World J Surg 2000; 24:208–15

Marusch F, Koch A, Schmidt U. Routine use of transrectal ultrasound in rectal carcinoma: Results of a prospective multicenter study. Endoscopy 2002; 34:385–90

McCaffrey J. Ultrasound in surgery: introduction. World J Surg 2000; 24:133

Meire H, Cosgrove D, Dewbury K. Clinical ultrasound. Abdominal and general ultrasound, 2nd edn. Harcourt, London, 2000

Nickl NJ, Bhutani MS, Catalano M et al. Clinical implications of endoscopic ultrasound: the American Endosonography Club Study. Gastrointest Endosc 1996; 44:371–7

Obermaier R, Benz S, Asgharina M et al. Value of ultrasound in the diagnosis of acute appendicitis. Eur J Med Res 2003; 8:451–6

Odegaard S. High-resolution endoluminal sonography in gastroenterology. Eur J Ultrasound 1999; 10:85–91

Poortman P, Lohle P, Schoemaker CM et al. Comparison of CT and sonography in the diagnosis of acute appendicits: a blinded prospective study. AJR 2003; 181:1355–9

Rettenbacher T, Hollerweger A, Gritzmann N et al. Appendicitis: should diagnostic imaging be performed if the clinical presentation is highly suggestive of the disease? Gastroenterology 2002; 123:992–8

Rieger NA, Sweeney JL, Hoffmann DC et al. Investigation of fecal incontinence with endoanal ultrasound. Dis Colon Rectum 1996; 39:860–4

Rifkin MD, Ehrlich SM, Marks G. Staging of rectal carcinoma: prospective comparison of endorectal US and CT. Radiology 1989; 170:319–22

Rumack CM, Wilson SR, Charboneau JW. Diagnostic ultrasound, 2nd edn. Mosby, St Louis, 1998

Sivit C, Siegel MJ, Applegate KE, Newman KD. When appendicitis is suspected in children. Radiographics 2001; 21:247–62

Sivit CJ, Applegate KE, Stallio A et al. Imaging evaluation of suspected appendicits in a paediatric population: effectiveness of sonography versus CT. AJR 2000; 175:977–80

Sultan AH, Kamm MA, Talbot IC et al. Anal endosonography for identifying external sphincter defects confirmed histologically. Br J Surg 1994; 81:463–5

Magnetic resonance imaging 6

J. Taylor, K.L. Gormly

Background

MRI is an imaging technique that uses the electromagnetic properties of body tissues rather than ionising radiation. It provides much better soft-tissue definition than other imaging modalities (such as CT) and has the advantage of multiplanar and volume acquisitions. While it is the optimum study for the assessment of many areas of the body, its use is limited by availability, cost, time and strict contraindications. As the images often take several minutes to be acquired the patient must be able to keep very still, and this will sometimes require sedation or a general anaesthetic.

BASIC PHYSICS OF MAGNETIC RESONANCE IMAGING

Magnetic resonance imaging (MRI) utilises the fact that spinning charged particles create an electromagnetic field. Hydrogen atoms contain one unpaired proton and thus have a net magnetic field. Any atom with an odd number of protons or neutrons will have a net magnetic field; hydrogen is used for MRI because it is extremely abundant throughout the body.

Normally, hydrogen protons spin around their own axes creating their own small magnetic fields, but as they are arranged randomly, the net magnetic field is zero. In MRI the body is placed inside a magnet with a strong external magnetic field. The most commonly used magnets are 1–1.5 Tesla, although low-field and high-field magnets are also available for different uses (0.1–4 Tesla). A 1-Tesla magnet has a field strength equal to 10 000 Gauss. By comparison, the earth's magnetic field is approximately 0.5 Gauss.

The placement of the body into the external magnetic field causes the protons to align along the axis of the external magnetic field, producing a net magnetisation vector with the same direction as the external magnetic field. A radiofrequency (RF) pulse is then sent into the body, which causes some of the protons to align with the applied magnetic field and precess 'in-phase', resulting in a 'flip' of the net magnetisation vector. When the RF pulse is turned off the protons will return to be aligned with the axis of the external magnetic field, giving up their excess energy. The relaxation of protons back into the equilibrium state occurs by T1 and T2 relaxation, providing the MR signal which is detected by an RF receiver placed over the patient's body.

Different tissues have different T1 and T2 relaxation times. By altering parameters such as the repetition time (TR) and echo delay time (TE), images can be produced that predominantly look at either the T1 or T2 relaxation of a tissue. Water has a long T1 relaxation, compared with fat, which has a short T1 relaxation and so on T1-weighted images water will appear dark (low signal intensity) and fat bright (high signal intensity). Comparatively, water also has a long T2 relaxation time and will appear bright on T2-weighted images, whereas fat has an intermediate relaxation time and will appear of intermediate signal intensity (Fig. 6.1). The appearance of different tissues on different sequences is complex and beyond the scope of this text (see Box 6.1).

Two techniques using this technology are chemical shift imaging and magnetic resonance angiography.

Chemical shift imaging

This technique relies on the variation in frequency of precess of hydrogen protons in different molecules (e.g. in fat and H_2O). Normally this is an artefact, but is exploited in 'in and out-of-phase' imaging to detect the presence of fat. If water and fat are in the same voxel, and the image is acquired at the time when they are precessing out of phase, the signals will cancel each other out and will appear dark on the images. This is used, for example, in imaging of adrenal adenomas, where on out-of-phase images a lipid rich adrenal adenoma will appear darker than the spleen. It is possible to tell an out-of-phase sequence by the black line

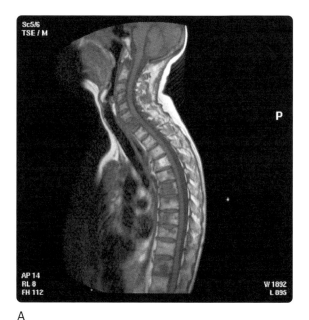

A

B

Fig. 6.1 (A) T1 and (B) T2 images of the spine. Note the CSF is dark on T1-weighted images and bright on T2-weighted images. Multiple metastatic deposits are present within the vertebral bodies.

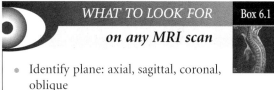

WHAT TO LOOK FOR | Box 6.1

on any MRI scan

- Identify plane: axial, sagittal, coronal, oblique
- Identify sequence:
  - T1: dark fluid, bright fat
  - T2: bright fluid
- Assess anatomy
- Assess pathology: lesions often contain fluid and so will appear bright on T2-weighted images

seen around the abdominal organs where they are adjacent to intra-abdominal fat, appearing as an 'Indian ink' border (Fig. 6.2).

Magnetic resonance angiography

There are currently three basic forms of magnetic resonance angiography (MRA). Time of flight (TOF) MRA suppresses signal from stationary tissue, while inflowing blood appears bright. However the level of signal from blood varies with the velocity and angle of the vessel. TOF MRA is now mainly used for peripheral run-off vessels. Phase contrast MRA is another technique, which relies on detecting changes in phase that result from motion. It is able to quantify blood flow, but requires long scan times, has problems in areas of turbulence and is not as commonly used. The third technique is contrast-enhanced MRA. This involves an intravenous bolus of gadolinium and dynamic imaging. On heavily weighted T1-weighted images the contrast will appear very bright against the background tissues. This is particularly useful for abdominal and peripheral MRA (Fig. 6.3).

Contrast-enhanced magnetic resonance imaging

The most commonly used MRI contrast agent is a gadolinium chelate, which has an intravascular and extracellular distribution similar to iodine. Gadolinium is a paramagnetic substance which causes increased signal on T1-weighted images. Contrast is less frequently used in MRI, as non-contrast imaging has good soft tissue contrast, unlike in CT. Intravenous gadolinium is most frequently used for cerebral tumours where enhancement indicates a higher grade, and for meningeal disease, spinal cord masses and liver lesions. It is also used in musculoskeletal imaging, injected intravenously for an indirect arthrogram, or directly into the joint prior to imaging. It is considered safe in patients with nephrotoxicity at the doses required for MRI.

Tissue-specific contrast agents have been developed, and are of increasing use. These include superparamagnetic iron oxide particles (e.g. Resovist®, Schering), which accumulate in the reticuloendothelial system and have been shown to have high sensitivity and specificity in lymph node imaging and liver lesion detection. Hepatocyte specific contrast agents such as mangafodipir trisodium (Teslascan®, Nycomed

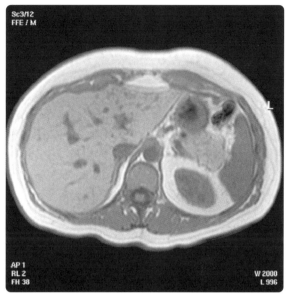

A

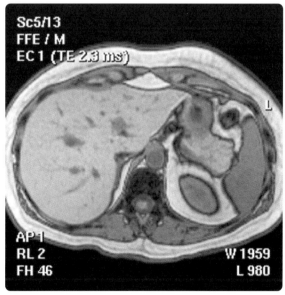

B

Fig. 6.2 (A) In phase T1-weighted image of the liver. (B) Out of phase T1-weighted image with an 'Indian-ink' border around the organs at the junction of fat and water.

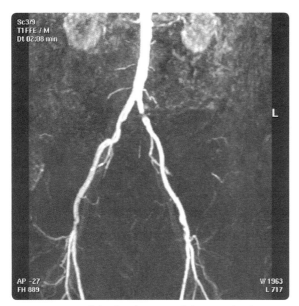

Fig. 6.3 MRA of the distal aorta and iliac vessels, showing a stenosis of the left common iliac artery.

Amersham) and gadobenate dimeglumine, (Multi-Hance®, Bracco Imaging) increase the sensitivity of liver lesion detection and allow differentiation of hepatocellular from non-hepatocellular lesions.

HAZARDS AND SAFETY ISSUES

MRI is contraindicated in patients with cardiac pacemakers, ferromagnetic intracranial aneurysm clips, ferromagnetic foreign bodies in the orbit, implanted neurostimulators and most cochlear implants. Metallic surgical prostheses may cause local artifact and degrade image quality. MRI is not believed to be harmful to the fetus. However its use in pregnant women should be limited to those clinical situations where it is essential to medical management. Claustrophobia can be a significant problem in clinical practice.

SURGICAL ROLES AND USES OF MAGNETIC RESONANCE IMAGING

Anorectal disease

With recent improvements in techniques, MRI has become an important modality in the assessment of anorectal disease (Fig. 6.4). It has an important role in the staging of primary and recurrent rectal tumours and complements endoluminal ultrasound in the classification of perianal fistula. It can also be used in the assessment of faecal incontinence.

Local staging of rectal cancer

The development of endoluminal coils and high resolution MR imaging has permitted detailed investigation of the rectal wall and tumour. High-resolution MRI has accuracies of up to 94% for T staging, and 97% in predicting involvement of the circumferential resection margin (Fig. 6.5). Accurate preoperative staging of tumours is of increasing importance as preoperative chemoradiotherapy regimens are being advocated for more advanced rectal cancers. MRI allows planning of sphincter saving surgery in low rectal tumours where appropriate. It is also sensitive in detecting rectal cancer recurrence.

The major limitations of imaging to stage rectal cancer are understaging due to microscopic invasion and overstaging due to adjacent desmoplastic reaction to the tumour.

Perianal fistula

The role of imaging in the management of patients with perianal fistula is to establish the relationship between the fistula track and the anal sphincter. This is particularly important in patients with complex fistula disease where there may be surgical concerns about postoperative faecal incontinence (see Chapter 14).

Biliary tract disease

Endoscopic retrograde cholangiopancreatography (ERCP) is still considered the procedure of choice for the obstructed biliary tree or pancreatic duct, where the aim is to decompress as well as diagnose. However, an MRCP can also provide clear images of the pancreatic-biliary ductal systems and in particular the state of the duct beyond the site of a complete obstruction (Fig. 6.6). In addition magnetic resonance cholangiopancreatography (MRCP) can be used to stage pancreatic tumours and cholangiocarcinoma (see Chapter 12). An MRCP can be used to document vascular invasion or lymph node spread.

If surgery is contemplated in the presence of duct obstruction, an MRCP may provide the required

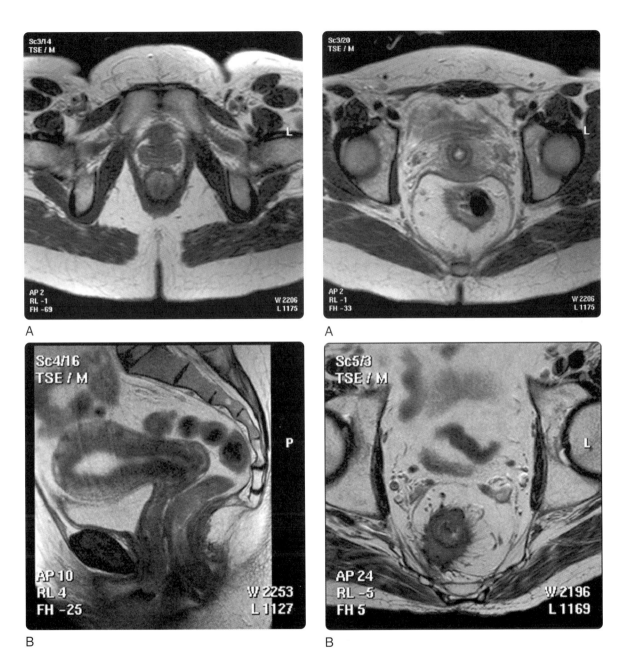

Fig. 6.4 Normal female pelvis T2-weighted images (A) axial and (B) sagittal demonstrate the high soft tissue resolution of pelvic structures on MRI.

Fig. 6.5 High resolution axial T2-weighted image of the rectum. (A) T3 tumour with desmoplastic reaction and mesorectal lymph nodes. (B) T3 tumour with involvement of the postero-lateral mesorectal fascia.

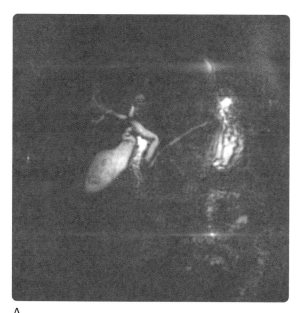
A

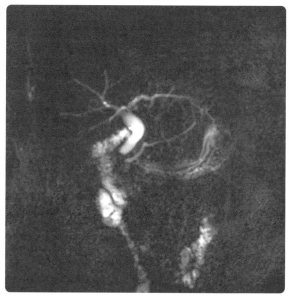
B

Fig. 6.6 Two MRCPs showing the gall bladder and normal common bile and pancreatic ducts (A) and a common bile duct obstructed at its lower end (B).

information on the site and nature of the obstruction without the inherent risk of a more invasive procedure such as ERCP. The latter may lead to contamination, decompression and possible compromise of the planned procedure.

MRCP has a further advantage over ERCP when bile duct visualisation is required and access to the ampulla may not be feasible. Such patients include those who have had upper gastrointestinal procedures such as gastric bypass.

Liver lesions

MRI is used in the characterisation of liver lesions, and detection of lesions prior to hepatic metastasectomy (see Chapter 12).

Prostate tumours

MRI has been advocated in the pre-operative staging of prostatic cancer in certain subgroups. It can demonstrate T3 and T4 extension beyond the prostatic capsule, into the seminal vesicles and adjacent structures (Fig. 6.7). It is also useful in the detection of pelvic lymph nodes. Continued research into new techniques such as MR spectroscopy should see further improvements.

Musculoskeletal sarcoma

MR imaging has dramatically influenced the treatment of patients with musculoskeletal sarcoma (Fig. 6.8). The high accuracy of local staging has made the introduction of reconstructive and limb salvage procedures instead of amputation or disarticulation available to the majority of patients with musculoskeletal sarcoma. Preoperative work-up with MRI is not only more accurate, but also much faster and cheaper than the conventional work-up. MRI is also a valuable investigation in suspected pelvic sarcoma.

FUTURE DEVELOPMENTS IN MAGNETIC RESONANCE IMAGING

Advances in the image sequences, the use of phase array coils and gadolinium based contrast agents have resulted in new applications for MRI imaging.

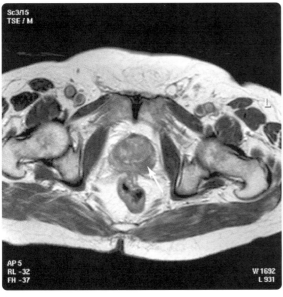

A

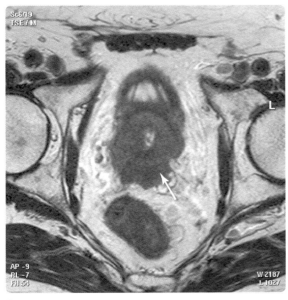

B

Fig. 6.7 Axial T2-weighted image of the prostate. (A) T2 tumour in left peripheral zone, (B) T3b tumour invading the seminal vesicles.

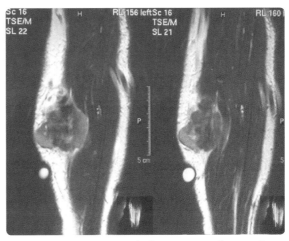

Fig. 6.8 Sarcoma of the right forearm. Note the use of an oil marker to define the anatomical extent of the tumour.

Magnetic resonance mammography

MR mammography is currently limited to major centres where it is predominantly a research tool. It is reported to offer a higher sensitivity than conventional mammography for the detection of multifocal cancer and has been promoted as a tool for screening in high-risk populations. MR mammography can also differentiate between scar tissue and tumour and may have a role in postoperative follow-up. It is also a useful investigation in patients who have breast implants. Despite the increased acceptance of MR scanning, it remains expensive. It is likely that the transition to widespread clinical acceptance will remain limited to certain subgroups of patients where an advantage can be demonstrated over conventional techniques.

Dynamic contrast magnetic resonance

Dynamic contrast enhanced MRI uses intravenous contrast media to assess vascular characteristics of tumours. The same technique has also been used to assess the microvascular characteristics of human tissue xenografts. The basis of this investigation is the correlation between microvessel density and tumour grade. Dynamic contrast MRI is currently being trialled in the assessment of response to anti-angiogenic drugs. It is currently a research tool but offers some promise for the assessment of clinical cancer treatments.

3T magnetic resonance imaging

Until recently, 3-Tesla MRI has been limited to use as a research tool and 1.5 Tesla has been considered the 'gold standard' for MR imaging. More recently more powerful 3T machines have been introduced into clinical practice. These offer a dramatic improvement in image resolution and decrease in scanning times. In addition angiography, perfusion, diffusion and functional studies are easier to perform. At present 3T MR is being used predominantly for neuroradiology but ongoing technological advances will no doubt impact on general surgeons in the future.

Further reading

Bellin MF, Roy C, Kinkel K et al. Lymph node metastases: safety and effectiveness of MR imaging with ultrasmall superparamagnetic iron oxide particles. Initial clinical experience. Radiology 1998; 207:799–808

Bloem JL, van der Woude HJ, Geirnaerdt M et al. Does magnetic resonance imaging make a difference for patients with musculoskeletal sarcoma? Br J Radiol 1997; 70:327–37

Botterill ID, Blunt DM, Quirke P et al. Evaluation of the role of pre-operative magnetic resonance imaging in the management of rectal cancer. Colorectal Dis 2001; 3:295–303

Brown G, Radcliffe AG, Newcombe RG et al. Preoperative assessment of prognostic factors in rectal cancer using high-resolution magnetic resonance imaging. Br J Surg 2003; 90:355–64

Curry TS, Dowdey JE, Murray RC. Christensen's physics of diagnostic radiology, 4th edn. Lea & Febiger, Philadelphia, 1990

Engelbrecht MR, Jager GJ, Severens JL. Patient selection for magnetic resonance imaging of prostate cancer. Eur Urol 2001; 40:300–7

Georgopoulos SK, Schwartz LH, Jarnagin WR et al. Comparison of magnetic resonance and endoscopic retrograde cholangiopancreatography in malignant pancreaticobiliary obstruction. Arch Surg 1999; 134:1002–7

Hashemi RH, Bradley WG. MRI the basics. Williams and Wilkins, Baltimore, 1997

Herbst F. Pelvic radiological imaging: a surgeon's perspective. Eur J Radiol 2003; 47:135–41

Holzer B, Urban M, Holbling N et al. Magnetic resonance imaging predicts sphincter invasion of low rectal cancer and influences selection of operation. Surgery 2003; 133:656–61

Mann GN, Marx HF, Lai LL, Wagman LD. Clinical and cost effectiveness of a new hepatocellular MRI contrast agent, magnafodipir trisodium, in the preoperative assessment of liver respectability. Ann Surg Oncol 2001; 8:573–9

Meyenberger D, Huch Boni RA, Bertschinger P et al. Endoscopic ultrasound and endorectal magnetic resonance imaging: a prospective comparative study for preoperative staging and follow-up of rectal cancer. Endoscopy 1995; 27:469–79

Sahani DV, O'Malley ME, Bahat S et al. Contrast-enhanced MRI of the liver with mangafodipir trisodium: Imaging technique and results. J Comput Assist Tomogr 2002; 26:216–22

Stoker J, Rociu E, Wiersma TG, Lameris JS. Imaging of anorectal disease. BJS 2000; 87:10–27

Summers PE, Jarosz JM, Markus H. MR angiography in cerebrovascular disease. Clin Radiol 2001; 56:437–56

Tatli S, Lipton MJ, Davison BD et al. From the RSNA refresher courses: MR imaging of aortic and peripheral vascular disease. Radiographics 2003; 23:S59–78

Vitellas KM, Keogan MT, Spritzer CE, Nelson RC. MR cholangiopancreatography of bile and pancreatic duct abnormalities with emphasis on the single-shot fast spin-echo technique. Radiographics 2000; 20:939–57

Nuclear medicine

B.E. Chatterton

Background

Nuclear medicine uses the nuclear properties of elements (predominantly radioactive) in diagnosis or therapy of diseases. Common uses of radioisotopes are listed in Box 7.1.

PROPERTIES OF RADIONUCLIDES

Many of the radionuclides in clinical use are delivered to their intended site by linking them to complex organic or biological molecules ('molecular imaging'). The combination is referred to as a radiopharmaceutical. The most commonly used radionuclide used in conventional nuclear medicine is technetium 99m (^{99m}Tc), the chemistry of which allows its attachment to many molecules, allowing, in turn, concentration at

different sites (e.g. bone, heart, liver, kidney, lung). It has an ideal γ-ray energy for imaging; a half-life long enough to allow preparations to last a working day but short enough to minimise patient radiation exposure (typically similar to an X-ray of the corresponding region). Knowledge of the physiological handling of these radiopharmaceuticals is essential for the interpretation of nuclear medicine studies, When a radiopharmaceutical has been used for diagnostic (not therapeutic) purposes there is no need for a surgeon to delay a planned procedure, as the radiation dose received from the patient will be negligible.

Radioactivity is a property of the nucleus of the element in which the ratio of protons and neutrons in the element is such that an adjustment has to be made for the nucleus to be at the lowest energy state. This can be done by the release of an α particle (two protons and two neutrons). α-emitters (such as uranium or radium) are of potential use in therapy, but are of little use in diagnostic applications as the radiation causes marked tissue damage, but is not sufficiently penetrating to be detected from outside the body. β-emission occurs from many of the frequently used radionuclides, and accompanies the transmutation of a neutron to a proton (β⁻) from radioactive isotopes produced in a nuclear reactor, or proton to neutron (positron β⁺) from isotopes produced in cyclotrons. These latter tracers are more usually used in positron emission tomography (PET) (see Chapter 8).

The radiotherapeutic effects of many radionuclides (e.g. ^{131}iodine) are caused by their β-emissions. γ-rays are electromagnetic waves, physically indistinguishable from X-rays, which pass relatively freely through tissue and give a small radiation dose to the patient. They can

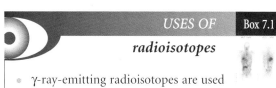

- γ-ray-emitting radioisotopes are used to produce images (scans)
- In vivo non-imaging diagnostic methods (e.g. breath tests)
- In vitro diagnostic tests (radioimmunoassay)
- γ, β and α radiation are used as therapeutic agents

be easily detected and are of most use in non-invasive imaging using gamma cameras.

Quantitative and computer-tomography-augmented studies

Nuclear medicine particularly lends itself to quantitative studies. Frequently, the distribution of tracer in the process of interest at one time point 'static image' is all that is required (e.g. to demonstrate the presence or absence of a tumour). The time–activity relationship of uptake or transit of tracer in or through an organ may be determined with dynamic studies (e.g. gastric emptying). CT is commonly performed in conjunction with conventional tracers, single photon emission computed tomography (SPECT) and positron emission (computed) tomography (PET). These tomographic images may be viewed in any plane, and, in common with many other modern imaging techniques, are best viewed and manipulated on a computer workstation rather than diagnosed from film.

The localisation of radiopharmaceutical to allow production of images in nuclear medicine is often dependent on the function of the relevant organ. The resolution is generally poorer than the more anatomically based conventional imaging techniques.

SURGICAL APPLICATIONS OF NUCLEAR MEDICINE

Radiopharmaceuticals are used to:

- localise an organ or structure of interest
- detect aberrations in the anatomy or dynamics of the organ

- localise pathological process of interest (e.g. cancer, infection)
- perform localised therapy (e.g. thyroid ablation).

Bone disease

Bone metastases

Skeletal nuclear medicine images are commonly used in surgical practice to assess or monitor bony secondary deposits.

The whole-body bone scan is sensitive in screening the whole skeleton for metastases, although the yield may be so low as to be cost ineffective in the early stage of malignant disease. Some benign lesions also show increased uptake on the bone scan (e.g. osteoid osteoma). Primary or metastatic malignancies usually have bony remodelling at the periphery, which is seen as increased tracer uptake ('hot spots') (Fig. 7.1). Both lytic and sclerotic metastases are 'hot' on the bone scan (Fig. 7.2). An exception is multiple myeloma, which may have normal bone scan appearances.

The whole-body scan is useful in following progression of therapy for established metastatic disease. Awareness of the 'flare' phenomenon (increased visualisation of previously invisible, but successfully treated healing metastases) is needed.

Painful bony metastases can be treated with bone-seeking radiopharmaceuticals (e.g. ^{153}Sm EDTMP and ^{89}Sr) and these have been used to produce effective palliation.

Other bone pathology

Other commonly occurring pathologies (e.g. vertebral crush fractures, arthritis) will give an abnormal scan. In such circumstances a directed plain radiograph, CT or MRI may add specificity.

The whole-body bone scan is also abnormal in paraneoplastic phenomena. For example hypertrophic pulmonary osteoarthropathy shows typical distal limb uptake while in malignant hypercalcaemia there is increased lung, stomach and increased bone uptake.

Other uses in non-malignant disease include:

- osteomyelitis
- avascularity, e.g. post-trauma
- orthopaedic conditions where degree of bone involvement is questioned (or there is suspicion of a primary bone malignancy).

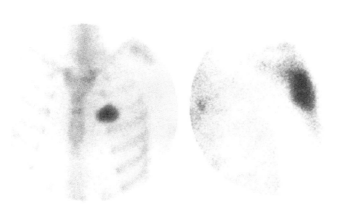

L

Fig 7.1 Osteosarcoma in proximal left humerus. Uptake in the left side of the chest is an ossifying pulmonary metastasis.

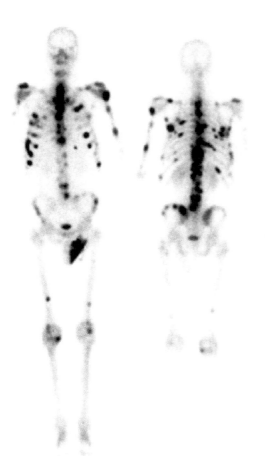

ANT   POST

Fig. 7.2 Whole-body bone scan of patient with widespread metastatic prostatic carcinoma (note urinary contamination).

Urinary tract

Nuclear medicine techniques are used in the assessment of:

- renal function
- renal artery stenosis
- vesicoureteric reflux
- obstruction
- renal transplantation.

Renal function studies

The uptake or clearance of radiopharmaceuticals in the kidney is in proportion to function in each kidney. Therefore their relative (percentage of total) contribution to renal function may be derived from the scan. Global GFR (total renal function) can be measured from plasma clearance of activity. The combination of the two then allows calculation of absolute individual renal function, e.g. a kidney with 25% of renal function with a total GFR of 40 mL/min is contributing 10 mL/min. Follow-up and surgical decisions may then be made on quantitative data. $^{99}Tc^{m}$ (dimercaptosuccinic acid) is used to assess renal parenchymal function but also provides information about the position, size and overall morphology of the functioning renal tissue.

Renal artery stenosis

Renal artery stenosis may be diagnosed and its treatment monitored by measuring reduced inflow into the affected kidney and its subsequent reduced function. These changes may be enhanced by prior administration of an angiotensin converting enzyme inhibitor

Fig. 7.3 Images obtained 10 minutes after injection of tracer on two separate occasions, one without, the other with administration of Captopril showing enhanced impairment of left renal function associated with renal artery stenosis.

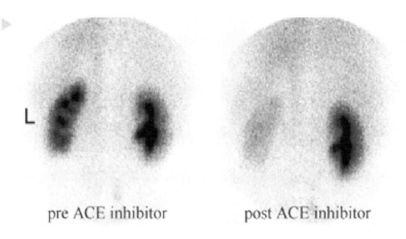

pre ACE inhibitor   post ACE inhibitor

(Fig. 7.3). Functional results of renal artery stenosis are shown by changes in size or function, rather than the anatomical arterial lesions shown by conventional imaging, which may not be associated with significant functional change.

Obstruction

Dilated renal collecting systems do not always indicate 'obstruction.' Interventional decisions may be assisted by use of a diuretic renogram, which uses a rapidly cleared radiopharmaceutical to fill the dilated system. When stressed with diuretic, the dilated, but not obstructed, system clears promptly.

Transplant

In the early postoperative period, perfusion of the transplant may be determined. Acute tubular necrosis is usual and rapid fading of filtered tracer will occur without excretion. Urinary leaks or obstruction may also be diagnosed and differentiated from lymphocele. Later, serial studies may be used to monitor rejection.

Gastrointestinal imaging

Static and dynamic studies are used in the investigation of gastrointestinal disorders.

Liver

Traditional colloid liver scans depend on phagocytosis of particles in liver Kupffer cells and splenic sinusoids. Their use is obsolete other than to confirm focal nodular hyperplasia (Fig. 7.4) (see Chapter 12).

Depending on the radiopharmaceutical, masses may have more uptake ('hot') or less ('cold') than the surrounding liver, or be invisible. Some of the typical patterns are shown in Table 7.1. Haemangiomata are common and, if they have typical appearances on ultrasound and CT scans, further imaging is not needed. If atypical, and if not thrombosed and confirmatory imaging is needed, they may be shown to slowly fill their vascular spaces with labelled red cells (Fig. 7.5). Very few other lesions (apart from vascular haemangiosarcomata) show similar activity. For these and most other liver lesions, a diameter of >1.5 cm is needed to make a confident diagnosis. SPECT improves the accuracy.

Liver metastases derive their blood supply from the hepatic artery, whereas the normal liver tissue is supplied predominantly through the portal venous system. This can be used to advantage by therapeutic radiopharmaceuticals, which embolise a capillary circulation and will preferentially localise in metastatic tissue after injection into the hepatic artery. ^{90}Y-labelled ceramic microspheres (SIR-Spheres) have had some success in this indication (Fig. 7.6); as has ^{131}I-labelled lipiodol in hepatocellular carcinoma.

Biliary function

[99m]Tc IDA derivatives might be of help in the assessment of biliary tract disease. Visualisation of the gall bladder an hour after injection (enhanced if needed by 2 mg IV morphine to cause contraction of the sphincter of Oddi) virtually excludes acute cholecystitis (see Chapter 12) (Fig. 7.7). Quantitative studies can also be

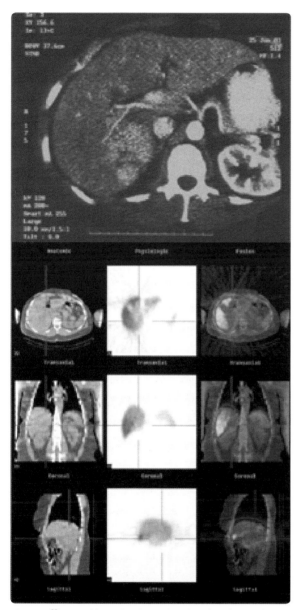

Fig. 7.4 ^{99m}Tc-sulfur colloid SPECT (fused with simultaneously acquired CT) scan in a patient with enhancing liver mass. Colloid uptake in mass typical of focal nodular hyperplasia.

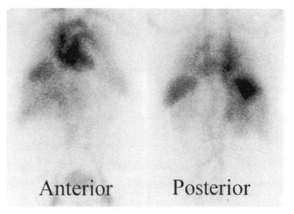

Anterior   Posterior

Fig. 7.5 Planar anterior and posterior images 3 hours after administration of ^{99m}Tc-autologous red cells showing mass posteriorly in right lobe of liver (segment 7) in a patient with a large haemangioma. Note physiological activity in heart and spleen.

useful in patients with biliary dyskinesia (gall bladder ejection fraction following fatty meal or intravenous cholecystokinin is normally >40%). Post-traumatic and postsurgical biliary leaks are readily assessed. Following liver transplantation nuclear scanning can show perfusion, uptake by liver parenchyma, excretory function and patency of biliary channels. Serial imaging is particularly useful. The technique is not generally of diagnostic value in obstructive jaundice.

Spleen

Autologous red cells labelled with ^{99m}Tc and damaged by heating to 49°C for 20 minutes are taken up very avidly by splenic tissue. This is the procedure of choice to confirm the nature of splenic 'rests' or splenunculi following relapse of conditions treated by splenectomy, (spherocytosis, idiopathic thrombocytopenic purpura) (Fig. 7.8).

Apart from the exclusion of splenic infarction (wedge-shaped defects often in an enlarged spleen), most indications for splenic colloid imaging are obsolete. It has no role in trauma.

Gastrointestinal motility and transit studies

Radionuclide tests lend themselves to quantitation, and assessment of gastrointestinal motility is an ideal indication. Pharyngeal clearance studies are seldom performed, but quantitative oesophageal clearance

Table 7.1 The patterns of uptake of radiopharmaceuticals by liver and splenic lesions

	Colloid	Red Cells	IDA derivatives	Octreotide	MIBG	Labelled anti-CEA antibody	FDG
Hepatocellular carcinoma	−	−	−	±	−	−	++
Adenoma	−	−	±	−	−	−	+
Haemangioma	−	++	−	−	−	−	−
Focal nodular hyperplasia	+	+	+	+	−	−	+
Metastasis	−	−	−	++	±	++ (colorectal)	++
Cyst	−	−	−	−	−	−	−
Neuroendocrine tumour	−	−	−	++	±	−	±
Splenic tissue (splenuculus)	++	++	−	+	−	−	−

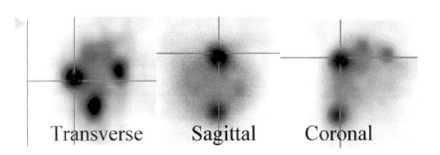

Fig. 7.6 SPECT views of SIR-Spheres accumulating in hepatic haemangiopericytoma after intrahepatic artery administration.

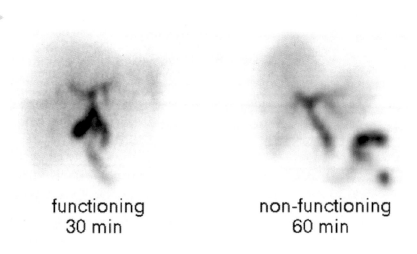

Fig. 7.7 Anterior images of the liver following ^{99m}TcDIDA showing functioning and non-functioning (consistent with acute cholecystitis) gall bladders in different patients.

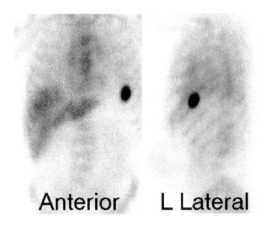

Anterior   L Lateral

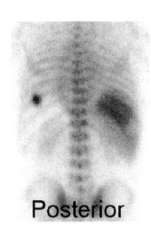

Posterior

Fig. 7.8 Images obtained 2 hours after administration of heat-damaged ^{99m}Tc-labelled autologous erythrocytes showing regenerating splenic tissue in splenic bed following splenectomy for ITP.

may be useful in the assessment of neuromuscular conditions (spasm, achalasia) or reflux.

Radionuclide gastric emptying is the gold standard in gastric emptying assessment. It is often useful to simultaneously follow the emptying of both solid and liquid components of a meal (Fig. 7.9). Indications include:

- assessment of gastroparesis
- unexplained nausea and vomiting
- gastro-oesophageal reflux.

Small bowel transit ('mouth–caecum transit time') is readily studied by radionuclide techniques, although the indications for this procedure are limited. Colonic transit studies are more commonly undertaken, particularly as part of the assessment of constipation. The study will provide a readily quantifiable assessment of bowel transit and any site of hold-up. The agent of choice is ^{67}gallium citrate because of its 72-hour half-life. Daily scans are performed and the rate of clearance measured. Obstructed defecation is readily distinguished from more generalised motility disturbances (Fig. 7.10).

Haemorrhage

In obscure anaemia, the faecal excretion of ^{57}Cr autologous red cells gives precision of gastrointestinal blood loss greater than 1 mL/day (the same technique can measure menstrual loss if this is a differential). This has no localising ability. If the bleeding is acute and rapid, then localisation of the bleeding site is feasible (see Chapter 15). Autologous erythrocytes are labelled with ^{99m}Tc and reinjected. Bleeding rates of 0.5–1 mL/min should be identifiable in the digestive tract. It is important that images are taken serially (at intervals of no more than a few minutes) to localise the bleeding (Fig. 7.11) If the patient is not imaged continually, then the extravasated activity may have moved distally, and redundantly confirm only that the patient has been bleeding with no localising information.

In the paediatric or young adult population, if a Meckel's diverticulum is considered then Na ^{99m}TcO$_4$ may be used. This is taken up by secretory epithelium, (particularly gastric mucosa) and will localise within a few minutes in native and ectopic gastric mucosa, adjacent to the ulcer causing bleeding.

Inflammatory bowel disease

The extent or activity of inflammatory bowel disease may be difficult to assess by conventional radiological techniques. Leucocytes (mixed or granulocytes) localise at sites of active bowel inflammation and are shed into the lumen. Imaging the abdomen (Fig. 7.12) and counting excreta can both localise and score disease activity.

Absorption disorders

Non-imaging nuclear techniques may be used in the investigation of absorption: The Schilling test (vitamin B$_{12}$) is affected both by gastric (intrinsic factor) or terminal ileal (specific receptors) disease, either medical or post surgical. Breath testing for malabsorption of fat (triglycerides, triolein) is also well established.

Fig. 7.9 Normal simultaneous solid and liquid emptying study, showing anterior images of the stomach (below) and derived time-activity curves (above).

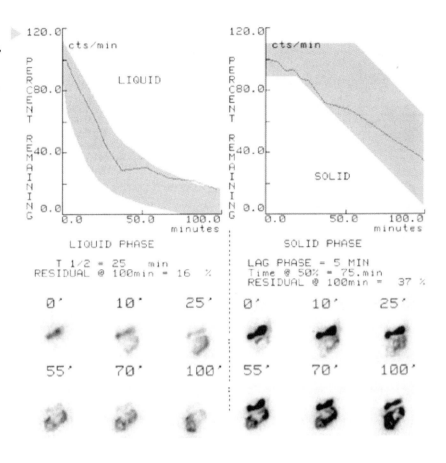

LIQUID PHASE

T 1/2 = 25   min
RESIDUAL @ 100min = 16   %

SOLID PHASE

LAG PHASE = 5 MIN
Time @ 50% = 75.min
RESIDUAL @ 100min =   37 %

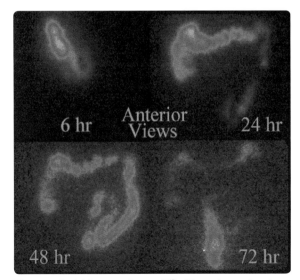

Fig. 7.10 Serial images after oral ^{67}gallium citrate showing normal transit through the colon.

Metastatic colon cancer

^{99m}Tc-monoclonal antibody (CEA scan) has been shown to be useful in the localisation of recurrent and metastatic colon cancer both within the liver and elsewhere. It is less accurate than ^{18}FDG PET.

Inflammation and infection

Several radiopharmaceuticals are available, although none are specific. Labelled granulocytes may be visualised accumulating in areas of leucocytic infiltration. Particular use has been made in determining infection in 'violated' bone, and inflammatory bowel disease, but the technique is useful in localising acute inflammation anywhere. Abscesses are readily seen (Fig. 7.13), and acute appendicitis can be seen well (Fig. 7.14), although if indicated at all anatomical imaging is usually used first (see Chapter 10). Chronic inflammation (infection) is less likely to have leucocytic

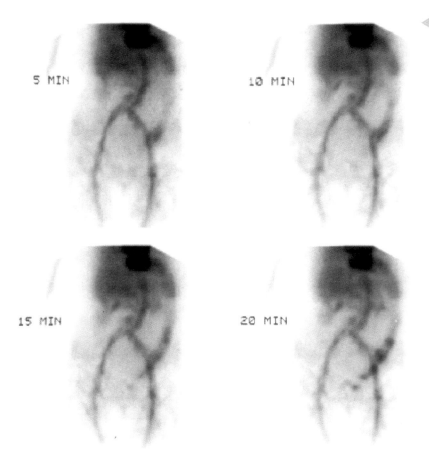

Fig. 7.11 Serial images following administration of ^{99m}Tc-labelled autologous red cells showing appearance of activity in the left side of the colon due to haemorrhage.

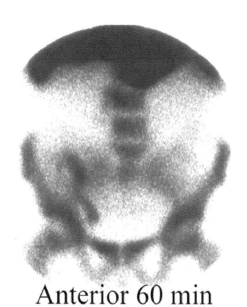

Fig. 7.12 Anterior abdominal image 60 minutes after administration of ^{99m}Tc-colloid labelled autologous leucocytes, which have localised in terminal ileal Crohn's disease (as well as liver, spleen and bone marrow).

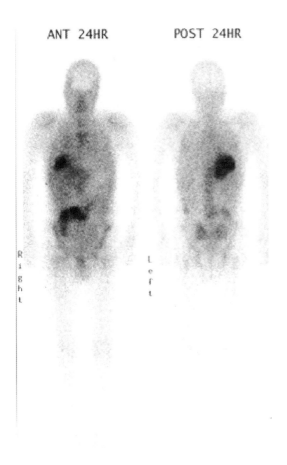

ANT 24HR POST 24HR

Right

Left

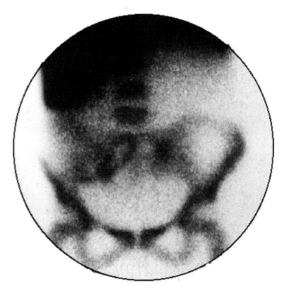

Fig. 7.14 Anterior abdominal wall image 60 minutes after administration of ^{99m}Tc-colloid labelled autologous leucocytes in the inflamed wall of an appendix abscess.

Fig. 7.13 Anterior and posterior whole-body images 24 hours after administration of ^{67}gallium citrate, which has localised in a liver abscess.

infiltration, and therefore labelled leucocytes may not reveal these. Gallium citrate is a more appropriate radiopharmaceutical in chronic inflammation. Pyrexia of unknown origin without a suspected focal sepsis has a poor yield with these investigations.

Endocrine disease

Thyroid

Nuclear medicine has both diagnostic and therapeutic roles in the management of thyroid disease. The structure of the thyroid and any morphological abnormalities is usually assessed in the first instance by ultrasound (often with FNAC). This may be complemented with

CT (see Chapter 20). Nuclear medicine techniques are usually used to assess thyroid global or local function, rather than demonstrate structural lesions.

Most thyroid scans are performed using ^{99m}TcO$_4^-$, with radioiodine (^{123}I, ^{131}I) used in limited circumstances. Isotope scans may be used in the following situations:

- assessment of activity within a solitary nodule (differential for malignancy)
- detection of an autonomously functioning hot nodule (as cause of hyperthyroidism)
- thyroiditis, usually hyperthyroid with tender neck (lack of uptake)
- whole-body scanning for metastatic spread of thyroid cancers.
- ^{18}FDG scanning in thyroid malignancy (often iodine non-avid tumour) (see Chapter 8).

Most 'cold' or non-functioning nodules will be benign. About 10% of cold nodules are shown to be malignant. The incidence of malignancy in functioning 'warm' or 'hot' nodules is typically much less than 1%, but they are a small minority of scanned lesions. In multinodular goitres shown on radionuclide scan, the scan is not discriminatory with malignancy found in 2–5% (often

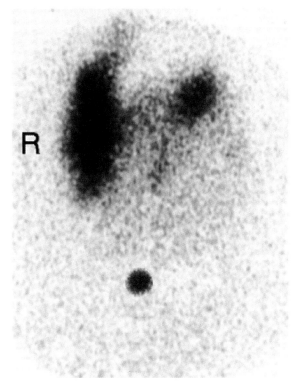

Fig. 7.15 Na ^{99m}TcO$_4$ image of the thyroid showing large left sided 'cold' nodule due to follicular thyroid carcinoma. Marker in midline overlies sternal notch.

remote from nodules), an incidence similar to the background autopsy incidence (Fig. 7.15).

Follicular and papillary cancers have less uptake than normal thyroid (i.e. show as 'cold' nodules). They have far more uptake than other tissues, and will usually concentrate radioiodine for diagnostic or therapeutic purposes. For whole-body iodine scanning (most usually ^{131}I) to be useful, prior radionuclide ablative treatment of remaining normal thyroid tissue should have been performed (this is also a requirement for follow up using thyroglobulin). Scanning is most appropriate in patients with a raised thyroglobulin, or if there is structural suggestion of metastasis. Satisfactory uptake on scan predicts a response to higher (therapeutic) doses of ^{131}I. For the scan to be effective, the tumour should be stimulated with adequate TSH. This can be either recombinant TSH parenterally, or more economically endogenous TSH released by ceasing thyroid hormone replacement.

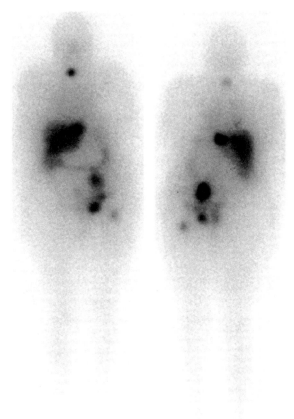

ANTERIOR   POSTERIOR

Fig. 7.16 Whole-body images obtained 7 days after therapeutic administration of ^{131}iodine demonstrating uptake in regenerating thyroid tissue in the root of the neck, and metastatic deposits in the liver, left pelvic bones and upper left femur from papillary thyroid cancer.

Medullary thyroid cancer arises from parafollicular 'C' cells and is not iodine avid.

Radioisotopes are a mainstay in the treatment of differentiated thyroid malignancy. Metastatic disease is treated by at least two doses of radioiodine (^{131}I). The first dose is needed to ablate the normal thyroid rests which remain, no matter how extensive the surgery. The metastases are usually less avid than normal thyroid tissue. Scanning should be performed after therapeutic doses, as sensitivity for thyroid metastases (Fig. 7.16) is greater. The patient should have an elevated TSH as for diagnostic scanning.

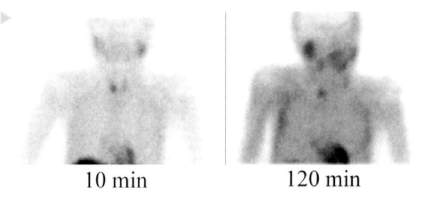

Fig. 7.17 Early and late images showing persistent uptake in a right lower parathyroid adenoma after administration of ^{99m}Tc-MIBI.

10 min   120 min

For hyperthyroidism as an alternative to medical or surgical therapy, the larger the dose of radioiodine administered, the more rapidly control is reached. Ultimately, most patients will become hypothyroid. Debate continues regarding the role of radioiodine in the therapy of multinodular goitre, but the reduction in goitre size is seldom great.

It is important that the patient not be pregnant when radioiodine is administered, because the fetal thyroid may be ablated. It is convention to recommend that conception (from male or female patients) be delayed for 12 months after radioiodine therapy, although there is no clear data regarding the magnitude of the risk. Again convention has favoured thyroid surgery over ^{131}I if thyroid eye disease is present, but there is no convincing data of a significant advantage.

Parathyroid

Although open surgery is very effective in locating and treating hyperparathyroidism, it may fail in 5–10% of operations. Minimally invasive parathyroid surgery is also becoming more common. Both of these are indications for pre-operative parathyroid imaging (see Chapter 20). The sensitivity of CT, MR, ultrasound and ^{99m}Tc sestamibi (MIBI) scanning is similar (70–90%). The nuclear scan is particularly useful in demonstrating mediastinal lesions and in the post-surgical situation, where conventional imaging is difficult because of scarring. Both the thyroid and parathyroid will take up the current agent of choice, MIBI, but the parathyroid lacks the P-glycoprotein mechanism that clears sestamibi from the thyroid, hence parathyroid tissue retains activity for several hours. Some thyroid nodules also lose this mechanism, and therefore they

may be a differential diagnosis for focal uptake in the neck (Fig. 7.17).

Adrenal

^{131}I or ^{75}Se cholesterol is incorporated into the steroid biosynthetic pathway in the adrenal cortex. In selected cases these tracers will confirm the function of a known mass, or localise a functioning lesion suspected biochemically. Commercial availability of these tracers is limited. Physiological uptake of these tracers in the normal adrenal is often suppressed by premedicating with dexamethasone or similar. Bilateral hyperplasia in Cushing's disease may be differentiated from a unilateral benign or malignant functional tumour. Similarly the lesion responsible for Conn's syndrome (hyperaldosteronism) may be localised. The indication for these studies has reduced with the availability of high resolution CT.

Meta-iodo-benzyl-guanidine (MIBG) (and usually labelled with ^{123}I) is a catecholamine precursor, which is taken up in phaeochromocytoma and some other malignancies (e.g. carcinoid, neuroblastoma). It may be used to confirm the nature of incidentally found lesions, as well as detecting those in hypertensive patients with appropriately abnormal biochemistry. Functioning metastases in these conditions can also be localised and may be treated with ^{131}I-MIBG.

Localisation of neuroendocrine tumours

Octreotide (a somatostatin analogue usually labelled with ^{111}In) is frequently taken up in primary and metastatic carcinoid tumours (Fig. 7.18) and other neuroendocrine tumours such as gastrinomas and pituitary neoplasms.

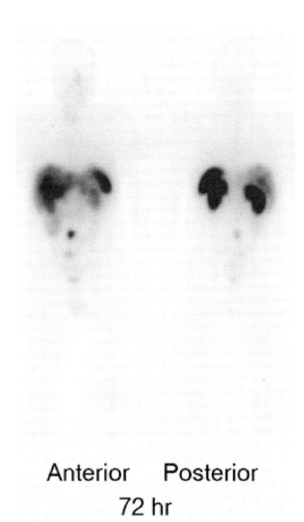

Anterior   Posterior

72 hr

Fig. 7.18 Whole-body images 72 hours after administration of ^{111}In pentetrotide (Octreotide) showing uptake in a primary appendiceal carcinoid tumour, and liver metastases.

Other uses

Other uses many radiopharmaceuticals will localise within tumours as a result of their intrinsic biodistribution. ^{99m}Tc-MIBI is initially distributed by blood flow and metabolic activity. It has been shown to be useful in the diagnosis of primary and recurrent breast cancer, particularly in mammographically dense breasts. The technique is not sensitive enough for local staging. Uptake has also been shown in sarcomata and lung cancers. ^{99m}TcDMSA(V) is a non-specific tumour

scanning agent, shown to be useful in medullary thyroid cancer and may detect recurrences indicated by calcitonin increases. Thallium 201 whole-body scans may detect iodine non-avid metastatic thyroid malignancy, sarcomas and brain tumours. Nevertheless it is likely that ^{18}FDG PET scanning is of equal or better utility in most of these indications (see Chapter 8).

Lymphoscintigraphy

Soluble or fine colloidal materials injected interstitially will be taken up into lymphatic vessels and subsequently particulate material will be taken up into draining lymph nodes, mimicking the presumed behaviour of micrometastases.

Sentinel lymph nodes receive direct drainage from the tumour, and are regarded as those most likely to be involved with (micro)metastases and thereby predict the status of the entire nodal basin. The technique has found most use in breast surgery and cutaneous melanoma (Fig. 7.19) although head and neck, vulval and internal cancers (injected endoscopically) have been studied by this technique. When staging the axilla in breast cancer, many studies have shown concordance between the sentinel node and axillary status of better than 95%. Localisation of lymph nodes for surgery is best performed with a combination of radioactive tracers, use of intraoperative scintillation probe and blue dye (see Chapter 23).

Pulmonary embolism

Both the ventilation-perfusion (V/Q) scan and the CT scan are important diagnostic modalities in cases of suspected pulmonary embolism. The V/Q scan has been a mainstay of diagnosis for many years, and continues to have a very high predictive value with normal or scans with mismatch (non-perfused but ventilated lung) (Fig. 7.20). There are no contra-indications to the V/Q scan. Corresponding ventilation and perfusion defects have lower specificity, and these tend to occur in the postoperative situation (e.g. postoperative atelectasis, pleural effusion, pneumonia and chronic obstructive pulmonary disease).

Performed with helical CT, pulmonary angiography (CTPA) is the preferred investigation where there is coexisting lung disease, which is frequent in the postoperative patient. Clot may be seen in the major pulmonary vessels (see Chapter 4). Some patients may

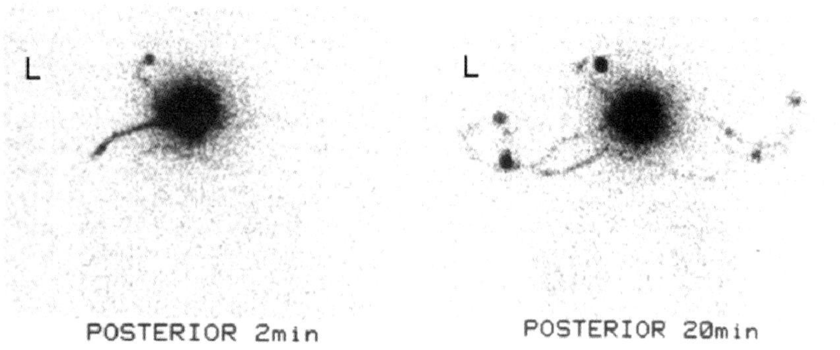

Fig. 7.19 Posterior trunk views following intradermal adminis-tration of ^{99m}Tc-antimony colloid around a biopsy scar in the midline of the back in a patient diagnosed with malignant melanoma. Note drainage to sentinel lymph nodes in both axillae and left supraclavicular region.

Fig. 7.20 Normal ventilation, with multiple bilateral segmental perfusion defects in a patient with post-hysterectomy pulmo-nary embolism.

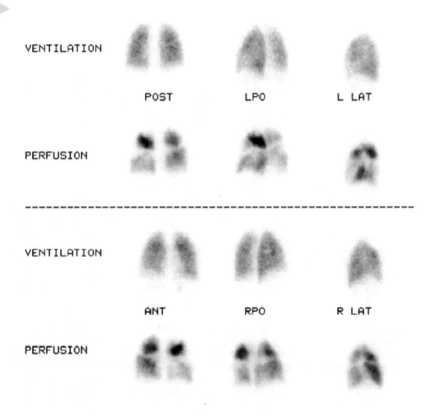

be allergic to the contrast used with a CT scan, and a contrast load may be inappropriate in a critically ill patient with renal impairment. Therefore a pragmatic approach is to use V/Q scanning if the chest X-ray is normal, and helical CTPA if the chest radiograph is abnormal unless contraindications exist to the use of contrast. If a patient presents with non-specific chest symptoms and a pulmonary embolus is only vaguely suspected, then a V/Q scan with its high negative predictive value may be more appropriate than a CTPA, which has an appreciable morbidity.

Further reading

Bajc M, Albrechtsson U, Olsson CG et al. Comparison of ventilation/perfusion scintigraphy and helical CT for diagnosis of pulmonary embolism; strategy using clinical data and ancillary findings. Clin Physiol Funct Imaging 2002; 22:392–7

Bartholomeusz D, Chatterton BE, Bellen JC et al. Segmental colonic transit after oral 67Ga-citrate in healthy subjects and those with chronic idiopathic constipation. J Nucl Med 1999; 40:277–82

Chatal JF, Le Bodic MF, Kraeber-Bodere F et al. Nuclear medicine applications for neuroendocrine tumors. World J Surg 2000; 24:1285–9

Chatterton BE. Assessment in renal transplantation. In: Peters AM (ed) Nuclear medicine in clinical diagnosis. Martin Dunitz, London, 2003 p 239–51

Chatterton BE. Gastric motility. In: Murray and Ell. Nuclear medicine in clinical diagnosis and treatment, 2nd edn. Churchill Livingstone, Edinburgh, 1998, p 419–32.

Cook GJ, Fogelman I. The role of nuclear medicine in monitoring treatment in skeletal malignancy. Semin Nucl Med 2001; 31:206–11

Focacci C, Lattanzi R, Iadeluca ML, Campioni P. Nuclear medicine in primary bone tumors. Eur J Radiol 1998; 27 Suppl 1:S123–31.

Gray B, Van Hazel G, Hope M et al. Randomised trial of SIR-Spheres plus chemotherapy vs. chemotherapy alone for treating patients with liver metastases from primary large bowel cancer. Ann Oncol 2001; 12:1711–20

Harris PE. The management of thyroid cancer in adults: a review of new guidelines. Clin Med 2002; 2:144–6

James C, Starks M, MacGillivray DC, White J. The use of imaging studies in the diagnosis and management of thyroid cancer and hyperparathyroidism. Surg Oncol Clin N Am 1999; 8:145–69

Kinkel K, Lu Y, Both M et al. Detection of hepatic metastases from cancers of the gastrointestinal tract by using noninvasive imaging methods (US, CT, MR imaging, PET): a meta-analysis. Radiology 2002; 224:748–56

Kinnard MF, Alavi A, Rubin RA, Lichtenstein GR. Nuclear imaging of solid hepatic masses. Semin Roentgenol 1995; 30:375–95

Kollias J, Gill PG, Chatterton BE et al. Reliability of sentinel node status in predicting axillary lymph node involvement in breast cancer. Med J Aust 1999; 171:461–5

Lawrence W Jr, Kaplan BJ. Diagnosis and management of patients with thyroid nodules. J Surg Oncol 2002; 80:157–70

O'Sullivan JM, Cook GJ. A review of the efficacy of bone scanning in prostate and breast cancer. Q J Nucl Med 2002; 46:152–9.

Reinhardt MJ, Moser E. Diagnostic methods in the investigation of diseases of the thyroid. Eur J Nucl Med 1996; 23:587

Rubello D, Bui C, Casara D et al. Functional scintigraphy of the adrenal gland. Eur J Endocrinol 2002; 147:13–28

Serafini AN. Therapy of metastatic bone pain. J Nucl Med 2001; 42:895–906

Taillefer R. The role of 99mTc-sestamibi and other conventional radiopharmaceuticals in breast cancer diagnosis. Semin Nucl Med 1999; 29:16–40

Taylor A. Renovascular hypertension: nuclear medicine techniques. Q J Nucl Med 2002; 46:268–82

Uren RF, Thompson JF, Howman-Giles R. Sentinel lymph node biopsy in patients with melanoma and breast cancer. Intern Med J 2001; 31:547–9

Vasquez TE, Rimkus DS, Hass MG, Larosa DI. Efficacy of morphine sulfate-augmented hepatobiliary imaging in acute cholecystitis. J Nucl Med Technol 2000; 28:153–5

Positron emission tomography 8

I. Kirkwood

Background

A positron emission tomographic (PET) scan is a non-invasive nuclear medicine imaging technique that creates tomographic images of the distribution of an intravenously administered positron-emitting radiopharmaceutical. The information obtained is 'metabolic' and complementary to 'anatomic' imaging modalities.

BASIC PRINCIPLES OF FDG-PET

The radiopharmaceuticals are labelled with positron-emitting isotopes such as ^{11}C ($[^{11}$C]-acetate, $[^{11}$C]-methionine), ^{13}N ($[^{13}$N]-ammonia), ^{15}O ($[^{15}$O]-water), and ^{18}F ($[^{18}$F]-2-deoxyglucose, L-2-$[^{18}$F]-tyrosine) produced by a cyclotron. Coincident 511 keV γ-rays are produced by annihilation of a positron from the nucleus by an electron. The scanner contains a ring of crystals, which surround the patient, and electronics that detect the coincident γ-rays. A computer converts the lines of coincidence detected by the scanner into a three dimensional image that can be viewed on a dedicated workstation. Attenuation correction is performed and images can be viewed in attenuation corrected (AC) and non-attenuation corrected (NAC) modes. This is important for quantifying radiopharmaceutical uptake by tissue.

PET radiopharmaceuticals can be used to measure carbohydrate metabolism, cell proliferation, amino acid transport, receptor density, cell oxygenation, blood flow and bone metabolism.

When a CT scanner is integrated with the PET scanner it is known as PET-CT. The CT is usually used for performing attenuation correction and anatomical localisation of abnormalities seen on PET and therefore no IV contrast is given.

Uses of FDG-PET

The radiopharmaceutical typically used for tumour imaging is $[^{18}$F]-fluoro-2-deoxyglucose (FDG), a synthetic radioactive glucose analogue. ^{18}Fluorine has a physical half-life of 109.5 minutes, therefore FDG can be manufactured on a daily basis and distributed to PET centres without a cyclotron on site.

FDG is actively transported into cells via glucose transporter proteins (Fig. 8.1). It is phosphorylated by the enzyme hexokinase to FDG-6-phosphate but cannot continue metabolism via the glycolytic pathway due to a missing oxygen at the C-2 position (unlike glucose-6-phosphate). The FDG-6-phosphate is therefore trapped within the cell. In general, tumour cells

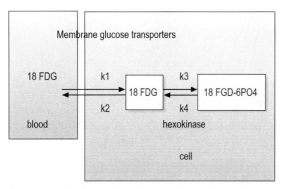

Fig. 8.1 Mechanism of uptake of FDG into the cell.

---

overexpress glucose transporter proteins and have high glucose utilisation rates. This results in increased FDG uptake compared to normal cells. Delayed imaging (typically 60 minutes after injection) provides a higher tumour-to-background uptake ratio but time is limited by the radioactive decay of ^{18}F. Recognised uses of FDG-PET are listed in Box 8.1.

For tumour imaging, FDG is administered intravenously after a minimum 6-hour fast under resting conditions. Patients with diabetes mellitus and poorly controlled blood glucose levels will have reduced FDG uptake due to competition with endogenous glucose. The sensitivity of FDG-PET may be reduced if insulin is administered within 2 hours of FDG or if plasma glucose is less than 8.0 mmol/L at the time of FDG injection.

To maximise the effectiveness of FDG-PET, the following additional procedures are considered:

- Midazolam oral sedation prior to FDG injection (reduces physiological muscle and brown adipose tissue uptake, which may otherwise lead to false positive results).
- Frusemide ± bladder catheterisation (improves visualisation of pelvic tissues by diluting or draining radioactive urine from the bladder).

A standardised uptake value (SUV) is a quantitative measure of tissue FDG uptake normalised to body weight or lean body mass. It can be used to compare tumour FDG uptake between serial scans in the same patient for monitoring treatment or for characterising a pulmonary nodule as likely to be benign or malignant.

Interpreting FDG-PET scans

Non-attenuation corrected (NAC) PET images can be recognised by accentuation of skin uptake and increased apparent lung uptake relative to normal soft tissue. Attenuation correction normalises these artefacts although the images may appear 'noisier' particularly in large patients. Other artefacts are occasionally produced by the attenuation correction process. The attenuation corrected images are usually interpreted with reference to CT or MRI. Normal sites of high uptake of FDG include:

- brain (grey matter)
- left ventricular myocardium
- bladder and urinary tract due to urinary excretion of FDG
- bowel (variable) (Fig. 8.2).

Normal sites of low grade FDG uptake include:

- liver
- skeletal muscle
- bowel
- bone marrow
- testis
- gastro-oesophageal junction
- stomach.

Abnormal FDG uptake is seen in many malignancies, but also in benign diseases such as tuberculosis, sarcoidosis, infection or inflammation (including surgical wounds). Tumours with low FDG uptake include:

- carcinoid
- bronchoalveolar carcinoma
- mucinous adenocarcinoma

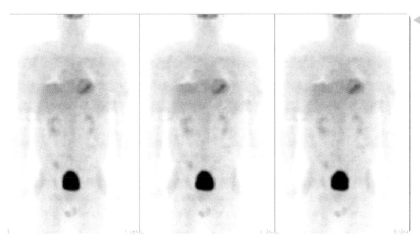

Fig. 8.2 A normal FDG PET scan. The area of maximum activity is the bladder. The myocardium also shows increased activity.

- renal cell carcinoma
- hepatocellular carcinoma
- prostate carcinoma
- MALT lymphoma.

Safety/efficacy issues

The radiation dose from an FDG-PET scan is between 3.5 mSv and 8 mSv (two to four times annual background radiation), depending on the type of PET scanner used. There are no side effects from the tracer amount of FDG administered for the scan. Depending on the type of PET scanner used, the resolution (FWHM) ranges from 4 mm to 7 mm, which compares with submillimetre resolution on CT. Tumours that are less than twice FWHM in size will have reduced apparent uptake limiting their detection. Microscopic malignant disease clearly cannot be detected using PET.

CLINICAL APPLICATIONS OF FDG-PET SCANNING IN SURGICAL DISEASE

- Characterisation of tissue as probable benign or malignant lesion (e.g. solitary pulmonary nodule).
- Grading of malignancy or for biopsy guidance.
- Staging of a malignancy prior to treatment (e.g. non-small-cell lung cancer).
- Monitoring of therapy.
- Restaging for suspected or proven recurrent or residual malignancy.

Role of PET in staging of gastrointestinal malignancies

The sensitivity of PET scans in detection of metastatic disease varies with the tumour type. It is generally reliable in detecting disease foci over 1cm but sensitivity decreases with smaller lesions. A high background uptake of FDG near to an area of a suspected metastasis (e.g. bladder) may obscure disease activity, resulting in a false negative scan. PET can be useful to assess questionable lymphadenopathy or other findings identified by CT, where potentially curative surgery is proposed.

Proponents of PET staging argue that a whole body PET scan is more cost effective than other staging modalities, particularly when imaging of multiple organ systems would be required e.g. CT scans of chest, abdomen, brain and pelvis.

Oesophageal cancer

PET has higher sensitivity (30%) than CT (11%) for detecting local nodal metastases but both modalities have lower sensitivity than endoscopic ultrasound. The high FDG uptake in the region of the primary tumour may mask interpretation of the adjacent lymph node basin.

PET is more sensitive than CT in detecting metastatic disease and therefore in guiding decisions about suitability for resection. PET after conventional imaging demonstrates undetected sites of metastatic disease in ~15% of patients (i.e. these patients are upstaged) (Fig. 8.3).

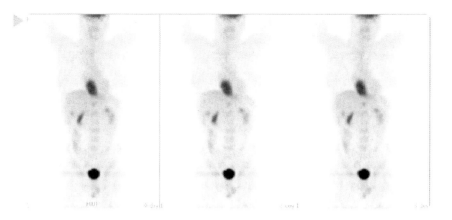

Fig. 8.3 A metastatic deposit in the liver in a patient with carcinoma of the oesophagus. The area of increased activity immediately above the diaphragm is the primary tumour.

Gastric cancer

PET has relatively low sensitivity and specificity due to the deficiency of Glut-1 receptors in signet ring cell carcinoma and mucinous adenocarcinoma which limit its role.

Pancreatic cancer

The PET scan has a sensitivity of 86–98% and a specificity of 78–84% in the differentiation of benign and malignant pancreatic masses. Sensitivity is decreased in the presence of hyperglycaemia (sensitivity 42%). False positive scans may be seen in chronic pancreatitis due to FDG uptake in inflammation. FDG-PET can influence surgical management in up to 43% of patients with pancreatic cancer by detecting distant metastases.

Neuroendocrine tumours of the pancreas have low FDG uptake and imaging with labelled somatostatin analogues (pentoctreotide) is more appropriate.

Colorectal cancer

The PET scan is of limited value in the detection of primary colorectal carcinomas and large adenomatous polyps. This is because the interpretation of the scan may be influenced by increased uptake associated with:

- physiological activity (bowel and urinary)
- inflammatory conditions (abscesses and postirradiation).

In addition, there may be low uptake associated with:

- the tumour type (mucinous adenocarcinomas)
- micrometastatic disease and small metastases. These are beyond the resolution of the scanner and will also escape detection.

The PET scan is of most use in the management of patients with suspected or proven recurrent disease. It has high sensitivity for the detection of recurrent colorectal carcinoma and is superior to conventional imaging particularly in detecting metastases (Fig. 8.4).

In recurrent colorectal carcinoma, FDG-PET provides additional information that can alter patient management in 59% of cases. Surgical treatment decisions may be influenced in 60% of patients because of positive PET findings. Inappropriate local therapy can be avoided if widespread disease is documented with PET. PET is useful for the evaluation of suspected recurrent colorectal cancer when conventional imaging is equivocal or negative but the CEA is increased.

Detection of liver metastases

PET has a sensitivity of 97% for liver metastases over 1 cm in size. False positive results occur in the presence of marked intrahepatic cholestasis. The addition of PET scanning to more conventional imaging will help better define patients with metastatic liver lesions suitable for resection. The PET scan will often detect lesions missed by the CT scan.

Use of PET to monitor response to treatment

Changes in FDG uptake can predict disease-free and overall survival after neoadjuvant therapy and resection. PET imaging may differentiate responding and non-responding tumours early in the course of therapy. By avoiding ineffective and potentially harmful treatment, PET may facilitate preoperative therapy, especially in patients with potentially resectable tumours.

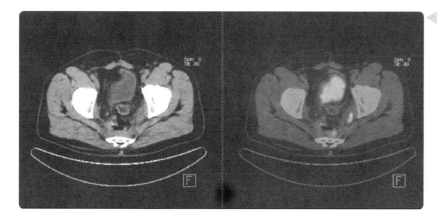

Fig. 8.4 A coregistered CT and PET showing two deposits of rectal cancer in the pelvis. The major area of activity is in the bladder (normal).

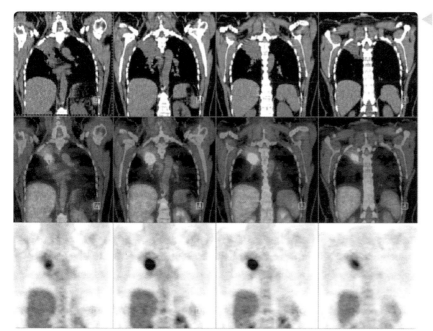

Fig. 8.5 A coregistered CT-PET image of recurrent lung cancer. The CT alone failed to identify the tumour and even with a CT-guided biopsy only inflammatory tissue was obtained. The PET images show malignant activity in the centre of the mass.

Changes in FDG uptake may precede imaging responses by other modalities, making it a useful tool in assessing response to treatment. For example, in patients treated with the tyrosine kinase inhibitor imatinib, PET responses correlate well with symptom improvement and precede objective tumour shrinkage on CT and MR by several weeks. PET may therefore have a role in detecting 'responders' early in the treatment course.

After neoadjuvant therapy, PET does not add to the estimation of locoregional resectability and does not detect new distant metastases.

Restaging or evaluation of disease recurrence

PET also has an established role in the re-staging and evaluation of tumour recurrence due to its higher accuracy compared to CT for detecting metastatic disease (Fig. 8.5). In follow-up, PET has a higher accuracy than CT in the detection of metastases within the abdomen, but CT is more sensitive than PET in detection of small pulmonary metastases.

Restaging of breast cancer patients with PET has been shown to change their treatment in up to 60%. This includes changing the existing treatment regimes (e.g. change from hormone therapy to chemotherapy). In re-staging patients with breast cancer approximately 30% will be upstaged due to detection of previously unsuspected metastases and up to 8% will be downstaged.

PET in non-gastrointestinal tumours

Melanoma

In the primary staging of melanoma, lymphoscintigraphy and sentinel node biopsy is more sensitive than PET in the detection of lymph node metastases due to the ability to localise involved nodes and detect micrometastases pathologically.

The major role of PET scanning in melanoma is to evaluate the extent of disease in patients with stage III and IV disease. Due to the unpredictable nature of melanoma metastases, multiple imaging with CT and MRI is often required. This is time consuming, expensive, subjects the patient to a significant radiation exposure and has limited sensitivity. PET scans have been shown to influence the management in up to 49% of patients with melanoma. PET responses may also be predictive of response to chemotherapy. One study has demonstrated that patients with high metabolic tumour activity on PET had a greater response to chemotherapy than patients with low metabolic activity. This is the subject of ongoing research.

Lymphoma

Both Hodgkin's disease and most types of non-Hodgkin's lymphoma are hypermetabolic and concentrate FDG. Low-grade non-Hodgkin's lymphomas generally show reduced FDG uptake except in areas of transformation. In the primary staging of lymphoma, PET complements CT as it is able to detect involved lymph nodes that may be normal in size. PET is also able to detect sites of extranodal involvement such as bone marrow, liver and spleen. Compared to gallium, PET has a lower radiation dose, is more sensitive for disease and is completed in 1 day. Occasionally lymphomas are not gallium avid but will be shown on PET.

As lymphomas are generally highly sensitive to chemotherapy and radiotherapy, a poor response as seen on PET after the completion of first line chemotherapy, suggests that more aggressive treatment should be considered. In the presence of suspected relapse of lymphoma, PET is useful for restaging and

provides a baseline for monitoring aggressive therapy. PET can be used to differentiate between viable residual lymphoma and scar tissue in patients with residual nodal masses after completion of therapy.

Breast cancer

FDG-PET currently does not have a role in the diagnosis or primary staging of early breast cancer due to its limited sensitivity for small tumours, invasive lobular carcinoma, micrometastases and involved lymph nodes with small tumour load.

In locally advanced breast cancer, PET has high accuracy for the detection of loco-regional lymph node metastases. It also has a higher sensitivity in detecting nodal and lytic bone metastases than conventional staging. However, PET is a recent imaging tool and should be considered as complementary to conventional methods of staging rather than a substitute for conventional staging studies, including computed tomography and bone scintigraphy.

NEW DEVELOPMENTS: PET-CT

Although PET scanning has been developed over the last 25 years, the more recent development of fused PET and CT images (PET-CT) has the potential to revolutionise imaging of cancer. One of the key advantages of PET-CT is the ability to merge anatomic with molecular image information (Fig. 8.6). This is particularly appealing to surgeons who are more comfortable dealing with anatomical imaging. Further, it provides functional information about the anatomical abnormalities, improving the diagnostic accuracy of imaging.

Experience with PET-CT is limited and its clinical efficacy has yet to be demonstrated. Despite this, the intrinsic appeal of this novel fusion of technologies means that it is anticipated to grow rapidly over the next few years. A further advantage of PET-CT is that acquisition times are reduced (compared to PET alone) and it is also possible to scan patients without the use of intravenous contrast. Accurate lesion localisation with PET-CT may also reduce the number of false-positive and false-negative PET findings due to underlying high FDG uptake.

In one study comparing PET-CT with PET and CT performed separately in chest malignancy, the accuracy of PET-CT was superior to that of 'visual' image

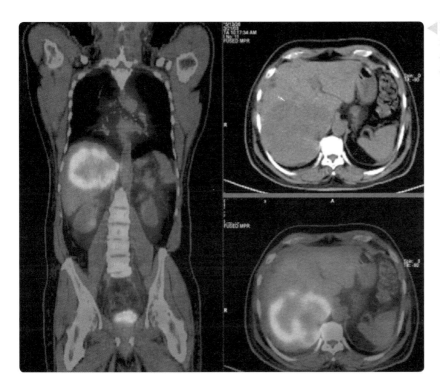

Fig. 8.6 Coregistered CT-SPECT images showing a large metastatic deposit in the liver from a colorectal primary.

fusion. PET-CT reduced the number of 'equivocal' lymph nodes, provided additional important information in 41% of patients, including localisation of lymph nodes, identification of chest wall infiltration, differentiation between tumour and inflammation, and localisation of distant metastases.

One area of particular interest is the potential for PET-CT to characterise response to chemotherapy or other cancer treatments. The differentiation of residual/ recurrent masses on CT images in patients treated for cancer is often problematic. For example, such a mass may represent active residual tumour, necrotic tumour with no viable cells or scarring. PET-CT may have a role in differentiating these lesions. It may also have a role in guiding radiation therapy to target boost the metabolically active component of the tumour, rather than encompass the entire tumour mass.

SUMMARY

FDG-PET can detect metabolic abnormalities before structural anatomical changes occur permitting earlier detection of metastatic disease. This results in more accurate staging leading to more appropriate manage-ment decisions. Cost savings can be realised by avoiding unnecessary surgery. Those treated by potentially curative resection based on FDG-PET have higher 5-year survivals.

Further reading

Antoch G, Vogt FM, Freudenberg LS et al. Whole-body dual-modality PET/CT and whole-body MRI for tumor staging in oncology. JAMA 2003; 290:3199–206

Brucher BL, Weber W, Bauer M et al. Neoadjuvant therapy of esophageal squamous cell carcinoma: response evaluation by positron emission tomography. Ann Surg 2001; 233:300–9

Chin BB, Wahl RL. (18)F-fluoro-2-deoxyglucose positron emission tomography in the evaluation of gastrointestinal malignancies. Gut 2003; 52(Suppl IV):23–9

Cohade C, Osman M, Leal J, Wahl RL. Direct comparison of (18)F-FDG-PET and PET/CT in patients with colorectal carcinoma. J Nucl Med 2003; 44:1797–803

Czernin J, Schelbert J. PET/CT imaging: facts, opinions, hopes and questions. J Nucl Med 2004; 45:S5

Downey RJ, Akhurst T, Ilson D et al. Whole body 18FDG-PET and the response of esophageal cancer to induction therapy: results of a prospective trial. J Clin Oncol 2003; 21:428–32

Edhayan E, Lloyd L. PET scans in general surgery: current status in their use for general surgery. Curr Surg 2004; 61:263–6

Gulec SA, Faries MB, Lee CC et al. The role of fluorine-18 deoxyglucose positron emission tomography in the management of patients with metastatic melanoma: impact on surgical decision making. Clin Nucl Med 2003; 28:961–5

Kalff V, Hicks RJ, Ware RE et al. The clinical impact of (18)F-FDG-PET in patients with suspected or confirmed recurrence of colorectal cancer: a prospective study. J Nucl Med 2002; 43:492–9

Lardinois D, Weder W, Hany TF et al. Staging of non-small-cell lung cancer with integrated position-emission tomography and computed tanography. N Engl J Med 2003; 348:2500–2507

Schoder H, Earson SM, Yeung H. PET/CT in oncology: integration into clinical management of lymphoma, melanoma and gastrointestinal malignancies. J Nucl Med 2004; 45(suppl):72S–81S

Strasberg SM, Dehdashti F, Siegel BA et al. Survival of patients evaluated by FDG-PET before hepatic resection for metastatic colorectal carcinoma: a prospective database study. Ann Surg 2001; 233: 293–9

Stroobants S, Goeminne J, Seegers M et al. 18FDG-Positron emission tomography for the early prediction of response in advanced soft tissue sarcoma treated with imatinib mesylate (Glivec). Eur J Cancer 2003; 39:2012–20

Toloza EM, Harpole L, McCrory H. Non-invasive staging of non-small cell lung cancer. A review of the current evidence. Chest 2003; 123:137S–146S

Weber WA, Ott K, Becker K et al. Prediction of response to preoperative chemotherapy in adenocarcinomas of the esophagogastric junction by metabolic imaging. J Clin Oncol 2001; 19:3058–65

Yoon YC, Lee KS, Shim YM et al. Metastasis to regional lymph nodes in patients with esophageal squamous cell carcinoma: CT versus FDG-PET for presurgical detection prospective study. Radiology 2003; 227:764–70

Zimny M, Siggelkow W. Positron emission tomography scanning in gynecologic and breast cancers. Curr Opin Obstet Gynecol 2003; 15:69–75

Interventional radiology

W. Thompson

9

Background

The specialty of interventional radiology is rapidly developing. Advances in both the imaging and equipment used have allowed the development of minimally invasive techniques to replace or complement the traditional surgical approach to many conditions. Many of these procedures can be performed under local anaesthetic on an outpatient or day case basis. The focus of this chapter is to provide the practicing surgeon with an understanding of what interventional techniques are available and their appropriate use.

BIOPSY AND DRAINAGE

Percutaneous biopsy

This is probably the most common interventional radiological procedure and can be used to obtain material for cytology, microbiology or histopathology, enabling diagnosis of focal or diffuse processes involving practically any organ or body region.

Options for image guidance include fluoroscopy, ultrasound (Fig. 9.1) and CT (Fig. 9.2). Each of these modalities has advantages and disadvantages, with the choice of procedure depending on size, location and visibility of the lesion, as well as the experience and preference of the operator.

There are two basic categories of biopsy commonly performed, fine needle aspiration (FNA) and core biopsy. FNA uses a 20- to 25-gauge needle to aspirate material for cytology, whereas core biopsy needles range in size from 14 to 20 gauge and are equipped with a spring firing mechanism that cuts a core of tissue, enabling histological diagnosis. In general, FNA, being less invasive, is attempted initially, with core biopsy reserved for those instances where FNA has proven non-diagnostic or where assessment of tissue architecture is required. The assessment of diffuse liver disease, lesions of suspected hepatocellular origin, and the diagnosis and classification of lymphoma all fall into this latter category and require core biopsy.

In general adequate material to enable a diagnosis is obtained in 80–95% of biopsy cases, but in approximately 5–10% there will be a false negative result. The risks for a given procedure vary depending on the nature and location of the lesion, but the overall com-

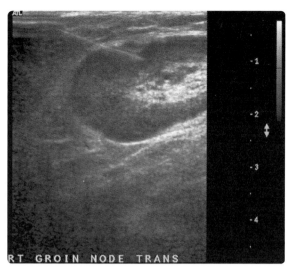

Fig. 9.1 Ultrasound-guided FNA of enlarged inguinal lymph node. The needle tip is seen in the cortex of the node. Cytology showed benign reactive changes.

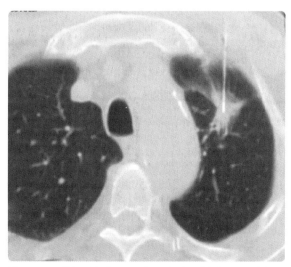

Fig. 9.2 A CT-guided FNA of a spiculated left upper lobe lesion.

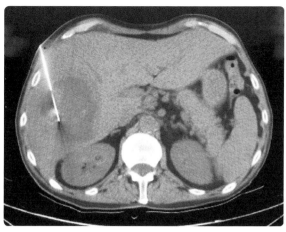

Fig. 9.3 CT-guided drainage of an abscess in the right lobe of the liver using the Seldinger technique.

plication rate should be <2%. The most common complication is haemorrhage, but this is rarely severe. Other reported complications include infection, organ injury (e.g. bowel perforation, bile leak or pancreatitis) and needle track seeding, all of which are extremely rare. Pneumothorax can occasionally occur after abdominal procedures, but is more frequent with lung biopsy (5–30%).

Percutaneous drainage

Fluid collections in a variety of organs or cavities throughout the body can be drained percutaneously. Drainage is indicated when an infected collection is suspected or when a non-infected fluid collection is causing significant symptoms (e.g. pancreatic pseudocyst causing gastric outlet obstruction).

Drainage may be performed using either CT or ultrasound guidance, the choice depending on the site and nature of the collection and the operator's preference. When ultrasound is used it is frequently combined with fluoroscopy, allowing real time visualisation at all stages of the procedure. Drain size is chosen depending on the viscosity of the fluid at initial needle aspiration and ranges from 8–14 F. Larger sizes, sump drains, or multiple catheters may sometimes be required for very thick or complex collections. The commonly used drainage catheters have a retaining pigtail, which can be secured by a string at the hub of the catheter and placed either using the trochar or Seldinger technique (Fig. 9.3). The trochar technique uses a catheter with an inner stylet and stiffener placed directly into the collection parallel to the aspiration needle, which is used as a guide. This technique is used for large or superficial lesions. The Seldinger technique uses a guide wire advanced via the needle and curled within the cavity. The track is then dilated and the drainage catheter placed over the wire.

Following drain insertion the collection should be aspirated to dryness or until the fluid becomes blood-stained. Regular saline flushes may be used to maintain catheter patency. Drain output should be monitored and removal considered when the patient is systemically well and output is less than 10–20 mL per day. Some advocate imaging with tube contrast study, CT or US prior to removal to ensure collection resolution. This is optional but should be considered if the patient remains febrile, if drainage is less than expected, or if output drops off suddenly as these may indicate catheter blockage or undrained locules. If output remains high a fistula should be suspected and a tube contrast study is recommended to delineate this. When removing the catheter the string holding the pigtail must be released. This can be most easily done by cutting the catheter as the locking mechanism at the hub will vary depending on the brand of catheter used.

Success rates in the region of 90% should be expected for simple collections, but this decreases in more complex cases. Re-accumulation of a fluid collection may occur in 10–20% and is usually due to early catheter removal, inadequate initial drainage or an unrecognised fistula. Multiloculated collections, and those that contain inspissated material are unlikely to be treated satisfactorily by a radiological approach alone. Complications occur in less than 10% and include haemorrhage, bacteraemia, septic shock, and injury to adjacent organs.

Most pancreatic pseudocysts will resolve spontaneously, but where appropriate, percutaneous drainage can achieve a satisfactory outcome. Large, thick-walled cysts (allow 4–6 weeks for maturation) and those free of debris, can be drained successfully. Indications for drainage include pain, upper gastrointestinal tract obstruction, infection and enlarging lesions >5 cm. Where possible, a transgastric approach should be used to prevent a pancreatico-cutaneous fistula from forming (Fig. 9.4A). After a period of drainage the option then also exists to place an internal plastic stent between the cyst and the stomach, effectively forming a cyst–gastrostomy (Fig. 9.4B). The stent is removed endoscopically after 2–3 months. Treatment of pancreatic abscess, phlegmon or necrosis is generally surgical, however percutaneous drainage can often be a useful temporising measure. Occasionally an aggressive approach with large or multiple catheters may prove definitive in these conditions.

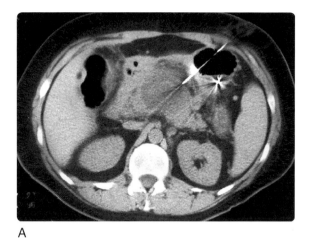

A

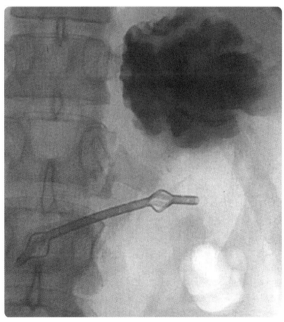

B

Fig. 9.4 (A) Percutaneous trans-gastric drainage of a pancreatic pseudocyst. (B) Insertion of a cyst–gastrostomy catheter 2 weeks after the initial drainage.

SPECIFIC SURGICAL APPLICATIONS OF INTERVENTIONAL RADIOLOGY

Hepatobiliary intervention

Liver biopsy and hepatic abscess drainage

The general principles outlined above apply to liver biopsy and hepatic abscess drainage. When planning these procedures, a route that crosses some normal liver tissue prior to entering any abscess or lesion should be chosen. A thorough non-invasive workup is recommended prior to liver lesion biopsy as specific imaging findings may permit accurate diagnosis and obviate the need for biopsy (see Chapter 12). Examples of lesions where such a diagnosis can often be made include simple cyst, haemangioma, focal nodular hyperplasia and hepatocellular carcinoma. When diagnosis of diffuse liver disease is required core biopsies are usually taken. When there is an increased risk of haemorrhage due to coagulopathy or ascites either a gelfoam plugged percutaneous biopsy or transjugular biopsy may be used to obtain tissue.

Percutaneous cholecystostomy

This is a treatment option in patients with acute cholecystitis or gall bladder empyema who are not fit for surgery. There is also evidence to support the use of this procedure in septic ICU patients where no other source of infection can be found. Even in the absence of any gall bladder abnormality on ultrasound, a significant number will improve after this procedure. Ultrasound guidance is used, either alone, in which case the procedure can be performed at the bedside, or preferably in combination with fluoroscopy. Where possible a transhepatic path is chosen to minimise the risk of intraperitoneal leakage and bile peritonitis. After a period of drainage a tube contrast study is performed to assess cystic duct patency. If the cystic duct is occluded then either long term tube drainage or interval cholecystectomy are required. If the cystic duct is patent and the infective episode has resolved the drain can be removed after the track has been allowed to mature.

Percutaneous transhepatic cholangiography (PTC)

This technique is now almost exclusively performed as the first step of percutaneous biliary drainage. The purely diagnostic role of PTC has been largely replaced by ERCP and non-invasive modalities such as MRCP. Opinions differ on the role of ERCP or MRCP as first-line imaging of the pancreatico-biliary systems. Although ERCP is invasive, it probably provides better definition of the extrahepatic bile ductal system, whereas MRCP will provide good imaging of the intrahepatic bile ducts and the pancreatic duct.

Decompression of the obstructed biliary system is indicated when there is cholangitis or symptomatic jaundice. This is best achieved endoscopically by ERCP and stent placement and this is feasible in most cases. Percutaneous biliary drainage is indicated where ERCP has failed or is not possible due to anatomical factors. Most often this is a previous partial gastrectomy with a Roux-en-Y reconstruction. A percutaneous approach is also favoured in high biliary obstructions, particularly where there is hilar or intrahepatic duct involvement. Sedation is often required for percutaneous biliary drainage; best delivered by an anaesthetist, with general anaesthetic occasionally necessary. Antibiotic prophylaxis is also routinely used.

Either a right- or left-sided approach to drainage can be used. With distal obstruction either approach is suitable, with the left side preferred by many due to the relative ease of ultrasound-guided puncture. In treating hilar lesions, however, the largest volume of liver possible should be drained with a single catheter, normally implying a right sided approach. Bilateral drainage should not be routinely employed, being reserved for cases where a unilateral drain does not relieve the patient's jaundice or where the undrained portion of the biliary system becomes infected.

For biliary drainage a relatively peripheral intrahepatic duct should be punctured. This can be done with ultrasound guidance or under fluoroscopy after a blind puncture has been made into a more central duct and the biliary tree opacified with contrast. Once a suitable duct has been punctured a guidewire is inserted through the needle into the biliary system (Fig. 9.5A). The catheter and guidewire are negotiated through any obstruction to the duodenum and a biliary drainage catheter is placed over the wire (Fig. 9.5B). This has a retaining pigtail, which is formed in the duodenum and has side holes extending along the shaft of the catheter to above the level of obstruction. The catheter should be connected to a bag to allow external drainage for 24–48 hours, allowing any potentially life-threatening sepsis to settle. The catheter is then clamped and bile drains internally to the duodenum. External drainage should be reinstated and a tube cholangiogram obtained if there is any sign of internal catheter blockage (increasing pain, fever, bile leakage, rising bilirubin).

On occasion it is not possible to traverse a complete obstruction in a distended system at the initial attempt,

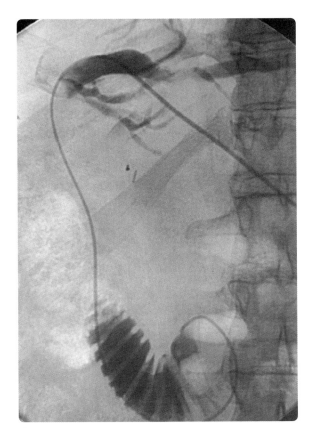
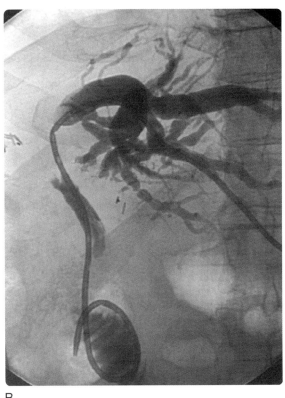

A   B

Fig. 9.5 (A) Previous right hepatectomy for metastases from carcinoma of the colon and subsequent presentation with obstructive jaundice due to tumour recurrence. An ultrasound-guided, segment 3 duct puncture was performed and catheter inserted. The cholangiogram showed complete obstruction of the left hepatic duct. A catheter was negotiated through the obstruction. (B) An external biliary drain has been placed over the catheter.

by waiting several days and re-attempting after the dilatation has subsided, most obstructions can be traversed.

With dilated ducts biliary drainage can be achieved in nearly all patients, with success decreasing slightly in a non-dilated system. Percutaneous biliary drainage is an invasive procedure with potential serious complications that include haemorrhage, haemobilia, septic shock, bile leak with peritonitis, and pneumothorax. Delayed complications include skin infection or irritation, tube blockage and cholangitis.

Benign biliary strictures can usually be treated successfully by repeated balloon dilatation and a temporary period of catheter drainage, although strictures may recur. In cases of malignant obstruction inter-

nal–external biliary drainage may be used as a long-term treatment strategy. This obviously involves the presence of an external catheter and requires catheter exchange three-monthly or sooner in cases of blockage. The alternative in these patients is internal biliary stenting, which is often preferred. Self-expanding metallic stents are the most commonly used devices (Fig. 9.6). Whilst these may be inserted at the initial procedure, a period of catheter drainage is often provided with stenting done at a subsequent sitting, particularly when there is cholangitis or significant haemobilia.

There are few additional immediate complications associated with stenting other than those encountered with percutaneous biliary drainage. In the longer term

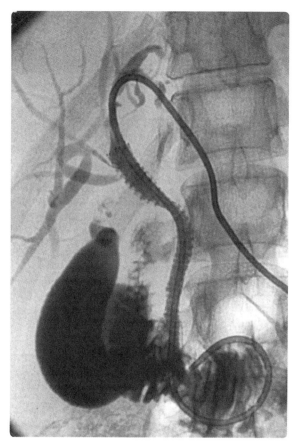

Fig. 9.6 Internal metallic stent in a patient with unresectable pancreatic cancer where ERCP was not possible.

however tumour ingrowth and overgrowth may occur, resulting in stent blockage. Mean patency for metallic stents is approximately 6 months. When stent blockage occurs a new procedure is required, usually in the form of a repeat percutaneous biliary drainage with a biliary catheter being passed through the blocked stent to the duodenum. In an attempt to prevent tumour ingrowth covered stents have been used in the bile duct, with mixed initial results. Because of their limited lifespan metallic stents are not recommended in benign biliary disease.

Radiofrequency ablation

Relatively new to most interventional radiology practices are the techniques used for local ablation of liver lesions. The most widespread of these is radiofre-quency ablation (RFA), which relies on heating of the tissues to such a level as to induce necrosis. This technique has been used for hepatocellular carcinoma and metastases where surgical resection is not an option. The probe may be placed percutaneously using CT or ultrasound guidance, or alternatively at an open surgical procedure. The size of the burn lesion created depends on the configuration of the probe used but is generally around 3 cm. This technique can successfully produce complete necrosis in small lesions but recurrence may occur either at the treatment site or elsewhere in the liver.

Gastrointestinal intervention

Radiological procedures have been developed to:

- provide access to the gut for feeding (gastrostomy)
- decompress an obstructed system.

Percutaneous radiological gastrostomy (PRG)

Gastrostomy tubes are used for long-term enteral feeding or decompression. The radiological approach to gastrostomy is most often requested when percutaneous endoscopic gastrostomy (PEG) has failed or is not possible. Patients referred preferentially for the radiological approach include those with upper digestive tract obstruction (e.g. head and neck malignancy and oesophageal strictures). Absolute contraindications to percutaneous gastrostomy (endoscopic or radiological) include:

- uncorrected coagulopathy
- lack of a safe access to the stomach
- interposed liver or bowel
- subcostal or intrathoracic gastric location.

Relative contraindications include:

- ascites
- portal hypertension
- previous gastric surgery
- tumour involvement of the stomach wall.

The procedure is generally performed under local anaesthetic and sedation. The stomach is distended with air via a nasogastric tube. A site for gastric puncture is chosen using ultrasound and fluoroscopy to avoid liver and bowel, generally over the mid to distal gastric body. Most radiologists prefer gastropexy, with potential advantages including a decreased risk of intraperitoneal tube misplacement and intraperitoneal leakage of gastric content. Between one and four T-fasteners are used to secure the anterior gastric wall to the abdominal wall. The stomach is then punctured between the T-fasteners and a guide wire curled within the gastric lumen. One-step dilatation of the track using a peel away sheath is preferred to minimise any pneumoperitoneum and a 14–18 F balloon gastrostomy tube placed. Radiological techniques using smaller calibre pigtail catheters or pull type gastrostomy tubes similar to those used in PEG have been described. If there is evidence of gastroesophageal reflux or gastric stasis it is a simple procedure to convert to a trans-gastric jejunostomy using radiological techniques.

Successful gastrostomy placement is achieved in approximately 99% of cases. The reported figures for the various forms of gastrostomy suggest that the radiological approach has a higher success rate than PEG and similar or fewer complications than PEG or surgical gastrostomy. These differences, however, are small and the technique of choice should depend on local expertise and resources, ideally with a cooperative approach between the groups involved. Complications are uncommon and include haemorrhage, tube misplacement or migration, peritonitis, sepsis and reflux with aspiration.

Gastrointestinal strictures

Benign gastrointestinal strictures are treated either by surgery or dilatation. The commonest example is an oesophageal stricture where dilatation is generally performed endoscopically. The endoscopist has the advantage of being able to place the guide wire under direct vision. However, if the stricture is tight and unable to admit the endoscope, it is safer to place the guide wire beyond the stricture under fluoroscopic control. Stenting, generally of malignant lesions, can be performed in the oesophagus, duodenum and colon.

Oesophageal stenting The usual indication for this procedure is palliation of dysphagia in patients with malignant oesophageal strictures. Stents do not provide ideal relief of symptoms, and where possible the patient should be considered for combination chemoradiotherapy. The stents may be placed endoscopically or radiologically. Covered stents are used when there is an associated perforation or fistula formation.

Before the procedure, the diagnosis must be confirmed (usually by endoscopy and biopsy) and the exact location and length of the stricture established. Radiological insertion of an oesophageal stent starts with the patient lying in a lateral position, using topical anaesthesia and sedation as required. A catheter is passed orally to the upper oesophagus and contrast is used to delineate the stricture, which is outlined on the skin with radio-opaque markers. The lesion is crossed and a stiff guidewire passed to the stomach (Fig. 9.7). Although not normally required, the stricture may be dilated prior to insertion of the mesh stent. Similarly, once the stent has been deployed, balloon dilatation may be employed to gain full expansion. Most malignant strictures are sufficiently pliable to allow spontaneous full expansion of the stent although this may take 24 hours to achieve. Two hours following insertion of the stent the patient can take clear fluids. A

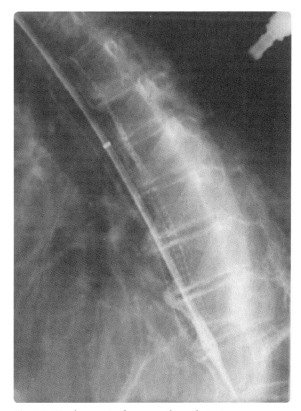

Fig. 9.7 Deployment of an oesophageal stent across a stenosing squamous cell carcinoma of the mid-oesophagus which had failed to respond to chemoradiotherapy.

barium swallow is performed at 24 hours to exclude perforation and ensure stent position, patency and expansion. After this a soft diet may be commenced. Long-term proton pump inhibitors are recommended when the stent crosses the gastroesophageal junction into the stomach to counter the expected reflux.

Technical success rates are high, approaching 100%, and improvement in dysphagia is reported in over 90%. Some chest pain is common as the stent expands, but this is rarely severe and should resolve within the first few days. Serious complications such as perforation and haemorrhage are rare. In the longer term stent migration, and tumour ingrowth or overgrowth may occur. Tumour ingrowth can be prevented by the use of covered stents, but this is at the expense of slightly higher migration rates. Nevertheless, most operators prefer covered stents.

Colonic stenting Mesh stents can also be used to relieve malignant obstruction either to allow stabilisation and bowel cleansing prior to elective single stage surgery or as a palliative procedure in unresectable or advanced metastatic disease. Stenting is absolutely contraindicated in cases of colonic perforation and relative contraindications include right sided or low rectal lesions, long strictures and lesions that lie close to an angulated segment of bowel. In cases of a proximal lesion or tortuous anatomy colonoscopic assistance may help to access the lesion and ultimately make the procedure possible.

The procedure is performed in a lateral position with sedation provided as necessary. Contrast is injected rectally and the lower edge of the stricture marked. The lesion is then crossed with a catheter and wire, and further contrast is injected to show the proximal extent of the lesion. A stiff guidewire is placed across the lesion and passed as far proximally as possible for added stability. Predilatation is generally not recommended in the colon due to a perceived increased risk of perforation. The stent is placed and deployed across the lesion, often followed by a gush of liquid faecal material, confirming success. Further contrast injection may however be performed to confirm stent position and patency and to exclude perforation. Either plain abdominal X-ray or preferably gastrografin enema should be performed at 24 hours to assess stent position and expansion.

Both technical and clinical success rates of between 80 and 100% are reported. Early failure may occur due to poor stent expansion, migration, or incomplete lesion coverage. Transient minor rectal bleeding and abdominal pain are not infrequently encountered and perforation is seen in between 0 and 16%. In the longer term faecal impaction, tumour ingrowth or overgrowth, or stent migration may be seen. The latter is more common with extrinsic lesions, covered stents and following chemo or radiotherapy.

Urological intervention
Nephrostomy
Insertion of a drainage tube into the renal pelvicalyceal system is a commonly performed procedure used to relieve urinary tract obstruction when retrograde ureteric stenting has failed or is deemed inappropriate. The retrograde approach is less invasive and should be considered in the first instance unless there is evidence of an infected system. Other indications for nephrostomy include access for further interventions such as stone removal or to provide urinary diversion in cases of ureteric leak, fistula or severe cystitis. The main contraindication is coagulopathy and hence the usual preprocedure blood tests are mandatory. Antibiotic prophylaxis is recommended and most patients will require conscious sedation in addition to local anaesthesia.

Several different nephrostomy techniques have been described. The technique favoured by most radiologists involves the use of a combination of ultrasound and fluoroscopic guidance. With the patient in a prone or prone oblique position a fine needle is passed through the relatively avascular posterolateral aspect of the renal parenchyma and into a posterior calyx, usually in the mid or lower pole. A specimen of urine is taken and a small amount of contrast injected to outline the collecting system. A fine guidewire is then advanced and either curled in the renal pelvis or passed down the upper ureter. This is followed by a coaxial dilator system that allows exchange to a thicker heavy-duty wire, over which the track is dilated and the nephrostomy tube placed (Fig. 9.8). An 8-F pigtail catheter is generally sufficient, with larger tubes sometimes used in cases of pyonephrosis.

Nephrostomy placement should be achieved in nearly all cases when the collecting system is dilated,

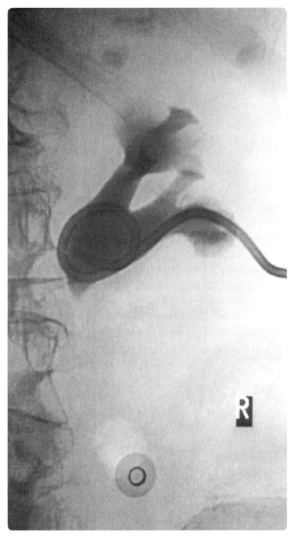

Fig. 9.8 A percutaneous nephrostomy tube in a woman with a urinary infection and hydronephrosis.

scanning is recommended. In cases of severe bleeding angiography and embolisation may be required. Bacteraemia or septic shock may be precipitated when draining an obstructed infected system. This risk can be minimised by the use of antibiotic cover and avoiding over-injection of contrast and excessive catheter manipulations.

Ureteric stenting

Antegrade stenting of a ureter may be undertaken to relieve malignant obstruction when retrograde stenting has failed or when there is already a nephrostomy tube in place. Stent insertion may be performed at the initial procedure; however, some people prefer a period of external drainage. This probably is only necessary when heavy haematuria is encountered or there is evidence of infection. In either case once access to the collecting system is secured a guidewire and catheter are directed down the ureter, passed through the obstruction and advanced to the bladder. A stiff wire is then placed in the bladder and a peel away sheath inserted. The stent-pusher assembly is advanced over the wire, through the sheath and deployed with distal pigtail in the bladder and proximal end in the renal pelvis. It is recommended that a covering nephrostomy tube be left in place for 24 hours, being removed after a nephrostogram shows adequate stent function.

Stent insertion is achieved in most cases. Occasionally the ureteric obstruction cannot be crossed, in which case long-term nephrostomy drainage is required. Stent patency is not indefinite and cystoscopic exchange is required at 3-monthly intervals. Significant complications other than those related to the initial nephrostomy are rare and include ureteric injury, stent malposition and early stent occlusion due to haematuria and clot.

Arterial intervention

Imaging is an integral part of diagnosis and therapy in major vessel vascular disease. The roles of the radiologist and vascular surgeon frequently overlap and many vascular surgeons are now acquiring both diagnostic and interventional radiological skills (see Chapter 21).

Angioplasty and stenting

These are two commonly performed procedures used to treat symptomatic vascular stenoses or occlusions.

with success rates decreasing slightly in non-dilated systems or those filled with stones. Minor haematuria is common post nephrostomy and this should clear within 48 hours. Complications are uncommon, occurring in approximately 5% of procedures. The most frequent complication is haemorrhage, with significant vascular trauma occurring in 1–2%. This is usually manifest by haematuria, which may be delayed in the cases of arteriovenous fistula or pseudoaneurysm. If there is flank pain and a fall in haemoglobin in the absence of haematuria, a subcapsular or perinephric haematoma should be suspected and CT

With developments in equipment, angioplasty can be performed and stents inserted through relatively small arterial punctures, with 5–7 F sheaths sufficient in most cases. Heparin is commonly used during angioplasty and stenting in doses of 3000–5000 units and long-term aspirin treatment is recommended thereafter. Haemostasis is usually easily achieved by manual compression, but a variety of closure devices are now available which may be used for larger sheath sizes, anticoagulated patients, or those unable to comply with bed rest requirements.

Percutaneous transluminal angioplasty is performed using balloon dilatation catheters that are inflated across the stenotic lesion. Balloon size is chosen so that diameter is equal to or slightly greater than the vessel being treated and the length just covers the lesion. The primary mechanism of action is thought to be plaque fracture and local dissection. Lesions most suited to angioplasty are short, focal, concentric and free of calcification.

The insertion of a stent adds considerable cost to the procedure and is usually reserved for failed angioplasty or restenosis at a previous angioplasty site. Primary stenting may be considered for some lesion types or at specific sites. Primary stenting has demonstrated better results in the carotid bifurcation, renal and common iliac arteries. Stenting is usually only of benefit in the external iliac and femoral arteries to repair a complication. Most stents are made of stainless steel or nitinol and are either balloon mounted or self-expanding. Covered stents may be used to treat traumatic or iatrogenic arterial rupture or aneurysmal disease. Technical and clinical success rates for stenting are similar or superior to angioplasty at most sites.

Complications are similar for both angioplasty and stenting, with significant groin haematomas seen in 2–8% and false aneurysms in <1%. Treatment site dissection is relatively common, although rarely flow limiting. Acute thrombosis and occlusion are seen in 5–8% and vessel rupture in 0.5%. Distal embolisation occurs in 1–5%. Late restenosis and occlusion rates vary with site and type of lesion being treated and this is usually due to neointimal hyperplasia. Drug eluting stents, which aim to prevent this, are currently close to market release. These may well revolutionise the treatment of peripheral vascular disease and the results of further trials are eagerly awaited.

Peripheral arteries

Patency rates for peripheral arterial interventions are usually defined in clinical terms, being based on a lack of symptom recurrence and comparison of non-invasive measurements to baseline. Technical success refers to relief of stenosis or occlusion angiographically, with no residual pressure gradient across the lesion. A residual narrowing of 20–30% is usually accepted.

Iliac lesions tend to respond well to angioplasty with technical success in excess of 90% and patency rates of around 90% and 70% at 1 and 5 years. Stenting does little to improve these results in most cases and generally should be reserved for failed angioplasty or restenosis. Many operators opt for primary stenting in long, irregular or eccentric lesions of the iliac arteries. Stenting improves results in common iliac arterial lesions, particularly those near the aortic bifurcation.

Angioplasty has a similar technical success rate in the femoropopliteal segment, but there is a higher incidence of neointimal hyperplasia at this site, resulting in poorer long-term patency. Figures are quite variable, depending on the type of lesion and clinical indication. Patency rates are in the range of 60–80% at 1 year and 20–60% at 5 years. Short, smooth focal stenoses and claudicants tend to do best, whereas long segment, irregular stenoses or occlusions and patients with critical ischaemia show poorer long-term patency. Subintimal angioplasty is an option advocated by some for the treatment of long-segment stenoses or occlusions of the superficial femoral artery, although results are variable. With this technique a dissection is deliberately created, the vessel lumen re-entered below the lesion and the resulting subintimal track dilated with an angioplasty balloon. Stents tend to perform poorly in the femoral artery and are rarely used, however drug-eluting stents show early promise in this region. Cutting balloons may also find a role in the treatment of resistant fibrotic strictures as are seen in femoropopliteal bypass grafts.

Randomised trials comparing angioplasty to surgical bypass in the lower limb have shown no significant difference in long-term outcome for selected patients with femoropopliteal disease. Five-year patency rates of around 55–60% were seen for both techniques. Surgery performs better than angioplasty in the iliac arteries with 5-year patencies of around

80% and 60%, respectively. This is at the cost of a far more invasive procedure.

Renal arteries

Renal artery intervention remains a controversial area with potential indications for treatment including renal artery stenosis associated with 'flash' pulmonary oedema, difficult to control hypertension or impaired renal function. Asymptomatic renal artery stenosis should not be treated except in solitary kidneys or renal transplants. Fibromuscular dysplasia and non-ostial stenoses tend to respond well to angioplasty alone, while atherosclerotic ostial lesions do better with primary stenting (Fig. 9.9); 5-year primary patency for renal stents is approximately 80%. When performed for hypertension about 80% show substantial improvement and when for renal impairment approximately 50–60% will obtain benefit.

Carotid arteries

Carotid artery stenting is an area of much recent interest and debate. There has been rapid improvement in equipment with several purpose-built carotid stents and cerebral protection devices now available, the use of which has become mandatory. Most recent reports focus on high surgical risk patients, but describe acceptably low stroke rates in the range of 1–4%, comparable to that of carotid endarterectomy. This procedure is in its infancy and results are likely to improve with further technical developments, however widespread acceptance is unlikely until superiority or equivalence to endarterectomy is shown in randomised trials, which are currently under way.

The abdominal aorta

Endoluminal repair of abdominal aortic aneurysms was first reported in 1991 and since that time the technique has developed rapidly with associated improvements in stent–graft technology. Currently accepted indications for this procedure are anatomically suitable aneurysms larger than 5 cm in elderly patients with comorbidities that would otherwise prevent surgical repair or make it of unacceptably high risk. With current devices and well-selected patients there is a technical success rate approaching 100%. This is a less invasive treatment option with morbidity and hospital

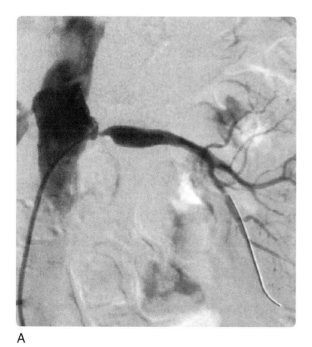

A

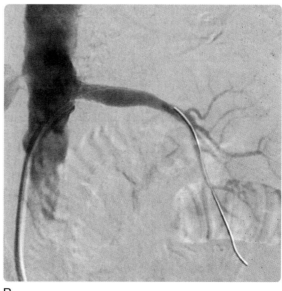

B

Fig. 9.9 (A) Renal artery ostial stenosis in a hypertensive. (B) After insertion of a stent, the hypertension became easier to manage.

stay less than for open repair. Long-term results, however, remain largely unknown and hence there is still significant controversy regarding the role of aortic stenting and its indications. Trials are underway in Europe with randomisation between endoluminal and open repair and endoluminal repair and no treatment. The results of these trials will help to determine the final role of the procedure.

Endoluminal repair can also be used to treat thoracic aortic aneurysms and traumatic rupture of this vessel.

Imaging workup of potential candidates for endoluminal repair is crucial, with CT angiography the mainstay. This enables multiple diameter and length measurements to be made to assess for anatomical suitability and to help with planning.

The procedure is best undertaken in a theatre-equipped angiography suite and may be performed with either general or spinal anaesthetic. The technique has previously involved surgical cut down on both femoral arteries. The introduction of suture closure devices has enabled a totally percutaneous approach with minimal complications. Stent grafts may be custom-made to fit the patient's anatomy or modular components of appropriate size may be purchased 'off the shelf.' They consist of a metal framework and fabric cover and are generally bifurcated, extending down each common iliac artery. A seal is achieved at the proximal neck and in the iliac artery, so excluding the aneurysm from the circulation and preventing rupture.

The presence of blood flow within the aneurysm sac external to the stent graft is termed 'endoleak'. This exposes the sac to systemic blood pressure and associated risk of rupture, which fortunately occurs only rarely. Endoleaks may be primary or delayed and are divided into four types depending on their origin.

- Type 1: occur around the graft at either proximal or distal attachment sites (Fig. 9.10).
- Type 2: fed by retrograde flow in aortic side branches e.g. inferior mesenteric or lumbar arteries.
- Type 3: occur through the fabric of the graft.
- Type 4: occur at joins between modular components.

Type 1 leaks should be treated when they are first diagnosed. Type 2 leaks only need to be treated when

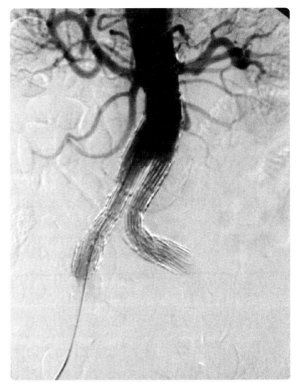

Fig. 9.10 A type 1 endoleak.

large or associated with an increase in the diameter of the sac. Many of these type 2 leaks will resolve spontaneously. Overall, endoleaks occur in up to 20% of grafts.

Therapeutic arterial embolisation

Embolisation is a catheter-directed technique used to occlude an artery or vascular bed. There are a variety of embolic materials available, which may be temporary, such as gelatin sponge, or may cause permanent vascular occlusion. Permanent embolic agents include coils, polyvinyl alcohol particles, glue, and liquid agents such as alcohol. These materials may be delivered through standard angiographic catheters or microcatheters in the case of smaller vessels. Embolisation is used to:

- control arterial haemorrhage (see Chapter 21)
- devascularise tumours.

The best recognised indications for embolisation include:

- trauma (e.g. pelvic fractures)
- iatrogenic bleeding (e.g. following biopsy or drainage procedures in the liver or kidney)
- gastrointestinal haemorrhage (see Chapter 21)
- massive haemoptysis
- intractable epistaxis
- postpartum haemorrhage.

Embolisation is successful in the vast majority of these cases, provided the site of bleeding can be identified angiographically and the offending vessel can be catheterised. These procedures should be performed only when intervention is absolutely necessary as potential complications, whilst uncommon, can be serious. For example, embolisation in the small intestine and colon carries a high risk (up to 20%) of ischaemic complications and infarction and should only be undertaken when the severity of the bleed is such that surgical intervention is being considered or where the patient is a poor surgical risk (see Chapter 21).

In other situations embolisation might not be the first-line treatment. For example, the bleeding associated with a fractured pelvis is usually controlled with external fixation (which facilitates tamponade) and radiological intervention is rarely required. In these circumstances embolisation is a relatively safe and simple procedure, which is probably underutilised.

Tumour embolisation

Another major use of embolisation is to occlude the blood supply and vascular bed of tumours. The aim may be to:

- improve survival
- control symptoms
- devascularise a lesion prior to surgery.

Despite lack of evidence of its efficacy, and based on uncontrolled case series, transarterial chemoembolisation (TACE) of liver tumours is a widely practised procedure. A recent randomised trial and meta-analysis has shown a survival advantage for TACE over palliative treatment when specific protocols and strict entry criteria are used.

Certain liver metastases respond well to embolisation. Symptoms related to hormone release from metastatic neuroendocrine tumours (e.g. carcinoid, insulinoma) can be well controlled. Relief is usually obtained for several months after which embolisation can be repeated as necessary. Unfortunately, metastases from more common tumours such as carcinoma of the colon, lung and breast are rarely responsive to this treatment.

Embolic agents fall into three groups:

- occlusive: i.e. the aim is to devascularise the tumour
- chemotherapeutic
- radiotherapeutic: radioactive particles deliver a relatively high and selective dose to vascular liver tumours.

Complications depend on the type and nature of the embolisation being performed and the embolic material used. Postembolisation syndrome consists of pain, fever, nausea, vomiting and general malaise. It is seen most commonly when a large amount of tissue is embolised. The manifestations of this syndrome are variable in severity and may last from a few days to two weeks. These symptoms should not be confused with infection of necrotic tumour tissue, which is seen far less commonly. Non-target embolisation is potentially the most serious complication and refers to ischaemia occurring in structures other than those in which embolisation was intended. This usually occurs when flow-directed particulate or liquid embolic agents reflux into adjacent vessels. The nature of the complication will depend on the site of embolisation. For example, potential complications of hepatic artery embolisation include gall bladder infarction, duodenal ischaemia and pancreatitis, although none of these are common.

Venous intervention

An increasing part of an interventional radiologist's workload is taken up by venous access procedures and insertion of various devices. These include:

- peripherally inserted central catheters ('PICC lines')
- tunnelled central catheters
- implanted ports (see Chapter 24)
- caval filters
- transhepatic shunts.

Peripheral venous catheters

PICC lines are used for medium to long-term venous access, typically to deliver antibiotics or chemotherapy agents. Blood products, parenteral nutrition and many other fluids can also be given through these lines. The catheters can be placed via an antecubital vein at the bedside. This approach results in failure or misplacement in at least a quarter of cases and insertion under radiological guidance has close to a 100% success rate. Ultrasound is used to localise and puncture a vein in the upper arm and fluoroscopy allows accurate tip placement in the superior vena cava. Catheters range in size from 3–5 French, are single or multi-lumen and have open or valved configuration tip. Insertion is quick, simple and well tolerated in most patients. Complication rates are acceptable, but these may include infection, venous thrombosis and catheter malfunction (blockage, fracture, dislodgement).

Central venous catheters

There are two general categories of tunnelled central catheters; tunnelled dialysis catheters (Permcath®), and Hickman lines, which are used mainly in haematology, oncology and TPN patients. These are inserted using both ultrasound and fluoroscopy. Placement into an internal jugular vein is preferred as there is a lower incidence of associated central vein occlusion. This is an important consideration in dialysis patients where future upper limb fistula creation may be required. A subcutaneous tunnel is created over the clavicle to the anterior chest wall where the catheter exits the skin. There is a Dacron cuff around the catheter within the tunnel that promotes in-growth of fibrous tissue, serving to anchor the catheter and provide a mechanical barrier to infection. There is a low infection rate with these catheters and they may be safely left in position for many months.

With only a small modification to technique a subcutaneous pocket can be formed and an implantable port placed. These devices are ideal for patients who require long-term intermittent access and have the cosmetic advantage of having no external component when not in use. The concern that port placement outside of the operating theatre would carry a higher infection risk has not been born out, with those placed in the angiography suite carrying a similarly low infection rate.

Caval filters

Inferior vena cava filters are devices, which are placed in the IVC to prevent pulmonary emboli by trapping any embolic material. Accepted indications for IVC filter insertion include deep venous thrombosis or pulmonary embolism in patients who have a contraindication to anticoagulation and patients with recurrent PE or progressive DVT despite adequate anticoagulation. Other potential indications include iliac or caval thrombosis and prophylactic insertion in patients with past venous thromboembolic complications who are to undergo high-risk surgery.

Traditionally, filters have been permanent but temporary or retrievable filters are now available and may be used when the contraindication to anticoagulation is likely to be of a short duration. Temporary filters are generally attached to an external catheter and must be removed within 14 days (Fig. 9.11). Retrievable filters are a more attractive choice as they are totally internal and provide the option of retrieval using a snare and sheath up to 12 days after insertion or otherwise can be left as a permanent device.

Access for filter insertion is usually via femoral or jugular veins. A cavogram is performed to measure IVC diameter (most filters only suitable for IVC < 30 mm) and to localise renal veins. The filter is then positioned, in most cases infrarenally, and deployed. Complications are relatively uncommon and include:

* recurrent PE (5%)
* caval thrombosis (5%)
* access site thrombosis (2%)
* filter migration (<1%).

Intrahepatic shunting

Transjugular intrahepatic portosystemic shunt (TIPS) is a percutaneous procedure where a needle passed via the jugular vein is used to create a communication between hepatic and portal veins. The intrahepatic track is dilated with a balloon and held open with a metallic stent (Fig. 9.12). The prime indication for TIPS is the patient with portal hypertension and variceal haemorrhage, where the bleeding has not been controlled by medical or endoscopic measures. Massive ascites refractory to large volume paracentesis and medical therapy is also an accepted indication. TIPS can be used successfully in Budd–Chiari syndrome, however recanalisation of the narrowed or obstructed hepatic veins using balloons and/or stents is preferred in this condition. Hepatorenal and hepatopulmonary syndromes are more controversial indications.

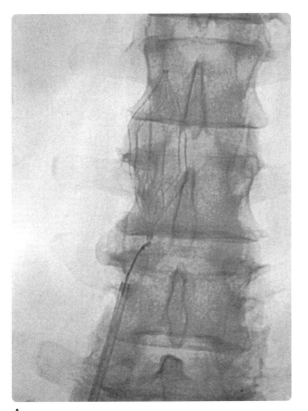

A

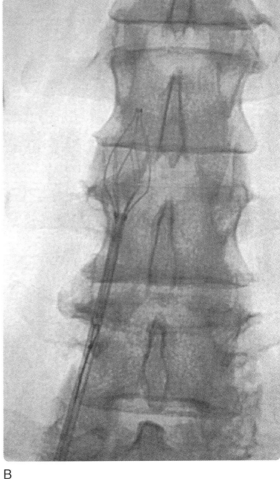

B

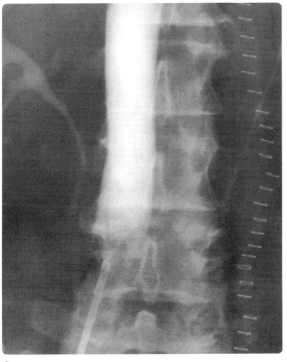

C

Fig. 9.11 (A) A retrievable IVC filter was placed prior to oesophagectomy in this patient with oesophageal carcinoma and recent pulmonary embolus. This allowed anticoagulation to be safely withheld in the perioperative period and the filter was removed after 10 days. The filter is about to be retrieved and the hook on the end of the filter has been snared. (B) The filter has been snared and is being withdrawn into the sheath. (C) The completion venogram shows normal flow in the IVC.

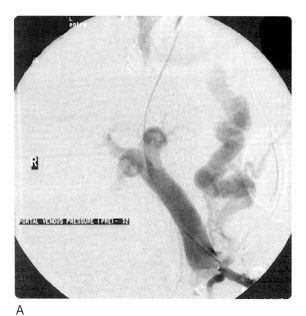

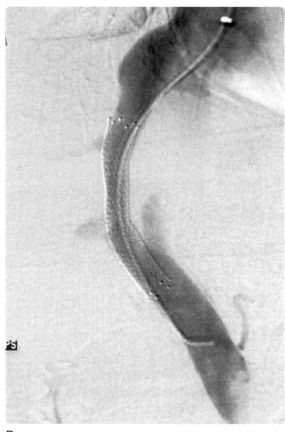

A   B

Fig. 9.12 TIPS procedure (A) Identification of the portal vein. A large gastro-oesophageal varix is visible. (B) The stent is in position and the varix has been decompressed.

Absolute contraindications to TIPS include:

- severe liver failure
- severe or uncontrolled encephalopathy
- congestive heart failure.

Relative contraindications to the procedure include:

- Biliary obstruction
- venous thrombosis (portal, hepatic, IVC)
- hepatic tumour
- polycystic liver disease.

In experienced hands technical success and reduction in portosystemic gradient can be achieved in approximately 95%. Bleeding will be controlled in 80–95% but will recur in 18–30%. There is a procedural mortality of only 1–3% but the 30-day mortality is significantly higher at 3–42%. Outcome and mortality is largely dependant on the patient's pre-procedure condition and can be predicted by Child–Pugh and APACHE II scores. Complications related to the procedure include haemorrhage due to transcapsular or extrahepatic portal vein puncture, and arterial or biliary injury. Other complications such as cardiovascular decompensation, liver failure and hepatic encephalopathy relate to the shunt created.

The main current limitation of this technique is the high incidence of shunt dysfunction, in the form of stenosis or occlusion, occurring in 35–75% at 1 year. This may result in recurrent portal hypertension with associated rebleeding or reaccumulation of ascites. A programme of surveillance using ultrasound, venography and manometry is hence necessary to detect dysfunction before it becomes clinically significant. TIPS revision in the form of balloon dilatation or re-stenting is a simple and safe procedure that will allow a 1-year primary assisted patency rate of about 85%. Most restenoses are due to pseudointimal hyperplasia, thought to be due to bile leaking from the intrahepatic track into the stent. Preliminary results for covered stents, which prevent this, are very promising and will hopefully lead to a more durable procedure in the future.

Further reading

Becker GJ, Katzen BT, Dake MD. Noncoronary angioplasty. Radiology 1989; 170:921–40

Bosch JL, Hunink MG. Meta-analysis of results of percutaneous transluminal angioplasty and stent placement for aortoiliac occlusive disease. Radiology 1997; 204:87–96

Camma C, Schepis F, Orlando A et al. Transarterial chemoembolisation for unresectable hepatocellular carcinoma: meta-analysis of randomized controlled trials. Radiology 2002; 224:47–54

Charboneau JW, Reading CL, Welch TJ. CT and sonographically guided needle biopsy: current techniques and new innovations. AJR 1990; 154:1–10

Cox MR, Davies RP, Bowyer RC, Toouli J. Percutaneous cystgastrostomy for treatment of pancreatic pseudocysts. Aust NZ J Surg 1993; 63:693–8

Curley SA, Izzo F, Delrio P et al. Radiofrequency ablation of unresectable primary and metastatic hepatic malignancies: results in 123 patients. Ann Surg 1999; 230:1–8

Cwikiel W, Tramberg KG, Cwikiel M et al. Malignant dysphagia: palliation with oesophageal stents long-term results in 100 patients. Radiology 1998; 207:513–8

De Baere T, Chapot R, Kuoch V et al. Percutaneous gastrostomy with fluoroscopic guidance: single center experience in 500 consecutive cancer patients. Radiology 1999; 210:651–4

De Gregorio MA, Mainar A, Tejero E et al. Acute colorectal obstruction: stent placement for palliative treatment results of a multicentre study. Radiology 1998; 209:117–20

Dondelinger RF, Kurdziel JC, Gathy C. Percutaneous treatment of pyogenic liver abscess: a critical analysis of results. Cardiovasc Intervent Radiol 1990; 13:174–82

Farrell TA, Hicks ME. A review of radiologically guided percutaneous nephrostomies in 303 patients. J Vasc Interv Radiol 1997; 8:769–74

Ferral H. Transjugular intrahepatic portosystemic shunts (TIPS). In: Savader S, Trerotola K (eds) Venous interventional radiology. Thieme Medical Publishers, New York, 2000

Greenberg RK, Lawrence-Brown M, Bhandari G et al. An update of the Zenith endovascular graft for abdominal aortic aneurysms: initial implantation and mid-term follow-up data. J Vasc Surg 2001; 33:S157–64

Hastings GS. Angiographic localization and transcatheter treatment of gastrointestinal bleeding. Radiographics 2000; 20:1160–8

Henry M, Amor M, Henry I, et al. Stents in the treatment of renal artery stenosis: longterm follow up. J Endovasc Surg 1999; 6:42–51

Kandarpa K, Aruny JE. Handbook of interventional radiologic procedures. Lippincott Williams and Wilkins, Philadelphia, 2002

Laberge JM, Gordon RL, Kerlan RK, Wilson MW. Interventional radiology essentials. Lippincott Williams and Wilkins, Philadelphia, 2000

Lambiase RE, Deyoe L, Cronan JJ, Dorfman GS. Percutaneous drainage of 335 consecutive abscesses: results of primary drainage with 1-year follow up. Radiology 1992; 184:167–79

Lee MJ, Rattner DW, Legemate DA et al. Acute complicated pancreatitis: redefining the role of interventional radiology. Radiology 1992; 183:171–4

Llovet JM, Real MI, Montana X et al: Barcelona Liver Cancer Group. Arterial embolisation or chemoembolisation versus symptomatic treatment in patients with unresectable hepatocellular carcinoma: a randomised controlled trial. Lancet 2002; 359:1734–42

Mainar A, De Gregorio MA, Tejero E et al. Acute colorectal obstruction: treatment with self-expandable metallic stents before scheduled surgery: results of a multicentre study. Radiology 1999; 210:65–9

Morgan R, Adam A. Use of metallic stents and balloons in the esophagus and gastrointestinal tract. J Vasc Inter Radiol 2001; 12:283–97

Muradin GSR, Bosch JL, Stijnen T, Hunink MG. Balloon dilatation and stent implantation for femoropopliteal arterial disease: meta-analysis. Radiology 2001; 221:137–45

Parkinson R, Gandhi M, Harper J, Archibald C. Establishing an ultrasound guided peripherally inserted central catheter (PICC) insertion service. Clin Radiol 1998; 53;33–6

Ray CE. Central venous access. Lippincott Williams and Wilkins, Philadelphia, 2001

Rossi P, Bezzi M, Rossi M et al. Metallic stents in malignant biliary obstruction: results of a multicentre European study of 240 patients. J Vasc Interv Radiol 1994; 5:279–85

Tetteroo E, van der Graaf, Bosch JL et al. Randomised comparison of primary stent placement versus primary angioplasty followed by selective stent placement in patients with iliac artery occlusive disease. Dutch Iliac Stent Trial Study Group. Lancet 1998; 351:1153–9

van den Ven PJ, Kaatee R, Beutler JJ et al. Arterial stenting and balloon angioplasty in ostial atherosclerotic renovascular disease: a randomized trial. Lancet 1999; 353:282–6

Watkinson A, Adam A. Interventional radiology: a practical guide. Radcliffe Medical Press, Oxford, 1996

Welch TJ, Sheedy PF, Johnson CM, Stephens DH. CT guided biopsy: prospective analysis of 1000 procedures. Radiology 1989; 171:493–6

Wilson SE, Golf GL, Cross AP. Percutaneous transluminal angioplasty versus operation for peripheral arteriosclerosis: report of a prospective randomised trial in a selected group of patients. J Vasc Surg 1989; 9:1–9

Wollman B, D'Agostino HB, Walus-Wigle JR et al. Radiologic, endoscopic and surgical gastrostomy: an institutional review and meta-analysis of the literature. Radiology 1995; 197:699–704

Section two

Specific clinical perspectives

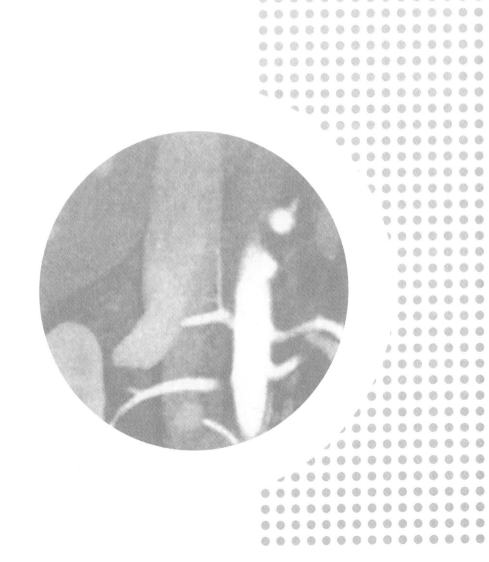

Radiology in the acute abdomen

10

P.G. Devitt, A. Aly, M. Thomas

Background

Although the management of the acute abdomen is still largely determined by clinical acumen, radiological assessment has a rapidly increasing influence. Reasons for this include community expectations, the rise of defensive medicine and the dramatic changes

in radiological technology. As few clinicians would now rely solely on their clinical judgement for the assessment of an intra-cranial lesion or a cardiac murmur, so imaging influences the management of a patient with an acute abdominal problem.

Although the emphasis remains with clinical judgement, imaging now has an important and often specific role to play. This starts with the diagnostic use of ultrasound for a patient on a trolley in the emergency room, through to CT scanning for a variety of acute abdominal conditions and on to therapeutic aspects such as TIPS, and embolisation.

Any radiological intervention will depend on the condition of the patient and the likely underlying problem. The haemodynamically unstable patient with a suspected ruptured aortic aneurysm will be taken straight to the operating room without any imaging studies. Likewise, a stable patient with clear-cut localising signs (e.g. right iliac fossa peritonitis) should not require any imaging as part of the diagnostic process. The patient with few physical signs or concurrent problems (e.g. head injury) is more difficult to assess. Most stable patients with an acute abdominal problem will undergo one or more imaging studies. The type of study will depend on the likely diagnosis.

This chapter will focus on the role of imaging in management whilst the patient is still based in the emergency department and concern problems based on acute abdominal pain. The term 'acute abdomen' is frequently used to encompass other conditions of which abdominal pain may be a component. The radiological aspects of these conditions are described in the appropriate chapters:

- nausea, vomiting (see Chapter 11)
- sudden change in bowel habit (see Chapter 13)
- sepsis, rigors and collapse (see Chapter 12)
- gastrointestinal haemorrhage (see Chapter 15)
- abdominal trauma (see Chapter 25).

RADIOLOGICAL INVESTIGATIONS

The plain abdominal film

The main purpose of the plain radiograph in the management of a patient with an acute abdominal problem is to assess the intestinal gas patterns in cases of suspected intestinal obstruction and to look for free intraperitoneal gas if perforation is suspected (see Box 10.1).

Ultrasound

Ultrasound has a number of specific roles in the management of the acute abdomen:

- to study the texture and integrity of solid organs (liver, spleen, kidneys)
- to look for free fluid (usually blood)
- alterations to blood vessels (abdominal aortic aneurysm, thrombosed portal vein)
- assessment of the biliary tree (dilatation, stones)
- the identification of inflamed structures (appendix, gall bladder, fallopian tubes).

The usefulness of this technique may be limited by:

- overlying gas-filled structures
- obesity
- inability of the patient to tolerate the procedure (pain)
- operator experience.

WHAT TO LOOK FOR Box 10.1

on the plain abdominal film

- Intraluminal gas distribution, volume and pattern
- Extraluminal gas
- Evidence of free fluid
- Unusual sites of calcification
- Foreign bodies

Computed tomography scanning

CT is increasingly used in the assessment of patients with acute abdominal problems, and can improve diagnostic accuracy of many conditions. Early use of CT may identify unforeseen serious abdominal problems and reduce the length of hospital stay. Whether more aggressive use of this investigative tool will have any impact on inpatient mortality is still unknown. The CT scan is used to provide information on the following:

- Solid organs: liver and spleen
- Gastrointestinal tract:
  - obstruction (e.g. gastric outlet)
  - perforation (e.g. peptic ulcer disease)
  - inflammation (e.g. diverticulitis)
  - ischaemia
- Retroperitoneal structures:
  - the renal tract and calculus disease
  - pancreas (inflammation, infarction, abscess, pseudocyst)
  - aorta (aneurysm, dissection, leak)
- The abdominal wall:
  - masses or defects
  - hernias
  - diaphragmatic defects (trauma)
- Miscellaneous:
  - omental infarction
  - epiploic appendagitis
  - gall bladder calculi or inflammation
  - free fluid
  - portal venous gas
  - free gas.

In addition to the diagnostic role of CT, it may also have a therapeutic place in the management of acute problems, e.g. aspiration of fluid collections.

Contrast studies

The pure contrast study has a limited role to play in the management of patients with acute abdominal problems (see Chapter 3). In renal tract disease, the intravenous pyelogram has given way to the spiral CT scan and few digestive tract problems require contrast alone for their elucidation. Where contrast is used, it is often in conjunction with a CT scan. Contrast studies may be used in the following circumstances:

- suspected ureteric obstruction (stone disease)
- unresolved small bowel obstruction

- distal large bowel obstruction (tumour, volvulus)
- angiographic intervention to control haemorrhage
- decompression of the biliary tree (ERCP, PTHC).

Isotope studies

Isotope investigations have a specific place in the management of certain abdominal emergencies. In some circumstances where there has been a negative ultrasound examination of a patient with right upper quadrant pain and suspected acute cholecystitis, a biliary scan will be undertaken to help determine what line of treatment should be followed (see Chapter 12).

Red cell scanning is used to help determine the site of bleeding when surgery is contemplated for what is thought to be uncontrolled haemorrhage arising from the lower part of the digestive tract (see Chapter 15).

Labelled white cell scans have been used to improve the diagnostic accuracy in suspected appendicitis where the clinical findings are equivocal.

THE CLINICAL PROBLEMS

Acute appendicitis

Measurable outcomes in acute appendicitis include the rates of negative appendicectomy and perforation and the overall length of stay. If ultrasound and CT scan are to be shown to be useful diagnostic tools, then they must have an impact on these outcomes. Arguments in favour of routine imaging include the observation that, even where there is a high clinical probability of appendicitis, imaging will reduce the negative appendicectomy rate and reduce the incidence of perforation. This is not a universally held view and there are many reports in the literature that do not show any improvements in these outcomes with imaging.

Figures of around 90% are reported for the sensitivity and specificity of CT and ultrasound in diagnosing appendicitis, but these are no different from those achieved by clinical diagnosis (Fig. 10.1). Similarly, the outcomes of adverse events (including negative appendicectomy) or length of hospital stay is not altered by imaging. The use of ultrasound in the diagnosis of acute appendicitis is discussed further in Chapter 5.

CT scanning subjects the patient to a substantial dose of radiation, may delay treatment and can only

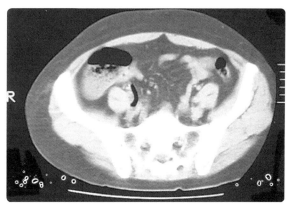

Fig. 10.1 This CT scan shows an inflammatory mass at the base of the appendix. There is a faecolith present.

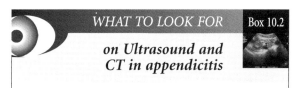

WHAT TO LOOK FOR Box 10.2

on Ultrasound and CT in appendicitis

- Inflammation of the appendix (Fig. 10.1)
- A non-compressible appendix greater than 6 mm diameter (US)
- Periappendicular fluid
- Evidence of abscess formation
- Other pathology that may be mistaken for appendicitis e.g. ruptured ovarian cyst

really be justified if it produces a significantly lower negative appendicectomy rate. Data from the literature is conflicting and imaging is probably best undertaken on a selective basis and reserved for the clinically equivocal cases (Box 10.2).

Scintigraphic scans are time-consuming and difficult to interpret. Where imaging is required, a helical CT scan or ultrasound is easier to perform and interpret.

Intestinal obstruction

The plain radiograph

The only imaging investigation required for the majority of cases of obstruction on initial presentation is the plain abdominal radiograph (see Chapter 2). A supine film will show the characteristic pattern of dilated loops of small bowel. The stretched mucosal folds (valvulae conniventes or plicae circulares) characterise small bowel, with a central distribution and an associated paucity of gas in the large bowel (Fig. 10.2). In such circumstances, any added value to be obtained from an erect film can be disputed and the additional view is probably superfluous. If performed, the erect or lateral decubitus film will show the gas–fluid interfaces in the obstructed loops as fluid levels, which may give a 'step-ladder' appearance. Taken in isolation, the radiological finding of air-fluid levels is of limited significance. The diagnosis of intestinal obstruction is a clinical one, backed up by the appropriate radiological changes.

The large bowel may be dilated because of:

- mechanical obstruction
- toxic megacolon
- adynamic states (pseudo-obstruction, megacolon).

Mechanical large bowel obstruction is most often a complication of malignancy, diverticular disease, volvulus or simple constipation (see Chapter 2).

Large bowel obstruction is characterised by:

- massively dilated loops of bowel with no transluminal mucosal pattern
- a peripheral distribution of the dilated intestine

- isolated dilated segments of bowel (volvulus) (Fig. 10.3)
- loss of gas pattern distal to the obstruction.

Serial plain radiographs may help in determining the likelihood of spontaneous resolution of any obstruction or progression of any toxic process. Progressive distension of small bowel with an absence of gas in the large bowel may encourage surgical intervention and similarly, grossly distended (>14 cm) large bowel in a pseudo-obstruction would suggest the need for decompression (Fig. 10.4).

Computed tomography

CT scanning is used with increasing frequency in the management of intestinal obstruction, particularly small bowel obstruction, and is of probable value where the cause of the obstruction remains obscure. CT has reported sensitivities of over 90% for both

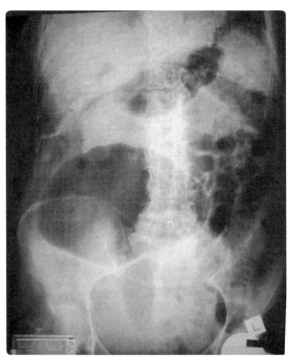

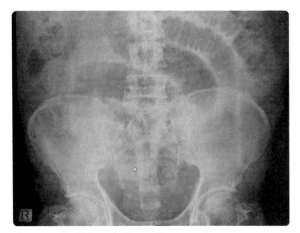

Fig. 10.2 Small bowel obstruction secondary to a stenosing carcinoid tumour of the distal jejunum. Note the plicae circulares on the dilated loops of small bowel.

Fig. 10.3 Caecal volvulus. There is an isolated and dilated segment of intestine in the right iliac fossa, with mild dilatation of the proximal small bowel.

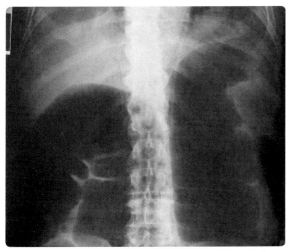

Fig. 10.4 Pseudo-obstruction that developed 1 week after joint replacement surgery. This resolved without the need for any intervention.

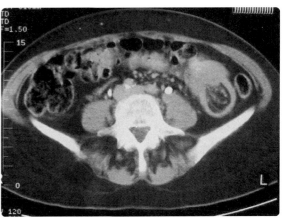

Fig. 10.5 CT slice from a patient with intermittent small bowel obstruction due to intussusception of a deposit of melanoma. The image shows contrast in the small bowel (the intussuscipiens) surrounding the intussusceptum.

the diagnosis of obstruction and the definition of a cause. It should be able to define the level of obstruction and detect complications such as ischaemia, which may alter any proposed conservative plans of management.

In assessing a CT in a case of intestinal obstruction, the presence and level of obstruction should be confirmed. This is best done on a workstation, where the loops of bowel may be more easily followed. Adhesions remain the most common cause of obstruction, and on CT are implied by the absence of any other cause at the site of calibre change, in a patient with an appropriate clinical history. Other causes which may be defined with CT include primary or secondary malignancy, hernia, volvulus and intussusception (Fig. 10.5). Strangulation of a closed loop obstruction may appear as thickening of the bowel wall, with increased or decreased enhancement and possibly intramural gas. Congestion of mesenteric vessels, portal venous gas and ascites may also be present (Box 10.3).

The use of oral contrast in CT for intestinal obstruction is debatable (see Chapter 4). Oral contrast will demonstrate the level and the passage of contrast through an obstruction indicates it is not complete. However, the increased density adjacent to the bowel wall makes assessment of bowel wall enhancement dif-

---

WHAT TO LOOK FOR | Box 10.3

on the CT scan for intestinal obstruction

- Dilated (and fluid-filled) loops of bowel
- Level of calibre change
- Presence of mass lesion (inside or outside the lumen of the bowel)
- Spiralling of mesenteric vessels to suggest a volvulus
- Gas-filled loops of bowel outside the abdominal wall (e.g. inguinal hernia)
- Bowel wall thickening or intramural gas (strangulation)
- Portal venous gas

---

ficult, decreasing the sensitivity of detecting strangulation (Fig. 10.6).

Contrast studies

If an initial plain AXR demonstrates a large bowel obstruction, a water soluble contrast enema may be performed and demonstrate an obstructing carcinoma, volvulus, diverticulitis or pseudo-obstruction

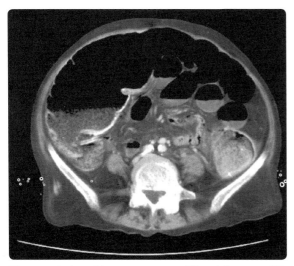

Fig. 10.6 A sigmoid cancer seen as a filling defect on a CT scan. The mass in the sigmoid colon has caused a closed loop obstruction. The caecum is dilated, and there is very little gas in the small bowel.

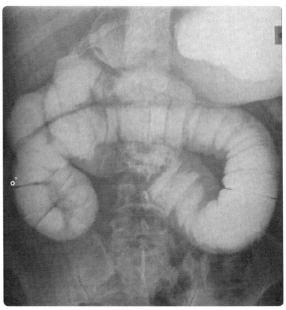

Fig. 10.7 A small bowel contrast study showing a high jejunal obstruction in a patient with a three week history of abdominal pain and vomiting. The cause of the obstruction was a lymphoma.

(see Chapter 3). In the setting of small bowel obstruction contrast studies have a limited role to play in the immediate management, but may be used during the course of a patient's illness, these studies may be used to:

- delineate the level of obstruction (oral or rectal administration) (Fig. 10.7)
- identify the cause of the obstruction
- help overcome partial small bowel obstruction.

The management of obstruction due to adhesions can be difficult. Even after an assessment of the clinical picture and interpretation of serial plain radiographs, in many instances problems remain, particularly in terms of the:

- totality of the obstruction
- stage and progress of the obstruction
- presence of any paralytic ileus.

In such circumstances a contrast study may provide answers as assessed by:

- any dilatation of the bowel
- the passage of contrast through to the caecum
- the length of time contrast takes to traverse the small bowel.

One technique is to use Gastrografin®. Such a study can accurately define complete obstruction and predict the need for surgery. The technique of the contrast study is discussed in detail in Chapter 3.

Peritonitis and perforation

If the patient has local or generalised abdominal signs of peritonitis and perforation, any imaging is likely to be superfluous to the decision-making process. In cases of diagnostic uncertainty a plain film will reveal free gas in 80–85% of cases of perforated peptic ulcer disease. It is less accurate in other important causes of generalised peritonitis such as diverticular perforation. If the patient is unable to sit upright to allow the diaphragms to be imaged, a left lateral decubitus film may reveal any free gas. Free gas on the supine film, as shown by demarcation of an intestinal wall by gas on either side can be subtle and difficult to identify. There are a number of subtle signs of free gas on the plain abdominal film. These are discussed further in Chapter 2.

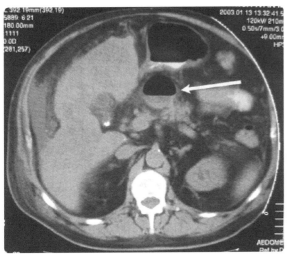

Fig. 10.8 A perforated peptic ulcer with a collection of air and fluid in the lesser sac (arrow).

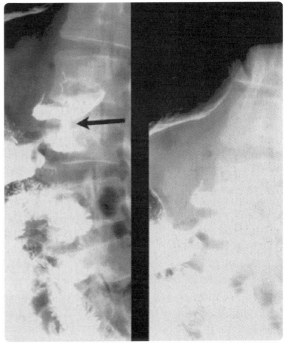

Fig. 10.9 A contained leak from a perforated duodenal ulcer (arrow). A non-operative policy was followed; dictated by the patient's general well-being.

CT scanning may be more useful in the detection of free gas, particularly if localised (e.g. retroperitoneal), but probably adds little to the plain film in terms of clinical decision making (i.e. is there a perforated viscus that requires operative intervention?) (Fig. 10.8).

Contrast studies have a limited role to play in the diagnosis of gut perforation (Fig. 10.9). Whilst a leak may be shown, the decision on surgical intervention is more often based on the patient's general condition and the abdominal physical signs.

Pneumoperitoneum

Although pneumoperitoneum is strictly speaking a radiological diagnosis, the underlying causes usually reflect an acute abdominal problem and hence its inclusion under a separate heading in this chapter.

The relevance of gas within the peritoneal cavity needs to be interpreted within the clinical setting. While spontaneous pneumoperitoneum usually indicates an acute abdominal surgical condition, free intraperitoneal gas can be found in association with a variety of benign conditions or as a result of air tracking from the chest. Common causes of pneumoperitoneum to consider include:

- perforated viscus:
  - duodenal or gastric ulcer
  - diverticula

- iatrogenic:
  - postoperative
- postintubation of the digestive tract:
  - gastrostomy
  - ERCP
  - colonoscopy
  - gynaecological manipulation with air via fallopian tube.

Less common causes of a pneumoperitoneum that should be considered include:

- penetrating trauma or rupture of a hemidiaphragm
- fallopian tube air entry following douching, intercourse or water skiing
- respiratory, e.g. mechanical ventilation, chronic obstructive pulmonary disease, pneumothorax
- tracheal intubation, head and neck surgery or trauma
- secondary to pneumatosis intestinalis.

141

Postoperatively, air should resolve within 3–7 days but can persist for several weeks. Carbon dioxide from laparoscopic procedures is absorbed rapidly, most disappearing within hours of the procedure. Of concern in the postoperative setting is a large or increasing volume of free gas.

The detection of free gas following perforation is dependent on site of perforation, visceral contents (more free gas is seen after colonic perforations than small bowel) and degree of localisation. Free gas is an uncommon radiological finding in perforated diverticulitis or appendicitis (Fig. 10.10), but can be identified in most cases of perforated peptic ulcer disease.

The detection of free gas on the plain abdominal radiograph has been described in Chapter 2, and only the important points will be repeated here. Large volumes of free gas within the peritoneal cavity are seen on the supine film; outlining the falciform ligament, collecting like a football centrally or outlining both sides of the bowel wall (Rigler's sign). Smaller quantities of gas are best identified on an erect chest radiograph.

While the plain AXR is often the initial investigation in suspected pneumoperitoneum, in practice the CT scan is the preferred investigation for the detection of small volumes of gas in unusual sites within the abdominal cavity. CT is extremely sensitive, especially if the images are viewed on lung window settings, and will usually detect most cases of gas outside the lumen of the digestive tract. This will include gas in the following sites:

- intraperitoneal greater and lesser sac (Fig. 10.11)
- retroperitoneum (Fig. 10.12)
- gas within or around other structures:
  - abscess (Fig. 10.13)
  - urinary bladder (Fig. 10.14)
  - gall bladder (emphysematous cholecystitis) (Fig. 10.15)
  - portal venous and biliary systems
  - bowel wall
  - mesentery.

Bowel ischaemia

Ischaemia and infarction may involve the small or large bowel and range in severity from mild superficial

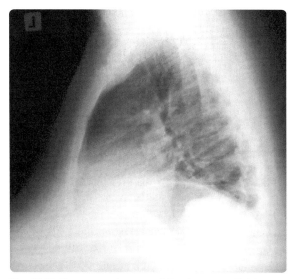

Fig. 10.10 Pneumoperitoneum following appendicitis. The silhouette of the spleen is clearly visible. The X-ray was taken 4 days post-partum, when it had still not been appreciated that the trigger for the patient going into premature labour was appendicitis.

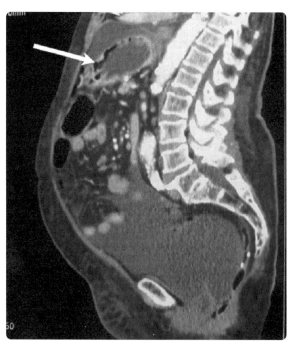

Fig. 10.11 Free intraperitoneal gas in a patient with a perforated duodenal ulcer. The free gas can be seen clearly around the liver (arrow). Free fluid is also visible in the pelvis.

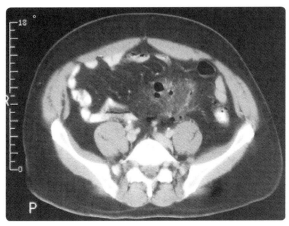

Fig. 10.12 Air in the mesentery of the sigmoid colon and adjacent retroperitoneal tissues in a patient with acute diverticulitis.

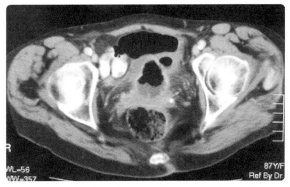

Fig. 10.14 Air in the urinary bladder in a patient with a colovesical fistula secondary to diverticulitis. There is also a large air-filled abscess cavity anterior to the bladder.

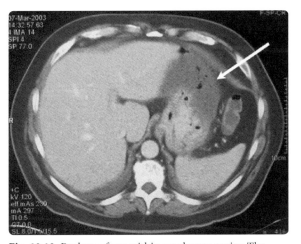

Fig. 10.13 Pockets of gas within an abscess cavity. The scan shows a localised collection of fluid (arrow) over the anterior aspect of the stomach that developed secondary to a perforated duodenal ulcer.

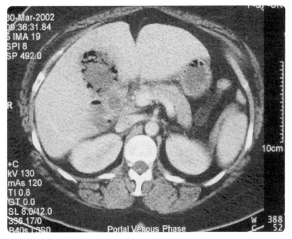

Fig. 10.15 Emphysematous cholecystitis. Gas in the wall of the gall bladder in a patient with acute cholecystitis.

partial ischaemia (often self limiting), to transmural infarction with a high mortality rate. Intestinal ischaemia has a variety of clinical and imaging presentations, which can make it a diagnostic challenge. The condition may be first suspected on the plain abdominal radiograph, with thickened and separated loops of bowel (Fig. 10.16). However, it is not uncommon for the plain AXR to appear normal, even in the presence of severe ischaemia. In more advanced cases where the ischaemic process has led to mucosal necrosis, air may

be visible in the bowel wall, mesenteric or portal veins (see Chapter 2).

The advent of multislice CT has seen an improvement in the radiological assessment of this condition, with the ability to perform CT angiography as required.

Acute bowel ischaemia can be due to occlusion of the arteries or veins, or non-occlusive reduction in intestinal perfusion. The most common cause is acute occlusion of the mesenteric artery due to thrombosis or embolism. The appearances on CT consist of abnormal thickening, attenuation and enhancement of the bowel wall, pneumatosis and portal venous gas, and demonstration of occlusion of vessels (Box 10.4). The

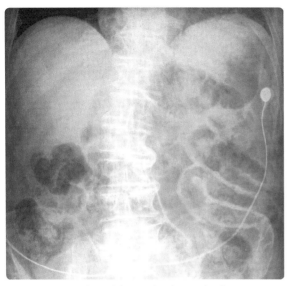

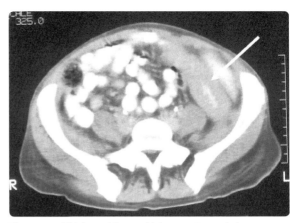

Fig. 10.17 Thickened loop of jejunum (arrow) due to ischaemia.

Fig. 10.16 The plain abdominal radiograph of a 78-year-old man with intestinal ischaemia. The film shows thickened loops of small bowel.

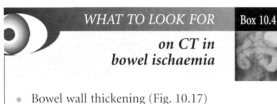

WHAT TO LOOK FOR **Box 10.4**

on CT in bowel ischaemia

- Bowel wall thickening (Fig. 10.17)
- Increased enhancement of bowel wall
- Gas in bowel wall, IMV/SMV, portal veins
- Thrombus in SMA/SMV
- Adjacent stranding and free fluid

most common finding is bowel wall thickening, which may be due to oedema, haemorrhage and/or super-added infection. Oedema also leads to decreased attenuation of the bowel wall, whereas haemorrhagic infarction may cause increased attenuation. Hyperaemia and hyperperfusion will produce increased contrast enhancement, which is best demonstrated if water has been used as the oral contrast agent. Intramural gas may be seen and followed into the mesenteric veins and portal venous system. Stranding of the adjacent fat and the presence of free fluid are supporting, although non-specific, findings.

Biliary disorders

Biliary-related problems that present acutely include:

- biliary colic
- acute cholecystitis
- cholangitis
- acute pancreatitis
- gallstone ileus.

Acute cholecystitis and biliary colic are common and are responsible for some 15% of all admissions to hospital with acute abdominal pain. The radiological aspects of management are covered in detail in Chapter 12. The main points include:

- Clinical suspicion of a gallstone-related problem as the cause of a patient's acute abdominal illness is usually rapidly confirmed by the ultrasonographic detection of stones in the gall bladder.
- The plain radiograph is of limited value in the management of biliary-related illnesses: few gallstones are radio-opaque and the preoperative diagnosis of gallstone ileus (gas in the biliary tree and radio-opaque stones in the digestive tract) is uncommon and usually fortuitous.
- ERCP is the preferred method of decompression of the common bile duct in a patient with cholangitis.
- Early ERCP may be advantageous in the management of severe, gallstone-related pancreatitis.

Acute pancreatitis

Imaging is of limited initial diagnostic value in acute pancreatitis. However, in cases where there is concern over the severity of the illness (made on clinical and biochemical assessment), CT scanning will provide information on the appearance of the organ and any likely complications (see Chapter 16). The CT findings to look for include:

- glandular enlargement
- stranding in the peri-pancreatic tissues
- changes within the pancreas (haemorrhage, necrosis, abscess formation)
- focal fluid collections.

Ureteric colic

The advent of spiral CT scanning has brought another dynamic into the method of investigation of stone disease affecting the renal tract (see Chapter 18). Whereas an intravenous urogram is time-consuming, invasive and subjects the patient to risks of allergic reaction to contrast material, the spiral CT scan can be performed without contrast and rapidly scans the whole renal tract. Intravenous urography and non-contrast CT scanning have a similar sensitivity and specificity for stone disease. Arguments have been made for early spiral CT scanning in suspected ureteric colic in terms of earlier discharge and cost savings, but this must be balanced against the higher radiation doses with CT and need for other investigations at some later stage in the management. Although CT scanning might represent time and cost saving in emergency departments, the overall benefit compared with conventional urography is not so clear.

Non-contrast CT is sensitive and can detect stones down to 5 mm diameter (Fig. 10.18). Even if the stone is not visible the scan may detect the dilated ureter proximal to the site of obstruction. Information to be sought from the CT scan includes:

- presence of calculi (pelvicalyces, ureter, bladder)
- evidence of obstruction (dilated ureters or pelvicalyceal systems)
- detection of extraurinary abnormalities that might mimic ureteric colic.

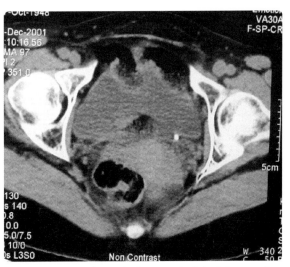

Fig. 10.18 A calculus at the lower end of the left ureter in a patient with acute left sided abdominal pain.

Diverticulitis

Acute diverticulitis is a clinical diagnosis. Early imaging may be undertaken to look for evidence of free perforation, but a visible pneumoperitoneum is not always evident on the plain abdominal radiograph. Immediate imaging in the emergency room is usually superfluous as management decisions will have been made on the basis of the clinical picture (i.e. does the patient have the physical signs that warrant surgical intervention?).

More useful is the CT scan, which with a greater than 90% sensitivity, is much more valuable than barium enema in the assessment of acute diverticulitis, particularly in the detection of pericolonic complications. A CT scan is performed with increasing frequency in the early assessment of acute diverticulitis (see Chapter 13). It may show:

- the presence of diverticula
- thickening of the wall of the colon
- an inflammatory mass (phlegmon)
- pericolic fat stranding (inflammatory streaking)
- free fluid
- gas pockets in adjacent tissues (mesentery, retroperitoneum)
- abscess formation.

A spiral CT scan with intravenous contrast may reveal characteristic rim enhancement of an abscess cavity.

The finding on CT scanning of abscess formation or extracolonic gas may be a predictor of failure of medical treatment of diverticulitis (see Fig. 10.12). Arguments in favour of early, routine CT scanning of all patients with acute diverticulitis include a more exact diagnosis, an earlier identification of any complications and the possibility of reducing length of hospital stay.

Trauma

Most patients who are haemodynamically unstable or who have penetrating abdominal injuries will go straight to the operating room without waiting for the niceties of abdominal investigation. Traditionally, otherwise stable patients who had sustained blunt abdominal trauma and who had a depressed level of consciousness were assessed by diagnostic peritoneal lavage (DPL). Many emergency departments are now equipped with mobile ultrasound equipment to help in assessment after the secondary survey (see Chapter 25). In such centres DPL is being replaced by a focussed assessment with ultrasonography for trauma (FAST) or CT scan. Sonography appears to be highly specific in its detection of haemoperitoneum and damage to solid organs in blunt trauma, but lacks the sensitivity of the CT scan. FAST examinations are likely to miss up to 50% of serious intra-abdominal injuries.

If the haemodynamically stable patient is thought to have blunt abdominal injury, a CT scan is the investigation of choice (Fig. 10.19; Box 10.5).

Splenic injury is graded radiologically according to the severity of the injury and the areas of the spleen affected (Fig. 10.20) (see Chapter 25). Similar criteria exist for the assessment of blunt liver injury and the

likelihood of success of non-operative management. Predictors of failure include capsular tears and pooling of contrast on CT scanning. Periportal tracking is no longer thought to be such a predictor.

If a vascular injury is suspected, then CT angiography is likely to provide as much essential information as an angiogram alone.

Gynaecological emergencies

Gynaecological problems that may present with acute abdominal pain and/or collapse include:

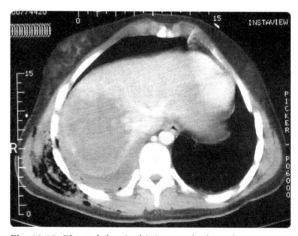

Fig. 10.19 Blunt abdominal injury and a large haematoma within the right lobe of the liver. This was managed conservatively. The patient also has a haemoperitoneum.

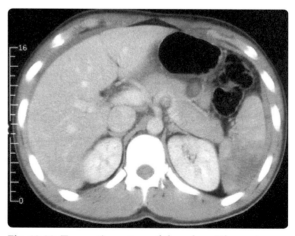

Fig. 10.20 Traumatic rupture of the spleen. The rupture involves the hilum of the spleen (grade III injury).

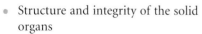

WHAT TO LOOK FOR | Box 10.5

on the trauma CT scan

- Structure and integrity of the solid organs
- Free intraperitoneal gas or fluid
- Damage to the abdominal wall, including the diaphragm

- ruptured ectopic pregnancy
- salpingitis
- torsion or rupture of an ovarian cyst.

Ultrasound examination in the emergency department will detect over 95% of all suspected ectopic pregnancies. The role of pelvic ultrasound in the female is discussed in Chapter 5.

Gynaecological conditions often masquerade as acute appendicitis and imaging may be undertaken to try and establish a diagnosis (Box 10.6). In the determination of either appendicitis or an acute gynaecological condition, CT scanning has positive and negative predictive values greater than 94%, but should not be performed if the patient may be pregnant.

Acute vascular problems

The vascular problems that present with acute abdominal pain can be categorised as follows:

- aneuryms:
  - leaking
  - frank rupture
  - dissection
- mesenteric ischaemia (see above)
- abdominal wall/ retroperitoneal haematoma.

Dissecting and leaking aortic aneurysms frequently mimic other more common problems and can present a diagnostic dilemma, particularly in the haemodynamically stable patient. About 10% of ruptured abdominal aortic aneurysms will be mistaken on presentation for an acute urological problem. The patient who presents with abdominal and/or back pain with haemodynamic instability should go straight to the operating room. Nearly half of all patients with a rupture of an aortic aneurysm die within an hour of

rupture and thus time is of the essence. Any delay for imaging is likely to prove fatal. In the stable patient the likely scenario will involve a bedside ultrasound examination to look for an aneurysm. Should one be found, further imaging will be undertaken (see Chapter 21).

With rapid improvements in image quality and a corresponding decrease in image acquisition time, CT scan is the investigation of choice for the evaluation of aortic aneurysms (Fig. 10.21) (Box 10.7). The proximal and distal extent of the aneurysm can be defined, and 3D reconstruction will allow vessels to be seen

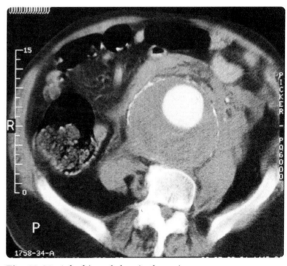

Fig. 10.21 A leaking abdominal aortic aneurysm.

WHAT TO LOOK FOR Box 10.6

on gynaecological ultrasound

- Free fluid in the pelvis
- The fallopian tubes (engorgement or a mass)
- The ovaries (texture and cyst formation)
- An empty uterus

WHAT TO LOOK FOR Box 10.7

on the CT scan aortic rupture

- Disruption of the calcium ring within the wall of the aorta
- Disruption of the aortic margins
- Retroperitoneal haematoma
- Mass lesions in the psoas muscles
- Loss of normal tissue planes
- Displacement of the kidneys
- Fluid collections

from any projection. If 3D angiographic reconstruction of the images is contemplated, oral contrast should be avoided.

SUMMARY

In summary, current imaging technology has allowed a more precise and immediate diagnosis to be made in many emergency room cases. Although it might not influence the decision making when prompt surgical intervention is required, the information obtained from spiral CT scan and ultrasound has undoubtedly helped with many early management decisions and made the surgeon's task much easier. These imaging modalities allow greater emphasis to be placed on non-operative management of the acute abdomen.

Further reading

Albrecht RM, Schermer CR, Morris A. Nonoperative management of blunt splenic injuries: factors influencing success in age >55 years. Am Surg 2002; 68:227–30

Assalia A, Schien M, Kopelman D et al. Therapeutic effect of oral gastrografin in adhesive partial small bowel obstruction: a prospective randomised trial. Surgery 1994; 115:433–7

Biondi S, Pares D, Mora L et al. Randomized clinical study of Gastrografin administration in patients with adhesive small bowel obstruction. Br J Surg 2003; 90;542–6

Brengman ML, Otchy DP. Timing of computed tomography in acute diverticulitis. Dis Colon Rectum 1998; 41:1023–8

Chen S, Chang K, Lee P et al. Oral urografin in postoperative small bowel obstruction. World J Surg 1999; 23:1051–4

Cho KC, Baker SR. Extraluminal air. Diagnosis and significance. Radiol Clin North Am 1994; 32:829–44

Douglas CD, MacPherson NE, Davidson PM, Gani JS. Randomised controlled trial of ultrasonography in diagnosis of acute appendicitis. BMJ 2000; 321:919–22

Durston WE, Carl ML, Guerra W et al. Ultrasound availability in the evaluation of ectopic pregnancy in the ED: comparison of quality and cost-effectiveness with different approaches. Am J Emerg Med 2000; 18:408–17

Field S, Guy PJ, Scourfield AE. The erect abdominal radiograph in the acute abdomen: should its routine use be abandoned? Br Med J 1985; 290:1934–6

Ianora AA, Midiri M, Vinci R et al. Abdominal wall hernias: imaging with spiral CT. Eur Radiol 2000; 10:914–19

Joyce WP, Delaney PV, Gorey TF, Fitzpatrick JM. The value of water soluble contrast radiology in the management of acute small bowel obstruction. Ann R Coll Surg Engl 1992; 74:422–5

McDonald GP, Pendarvis DP, Wilmoth R, Daley BJ. Influence of preoperative computed tomography on patients undergoing appendectomy. Am Surg 2001; 67: 017–21

Miller MT, Pasquale MD, Bromberg WJ et al. Not so FAST. J Trauma 2003; 54:52–9

Ng CS, Watson CJE, Palmer CR et al. Evaluation of early abdominopelvic computed tomography in patients with acute abdominal pain of unknown cause: prospective randomised study. BMJ 2002; 325:1387–40

Ochsner MG. Factors of failure for nonoperative management of blunt liver and splenic injuries. World J Surg 2001; 25:1393–6

Patel M, Han SS, Vaux K et al. A protocol of early computed tomography for the detection of stones in patients with renal colic has reduced the time to diagnosis and overall management costs. Aust N Z J Surg 2000; 70:39–42

Patrick DA, Janik JE, Janik JS et al. Increased CT scan utilization does not improve the diagnostic accuracy of appendicitis in children. J Pediatr Surg 2003; 38:659–62

Poletti PA, Kinkel K, Vermeulen B et al. Blunt abdominal trauma: should US be used to detect both free fluid and organ injuries? Radiology 2003; 227:95–103

Rao PM, Feltmate CM, Rhea JT et al. Helical computed tomography in differentiating appendicitis and acute gynaecologic conditions. Obstet Gynecol 1999; 93:417–21

Rekant EM, Gibert CL, Counselman FL. Emergency department time for evaluation of patients discharged with a diagnosis of renal colic: unenhanced helical computed tomography versus intravenous urography. J Emerg Med 2001; 21:371–2

Richards JR, Schleper NH, Woo BD et al. Sonographic assessment of blunt abdominal trauma: a 4-year prospective study. J Clin Ultrasound 2002; 30:59–67

Starnes S, Klein P, Magagna L, Pomerantz R. Computed tomographic grading is useful in the selection of patients for nonoperative management of blunt injury to the spleen. Am Surg 1998; 64:743–8

Urban BA, Fishman EK. Tailored helical CT evaluation of acute abdomen. Radiographics 2000; 20:725–49

Velmahos GC, Chan LS, Kamel E et al. Nonoperative management of splenic injuries: have we gone too far? Arch Surg 2000; 135:679–81

Weyant MJ, Eachempati SR, Maluccio MA et al. The use of computed tomography for the diagnosis of acute appendicitis in children does not influence the overall rate of negative appendectomy or perforation. Surg Infect 2001; 2:19–23

Williams N, Everson NW. Radiological confirmation of intraperitoneal free gas. Ann R Coll Surg Engl 1997; 79:8–12

Worster A, Haines T. Does replacing intravenous pyelography with noncontrast helical computer tomography benefit patients with suspected acute urolithiasis? Can Assoc Radiol J 2002; 53:144–8

Zalcman M, Sy M, Donckier V et al. Helical CT signs in the diagnosis of intestinal ischemia in small-bowel obstruction. Am J Roentgenol 2000; 175:1601–7

Imaging of the upper digestive tract

11

P.G. Devitt

Background

Endoscopy has largely replaced radiological studies in the management of gastro-oesophageal reflux and peptic ulcer disease. Cross-sectional radiology has become an important tool for the assessment and management of patients with oesophageal and gastric malignancy. Endoluminal ultrasound is also gaining wider use in the assessment of locoregional malignant disease. This chapter will discuss each of these imaging modalities and their application to surgical problems in the upper gastrointestinal tract.

THE RADIOLOGICAL INVESTIGATIONS

Plain radiology

Plain chest or abdominal radiographs are of limited value in the assessment of most patients with upper digestive tract problems. However, they may be useful to detect free gas in the chest or abdominal cavities, or to outline gas-filled structures.

Contrast studies

As a diagnostic modality, contrast studies have been largely superseded by endoscopy, but are still helpful to define anatomy, anatomical variants and the integrity of the upper gastrointestinal structures (see Chapter 3).

Ultrasound

Endoluminal ultrasound is used to stage cancers of the oesophagus and stomach, although it is subject to operator variability (see Chapter 5). It has proved particularly valuable in the T and N staging of oesophageal cancers, early gastric cancers and infiltrative gastric lesions where the overlying mucosa may be normal (e.g. lymphoma, linitus plastica). It is also useful in assessing the response to therapy of both gastric MALT tumours and oesophageal neoplasms treated with neoadjuvant therapy.

Computed tomography

Cross-sectional and reconstructed 3D CT imaging are used to facilitate tumour staging, particularly with regard to the size and extent of the primary tumour and distant spread. The CT is less effective in the assessment of endoluminal disease as it tends to overstate the degree of local tumour invasion. The accuracy of assessment will undoubtedly improve with the advances in technology and use of multidector row CT scanners. Volume-rendering techniques are being developed in an effort to enable simulated CT images to match those obtained by conventional contrast studies or gastroscopy.

Positron emission tomography

Preliminary data suggests that PET scanning is complimentary to CT in the staging of tumours of the oesophagus and stomach, but may not be any more sensitive (see Chapter 8). Little formal evaluation of this radiological tool in tumours of the upper digestive tract has been undertaken. A more important role is likely to be in the assessment of response to chemotherapy and radiotherapy.

THE CLINICAL PROBLEMS

Investigation of dysphagia

An accurate patient history will usually indicate the likely cause for the dysphagia. In most instances the first investigation will be endoscopy. Apart from direct visualisation of the upper digestive tract, any suspicious lesion may be biopsied and therapeutic manoeuvres, such as dilatation, performed. If the history is long-standing and malignancy thought unlikely, a contrast study will often yield more information than an endoscopy. Anatomical detail (hiatus herniation, pharyngeal bars, diverticula, extrinsic vascular compression, rings) is better defined and video studies help

assess motility disturbances. Oesophageal strictures can be well delineated on a contrast study.

These rules are not absolute, but Table 11.1 provides a guide to differentiation of benign and malignant strictures. A peptic stricture associated with severe oesophagitis and ulceration may have an irregular mucosal contour. Likewise, the mass effect of a (benign) leiomyoma may compress the oesophagus and produce irregular narrowing of the lumen.

Salivary gland disease

The surgeon's interest in the salivary glands is confined to:

* tumours (usually affecting the parotid gland)
* calculi (usually within the submandibular gland or duct).

Most salivary gland tumours occur in the parotid gland and at least 70% of these are pleomorphic adenomas. Whereas these tumours tend to be superficial, a precise knowledge of the relationship of tumour to the underlying facial nerve can help formulate management plans. A CT scan will give precise information of any extension through the branches of the nerve and into the so-called deep lobe of the gland (Fig. 11.3).

Salivary gland calculi may be the cause or consequence of chronic sialadenitis and may present acutely with duct obstruction. If they cannot be palpated, submandibular duct calculi can usually be seen on a plain radiograph. Sialography may be performed, looking for filling defects, duct obstruction or duct ectasia, the latter suggestive of chronic glandular tissue destruction.

Table 11.1 Radiological characteristics of benign and malignant strictures	Benign (Fig. 11.1)	Malignant (Fig. 11.2)
	Short (1–2 cm)	Irregular lumen
	Smooth mucosal contour	Shouldered transition from normal to stricture
	Lumen usually central	Lumen may be to one side of the oesophagus (mass effect)
	Tapered transition from normal to narrowed lumen	Associated fissures or fistulae
		Distortion of the normal axis of the oesophagus (mass effect)

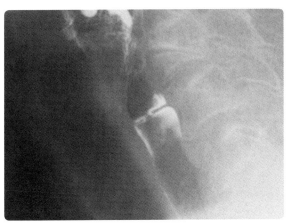

Fig. 11.1 A contrast study showing a postcricoid web. These rare lesions are often better defined radiologically than endoscopically.

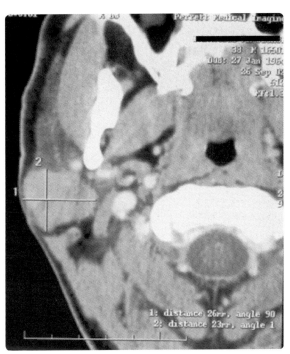

Fig. 11.3 A CT scan of a pleomorphic adenoma of the right parotid gland, showing some extension of the tumour into the deep component of the gland.

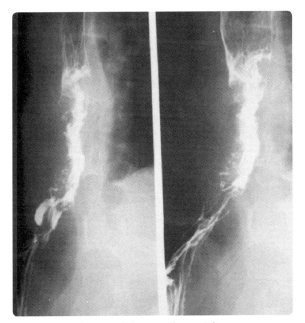

Fig. 11.2 Carcinoma of the oesophagus. The contrast study shows a long stricture with shouldered upper margins, an irregular mucosal outline and fissures.

Gastro-oesophageal reflux and hiatus hernia

Gastro-oesophageal reflux disease *per se* does not require radiological investigation, except where an anatomical defect (e.g. hiatus hernia) is a suspected component of the problem. A paraoesophageal hernia visible (and often first detected) on a plain radiograph of the chest may be better defined with a contrast study (Fig. 11.4). This will show the site of the gastro-oesophageal junction (above or below the diaphragm) and which parts of the stomach are in the hernial sac. Cross-sectional radiology does not provide any greater yield.

Hiatus herniae may be classified as:

- sliding (the gastro-oesophageal junction is above the diaphragm)
- paraoesophageal hernia (the gastro-oesophageal junction is in its correct anatomical position)
- mixed hernia (another component of the stomach, in addition to the gastro-oesophageal junction is above the diaphragm).

Large hiatal defects may allow other abdominal contents to herniate into the chest alongside the stomach. When this does occur, a section of transverse colon is the most common organ to herniate (Fig. 11.5).

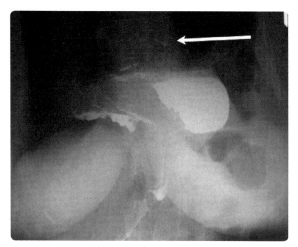

Fig. 11.4 A contrast study of a paraoesophageal hernia, showing the fundus, body and antrum of the stomach (inverted in the chest). The arrow points to where the greater curve of the stomach is uppermost in the hernial sac.

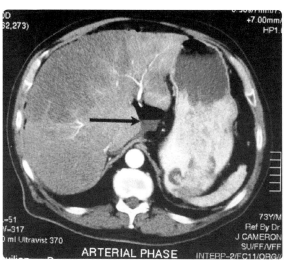

Fig. 11.6 A localised collection of free gas in the lesser sac (from a perforated duodenal ulcer) found during investigation of upper abdominal pain. The arrow points to the collection.

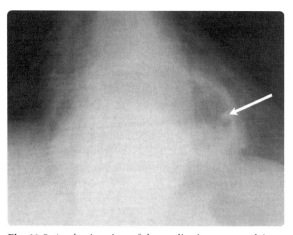

Fig. 11.5 A selective view of the mediastinum on a plain chest radiograph showing a large para-oesophageal hernia behind the cardiac shadow. Within the hernial sac lies a loop of transverse colon – identified by its haustra (arrow).

Peptic ulcer disease

Where endoscopic facilities are available, contrast studies are no longer used to diagnose uncomplicated ulcer disease. Even the diagnosis and management of gastric outlet obstruction and haemorrhage now fall preferentially in the realm of the endoscopist. Radiological intervention is occasionally required to help in the management of complex bleeding ulcers (see Chapter 15). At times, a localised perforation may be identified radiologically, by either CT (finding a pocket of free gas) or leakage of contrast, but such observations are more often serendipitous rather than planned (Fig. 11.6).

Oesophageal malignancy

There has been a dramatic increase in the incidence of adenocarcinoma of the cardia and lower oesophagus over the last two decades. This is probably related to an increase in reflux disease and Barrett's oesophagus. Most of these patients present with dysphagia and are referred for endoscopic assessment. Contrast studies offer little advantage in evaluating the primary lesion, except to delineate fistulae or leaks (Fig. 11.7).

Usually management decisions are only made in the light of radiological staging. Staging is critical given the relatively poor prognosis of oesophageal cancer as treatment often involves considerable morbidity and mortality. Radiological determination of the tumour size (Fig. 11.8) and nodal involvement (Fig. 11.9) may lead to some patients being offered neoadjuvant chemo-radiotherapy for down staging of the disease and others, palliative treatment only.

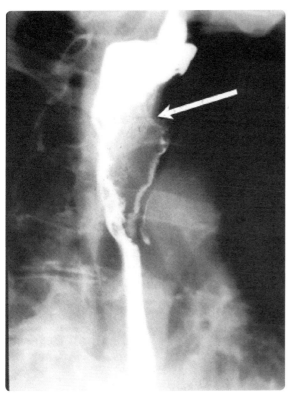

Fig. 11.7 The contrast study has outlined a long malignant stricture in the upper oesophagus, with a tracheo-oesophageal fistula (arrow) and contrast in the upper airways.

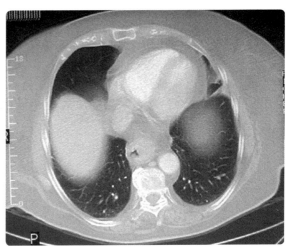

Fig. 11.8 A view of a squamous cell carcinoma of the mid third of the oesophagus. The scan shows that the tumour is occupying at least two-thirds of the cross-sectional area of the lumen. This is a bulky tumour and extends into the surrounding tissues medially.

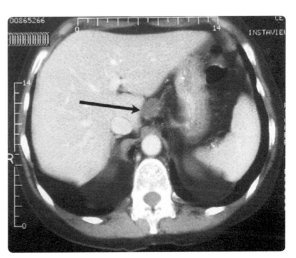

Fig. 11.9 A CT section from a patient with a squamous cell carcinoma of the mid-third of the oesophagus. There is an enlarged node at the coeliac axis (arrow).

Endoluminal ultrasound is used to determine the depth of invasion of the primary tumour and any involvement of adjacent lymph nodes (see Chapter 5). Correlation with T stage will provide an accuracy of over 80%, but the accuracy for N stage may be lower and in the region of 60%. CT scanning provides information about the site and size of the primary tumour, enlargement of regional lymph nodes and the presence of distant disease, but is less accurate than EUS in T and N staging.

As with malignancy at other sites, CT scanning may be used to target FNA biopsy, particularly of areas of suspicion of metastatic deposits from a known oesophageal primary lesion (Box 11.1).

The development of PET scanning has allowed this diagnostic modality to be applied to the staging of oesophageal cancer. Currently, PET is complementary to CT scanning and is most helpful where the CT scan has raised suspicion of nodal or distant disease (see Chapter 8). It has been suggested that PET may be more sensitive than CT in the detection of loco-regional nodal metastases, with sensitivities of 52% reported for PET compared with 15% for CT. PET may be more a more sensitive imaging tool (compared with endoscopic ultrasound and CT) in the

WHAT TO LOOK FOR Box 11.1

on the oesophageal CT scan

- Site and length of the primary tumour
- Degree of luminal involvement
- Local spread of disease
- Presence of distant disease (liver, lungs)

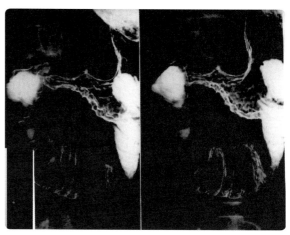

Fig. 11.10 A stenosing carcinoma of the antrum producing a fixed deformity in the distal stomach.

differentiation between responders and non-responders to neoadjuvant chemoradiation prior to oesophageal resection. On the assumption that non-responders have a worse prognosis, imaging with PET may help select out a group of patients for whom surgery would have little benefit.

A logical approach to the staging of oesophageal cancer once the diagnosis has been established is to use endoscopic ultrasound to assess the local tumour, CT to look for distant disease and PET to assess response to any neoadjuvant chemoradiation.

Gastric cancer

Although not common in Western communities, early gastric cancer is one form of gastric malignancy that is amenable to local resection for cure. Endoscopic ultrasonography has a clear role here in the differentiation of mucosal from more advanced disease. The accuracy for tumour staging with EUS is about 85%, but with nodal involvement the sensitivity drops to about 55%. Therefore, careful attention must be paid to histological examination of the resected specimen to ensure that there has been no submucosal invasion, where further and more formal gastric resection would be indicated. Recent reports have advocated the use of 3D computer tomography to help define the vascular anatomy of the stomach and adjacent organs in the preoperative planning of laparoscopic gastric cancer surgery. The images obtained from multi-detector-row helical CT leave minimal motion artefact and provide an accurate topography to facilitate a laparoscopic approach to the tumour.

Contrast studies are used occasionally in the diagnosis of more advanced forms of gastric cancer and can be helpful in showing the extent of the primary tumour, particularly those that produce distortion of

WHAT TO LOOK FOR Box 11.2

on the gastric CT scan

- Site and extent of the primary neoplasm
- Locoregional lymph node involvement
- Hepatic metastases
- Ascites
- Peritoneal and/or omental deposits

the stomach (Fig. 11.10). The role of imaging in gastric cancer is primarily to identify any disease spread, particularly in the abdominal cavity, which would preclude resection. A CT scan is often performed, looking for evidence of secondary disease. Whilst the CT scan can be useful in the detection of metastatic disease in adjacent lymph nodes, omentum and liver, its efficacy in detecting small peritoneal seedlings is low (Box 11.2).

Intraoperative (laparoscopic) ultrasonography

Another approach adopted by clinicians involved in the management of gastric cancer is to limit radiological investigation to ultrasound of the liver looking for hepatic deposits and, provided the liver is clear, to proceed to a laparoscopic assessment before considering resection. When this approach is combined with laparoscopic ultrasonography, up to 23% of patients with potentially resectable lesions may be found to have previously undetected intra-abdominal spread of their disease.

Endoscopic ultrasound

In the staging of gastric cancers, particularly those at the cardia, endoscopic ultrasound provides a more accurate assessment of the T stage than CT and this is most apparent for the T1 and T2 tumours. Similarly, endoscopic ultrasound excels over CT in the staging of locoregional disease.

Gastrointestinal stromal tumours

Previously classified as leiomyomas, these tumours arise from submucosal tissues and are often incidental findings. Small gastrointestinal stromal tumours of the upper gastrointestinal tract are most commonly detected endoscopically, however they produce a characteristic radiological pattern of:

- a soft tissue mass in the stomach, devoid of contrast
- a small 'puddle' of contrast in an apical ulcer (Fig. 11.11).

Endoscopic ultrasound (EUS) is increasingly being used to evaluate gastrointestinal lesions and may be a useful management tool in primary GIST allowing endoscopic biopsy. EUS may demonstrate a hypo-echoic mass contiguous with the normal muscle wall.

Radiological investigation with CT scanning plays an important role in helping determine the site and size of these lesions, since small tumours sited anteriorly may be amenable to laparoscopic resection. Contrast-enhanced CT/MRI provides staging information about intra-abdominal disease and can detect hepatic or other metastases. CT features vary with the size of the lesion. Small GIST (<5 cm) have sharp margins and a homogeneous appearance, often with evidence of intraluminal growth. In contrast, larger lesions (>10 cm) tend to have well-defined but irregular margins with a heterogeneous rim of soft tissue and central fluid attenuation (Fig 11.12) (see Chapter 16). Ascites is an unusual finding, although there may be evidence of metastatic disease, most commonly to the liver or peritoneum. The sensitivity of CT for small peritoneal nodules is low.

Imatinib is a new molecularly targetted treatment for GIST. FDG-PET has proven a useful imaging modality for assessing GIST response to imatinib as PET responses precede CT/MRI response by several weeks.

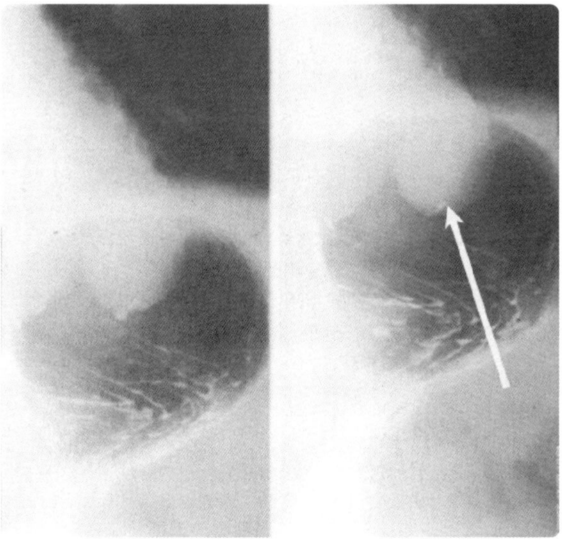

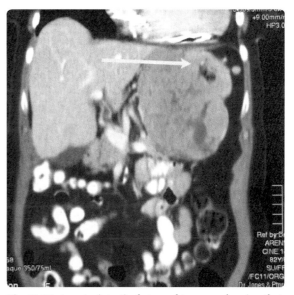

Fig. 11.11 A gastrointestinal stromal tumour seen on contrast study as a soft tissue mass with a small collection of barium in the apical ulcer (arrow).

Fig. 11.12 A gastrointestinal stromal tumour, showing that most of its growth is extramural. In this case the tumour is so large that the stomach has been almost completely compressed (arrow).

Achalasia and other motility disorders

In patients with long-standing dysphagia suggestive of a motility disturbance (contrast) radiology is often more valuable than an endoscopic examination. Whereas the diagnosis of achalasia is confirmed by the manometric findings, the radiological findings can be virtually diagnostic. The characteristic features include:

- tapering of the lower oesophagus, with a narrowed segment extending 3–6 cm around the lower oesophageal sphincter (Fig. 11.13)
- dilatation of the body of the oesophagus.
- An air–fluid level above the trapped contrast material (in advanced achalasia).

Video studies are often performed to illustrate the poor and uncoordinated peristalsis in this region. Other conditions associated with motility disturbances include:

- cricopharyngeal bar (Figs 11.14 and 11.15)
- pharyngeal pouch

- diffuse oesophageal spasm (Fig. 11.16)
- oesophageal diverticula.

These are best shown by contrast study, often combined with video examination. A pharyngeal pouch

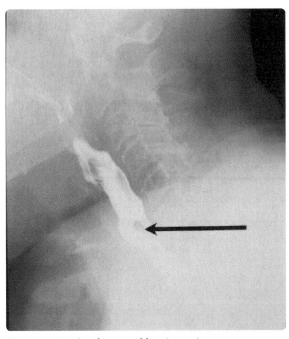

Fig. 11.14 A cricopharyngeal bar (arrow).

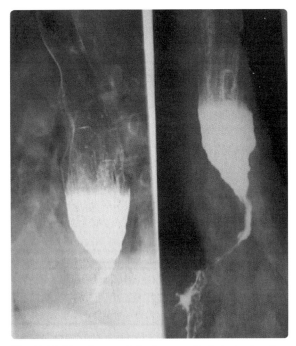

Fig. 11.13 The characteristic changes of achalasia, showing a tapered lower oesophagus and a dilated oesophagus with an air–fluid level.

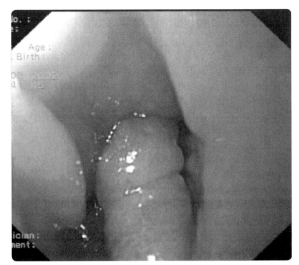

Fig. 11.15 The same cricopharyngeal bar shown endoscopically. The bar is seen as the vertical bulge in the middle of the photograph with the oesophageal lumen to the right.

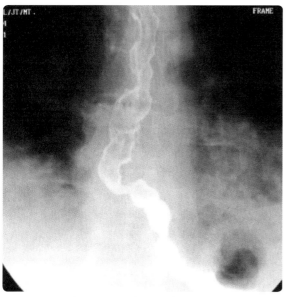

Fig. 11.16 Corkscrew oesophagus. The oesophagogram shows the characteristic areas of narrowing and curling of the oesophagus in an elderly patient with diffuse oesophageal spasm.

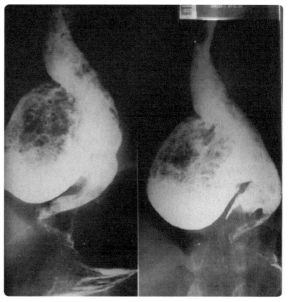

Fig. 11.17 Epiphrenic diverticulum. Apart from the contrast, the diverticulum contains a large volume of food matter.

and associated cricopharyngeal bar are often difficult to assess with the flexible endoscope and given the real risk of perforation, if a pouch is suspected, it is often safer to perform a contrast study as the initial investigation. Contrast studies, frequently combined with fluoroscopic imaging, assess the patient's ability to swallow, the effectiveness of deglutition, and any regurgitation into the trachea.

Other oesophageal diverticula may occur at any site, but are most often found immediately above the diaphragm (epiphrenic diverticulum). These may be large and are best defined with a contrast study (Fig. 11.17). While smaller diverticula tend to be asymptomatic, larger epiphrenic diverticula are usually associated with dysphagia and regurgitation.

Perforation of the oesophagus

Oesophageal perforation is a relatively uncommon condition and is usually the result of instrumentation (endoscopy, dilatation, transoesophageal echography). Whilst any free gas in the mediastinum and subcutaneous tissues may be readily visible on a plain film, a contrast study will be required to show the site of the perforation and the magnitude of the leak (Fig. 11.18)

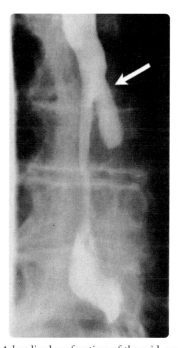

Fig. 11.18 A localised perforation of the mid-oesophagus, sustained after an attempted endoscopic dilatation of a peptic stricture. The arrow indicates the site of extravasation of contrast.

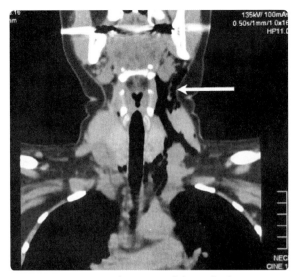

Fig. 11.19 Free gas in the tissues of the neck after an instrumental perforation. The CT scan will show the extent of a leak, but will not define the site of leak. The arrow points to a collection of free gas.

(see Chapter 3). Similarly, a CT scan may show free gas in the adjacent tissues and an associated pleural effusion, but will not show the site of perforation. It is the latter which is the critical piece of information sought by the surgeon planning operative intervention (Fig. 11.19).

Perforation of the oesophagus should not be confused with traumatic pneumomediastinum. Both may present with similar histories of chest pain and similar radiological findings of free air in the mediastinum. The latter is more likely to be a young male who has been weightlifting in the gymnasium or snorting cocaine. A contrast examination will rapidly exclude the former condition.

Further reading

Brucher BL, Weber W, Bauer M et al. Neoadjuvant therapy of esophageal squamous cell carcinoma: response evaluation by positron emission tomography Ann Surg 2001; 223:300–9

Burkill GJ, Badran M, Al-Muderis O et al. Malignant gastrointestinal stromal tumor: distribution, imaging features, and pattern of metastatic spread. Radiology 2003; 226:527–32

Chen CH, Huang HS, Yang CC, Yeh YH. The features of perforated peptic ulcers in conventional computed tomography. Hepatogastroenterology 2001; 41:1393–6

Horton KM, Fishman EK. Current role of CT in imaging of the stomach. Radiographics 2003; 1:75–87

Hulscher JB, Nievenn van Dijkum EJ, de Wit LT et al. Laparoscopy and laparoscopic ultrasonography in staging carcinoma of the gastric cardia. Eur J Surg 2000; 166:862–5

Kienle P, Buhl K, Kuntz C et al. Prospective comparison of endoscopy, endosonography and computed tomography for staging of tumours of the oesophagus and gastric cardia. Digestion 2002; 66:230–6

Kim K, Park SJ, Kim BT, Shim YM. Evaluation of lymph node metastases in squamous cell carcinoma of the esophagus with positron emission tomography. Ann Thorac Surg 2001; 71:290–4

Kim SH, Han JK, Lee KH et al. Computed tomography gastroscopy with volume-rendering technique: correlation with double-contrast barium study and conventional gastroscopy. J Comput Assist Tomogr 2003; 27:140–9

Lagergren J, Bergstrom R, Lindgren A, Nyren O. Symptomatic gastroesophageal reflux as a risk factor for esophageal adenocarcinoma. N Engl J Med 1999; 18(340):825–31

Lee SW, Shinohara H, Matsuki M et al. Preoperative simulation of vascular anatomy by three-dimensional computed tomography imaging in laparoscopic gastric cancer surgery. J Am Coll Surg 2003; 197:927–36

Richards DG, Brown TH, Manson JM. Endoscopic ultrasound in the staging of tumours of the oesophagus and gastro-oesophageal junction. Ann R Coll Surg Engl 2000; 82:311–17

Stroobants S, Goeminne J, Seegers M et al. 18FDG-Positron emission tomography for the early prediction of response in advanced soft tissue sarcoma treated with imatinib mesylate (Glivec). Eur J Cancer 2003; 39:2012–20

Imaging in hepatobiliary and pancreatic disease

12

S.J. Neuhaus

Background

Imaging investigations are pivotal in the assessment and management of patients with hepatobiliary and pancreatic disorders. The selection of patients appropriate for surgery and preoperative planning is particularly reliant on high quality imaging. Rapid advances in imaging technology have resulted in new non-invasive methods of evaluating the extrahepatic biliary tree, pancreas and liver such as CT cholangiography and MRCP. As a result, the role of traditional imaging methods such as ERCP is being redefined. Multiple imaging modalities are often required, particularly to characterise liver lesions. Therapeutic options include abscess drainage, biopsy and image guided tumour ablation (see Chapter 9).

THE RADIOLOGICAL INVESTIGATIONS

Ultrasound

With its versatility, ease of use and lack of ionizing radiation, the ultrasound examination is probably the single most useful investigation in hepatobiliary disease. The major limitation of ultrasound is obtaining adequate visualization in obese and non-fasted patients.

The development of microbubble contrast agents offers considerable promise in imaging liver lesions although this has yet to extend into routine clinical practice. In addition such agents can be used as potential targeting agents for ablative therapies. Colour Doppler is also useful to demonstrate arterial supply and further define tumours in the pancreas and liver.

Computed tomography cross-sectional imaging

With increased access to high resolution, high speed CT scanners with multiphase imaging, clear anatomical detail of the liver and pancreas is now feasible. With the advent of multislice spiral CT the current tendency is to scan the abdomen in 1–2-mm slices thus enabling multiplanar reformats. Pancreatic imaging can now be obtained with 3D reformations in a single breath-hold. Intravenous contrast can be used to enhance scans in arterial and venous phases and this provides optimal imaging of both the liver and pancreas. Water is usually used as oral contrast to distend the duodenum. CT is not limited by overlying bowel gas or obesity. It is

159

important to specify the purpose of a pancreatic CT study to the radiologist so that appropriate protocols can be used to obtain fine slices through the pancreas, particularly at the level of the pancreatic head.

Nuclear medicine

Hydroxyiminodiacetic acid isotope scan

HIDA is usually taken up rapidly by the liver, excreted in the bile and concentrated in the gall bladder. Scanning 30–45 minutes after an intravenous dose of technetium-labelled iminodiacetic acid will show a hot-spot in the region of the gall bladder (see Chapter 7). Failure of such a hot-spot to develop is indicative of absence of gall bladder function, which in the appropriate setting would match a diagnosis of acute cholecystitis. The use of HIDA scans has largely been supplanted by improvements in CT and MRI.

Contrast studies

Diagnosis in biliary tract disease: ERCP versus MRCP

The biliary and pancreatic ductal systems are best visualised by contrast. However, recent advances in cross-sectional radiology have allowed the biliary system to be clearly defined without the addition of contrast. The following imaging techniques are available:

- ERCP
- PTHC
- MRCP
- operative choledochography
- intravenous choledochography
- ultrasound.

Endoscopic retrograde cholangiopancreatography (ERCP) is considered to be the gold standard in the diagnosis and management of pancreaticobiliary diseases. One of the drawbacks of ERCP is that it does not provide any information about the extent of disease, which may be critical in planning management and it must be coupled with other imaging modalities. ERCP is an operator-dependent procedure that carries a risk of complications (particularly perforation and pancreatitis).

Percutaneous transhepatic cholangiography (PTHC) is an invasive procedure and has a limited role in biliary disease. It is used primarily when access to the obstructed biliary tree by ERCP is not feasible (e.g. after a gastrectomy with Roux-en-Y anastomosis). The technique is used for therapy (duct decompression) than diagnosis, where satisfactory information can usually be obtained by less invasive means (see Chapter 9).

Magnetic resonance cholangiopancreatography (MRCP) is non-invasive and not subject to operator variability. It provides high-quality images of the biliary and pancreatic ducts and can provide further information e.g. size and characterisation of a pancreatic tumour, evidence of vascular invasion or lymphadenopathy. The sensitivity of MRCP for choledocholithiasis is over 90% with a reported specificity of 94%. The sensitivity for malignancy is slightly lower (80–85%). This investigation provides an image of fluid within the duct (a 'luminogram'), but there is no functional information eg a dilated duct is not necessarily obstructed. In this sense it provides similar information to US. The advantages of MRCP include:

- no contrast is required
- images are obtainable in a completely obstructed system
- cross-sectional images of adjacent structures may be obtained simultaneously.

Recent advances in software technology have allowed development of 3D 'virtual' cholangiopancreatography. This is particularly useful in assessing the extrahepatic biliary tree and in planning resection of liver tumours.

The major drawback of MRCP is that it cannot be used therapeutically, e.g. for sphincterotomy or stent placement. MRCP however has an advantage in investigation of tumour where potential duct decompression and contamination of bile is viewed by some surgeons as a serious negative aspect of ERCP. MRCP also has a diagnostic role where ERCP has failed to provide satisfactory visualisation of the duct systems. ERCP and MRCP should be viewed as complimentary procedures. The relative advantages and disadvantages of each procedure are outlined in Table 12.1.

Oral cholecystography

This is now a rarely used technique and is mentioned for historical purposes only. Oral cholecystography has been superseded by ultrasound, which is a far more

Investigation	Advantages	Disadvantages
ERCP	Therapeutic options, e.g. stenting	Operator dependent Requires sedation Small but significant morbidity and mortality Theoretical risk of tumour seeding
MRCP	No contrast media required No sedation required Allows visualisation of extraductal anatomy, particularly for cholangiocarcinoma Provides a map of the biliary tree including segmental ducts not seen at ERCP Useful when ERCP fails, e.g. biliary–enteric anastomosis, complete ductal occlusion	No therapeutic options MRI not available in all centres

Table 12.1 Comparison of ERCP and MRCP

accurate and convenient investigation. With cholecystography, oral contrast is given the night before the planned investigation. It is taken up by the liver, excreted in the bile and concentrated in the gall bladder. Stones appear as 'filling defects'. The investigation requires a functioning gall bladder. Failure to opacify the gall bladder is not uncommon and may be due to patient non-compliance, failure to absorb the contrast material or gall bladder disease.

Computed tomography cholangiography

CT cholangiography is an uncommonly used modality for imaging of the biliary tree. However, with the advent of 3D imaging and newer contrast agents, it can be useful in some settings, particularly if MRI is not available. Oral and intravenous contrast agents are used which are concentrated in bile (see Chapter 3). CT cholangiography is non-invasive and has a diagnostic accuracy similar to ERCP in the detection of ductal pathology.

THE CLINICAL PROBLEMS

Gallstone disease

Gallstones are common in Western society although only 10–30% become symptomatic. The management

of asymptomatic gallstones is controversial but only 10% of patients develop symptoms over a 5-year period. Problems associated with gallstones include:

- biliary colic
- acute cholecystitis
- cholangitis
- jaundice
- pancreatitis
- bowel obstruction ('gallstone ileus')
- gall bladder cancer.

Radiological investigation of gallstones

Only 15% of gallstones are sufficiently radio-opaque to be visible on a plain abdominal radiograph. Ultrasound is the most appropriate radiological technique for the assessment of gallstones as it is quick, effective, accurate and non-invasive. Apart from showing stones which characteristically demonstrate an acoustic shadow, it can provide information about gall bladder wall thickness, pericholecystic collections and evaluate the liver and pancreas (Fig. 12.1, Box 12.1).

Ultrasonography is less effective in its detection of gallstones in obese patients or where there is bowel gas overlying the gall bladder. Whereas the sensitivity of ultrasound in its overall detection of gallstones exceeds 95%, it falls to less than 55% in its ability to detect stones in the bile ducts (Fig. 12.2).

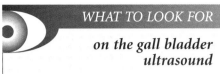

WHAT TO LOOK FOR | Box 12.1

on the gall bladder ultrasound

- Solitary or multiple stones
- Acoustic shadowing from stones
- Dilatation of extra or intrahepatic bile ducts (particularly CBD diameter)
- Thickness of the gall bladder wall
- Presence of any pericholecystic fluid
- Presence of adenoma or 'porcelain' gall bladder

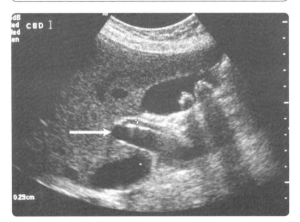

Fig. 12.1 An ultrasound examination showing two gallstones, with acoustic shadowing, a thin-walled gall bladder, a non-dilated common bile duct calibre and the portal vein (arrow).

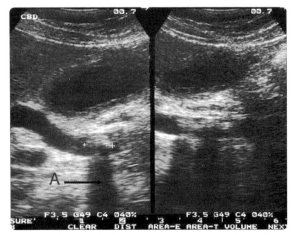

Fig. 12.2 Stones within a dilated common bile duct. The arrow points to the acoustic shadow created by the stone.

CT is less sensitive than ultrasound in the detection of gallstones with only 60–80% of stones visible, but MRI is highly sensitive, with a detection of almost 100%, including stones as small as 2 mm. MRCP and ERCP are more sensitive than both CT and US for detecting CBD stones.

Biliary colic

Biliary colic may occur as the result of impaction of a stone in the neck of the gall bladder. The obstruction is usually transient and the symptoms of severe right upper quadrant pain may only last a few hours. There are few, if any, associated physical signs. The diagnosis of biliary colic is a clinical one, supported by the ultrasonographic demonstration of gallstones. Occasionally a stone will be seen impacted in the neck, but more often the ultrasound will show stones mobile within the gall bladder.

Acute cholecystitis

Infection and inflammation of the gall bladder usually occurs in the presence of gallstones. The precipitating factor is obstruction of the cystic duct, with a chemical inflammatory reaction and then a superimposed infection. The diagnosis of acute cholecystitis is made on clinical grounds and supported by the ultrasound findings (Fig. 12.3, Box 12.2).

Occasionally the ultrasound examination will be negative and if the clinician is convinced that the underlying problem is acute cholecystitis, further confirmatory evidence may be sought. In such circum-

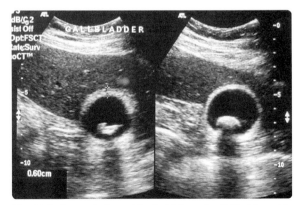

Fig. 12.3 Acute cholecystitis. A thickened gall bladder with stones and pericholecystic fluid.

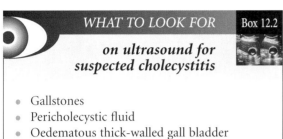
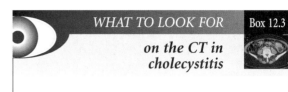
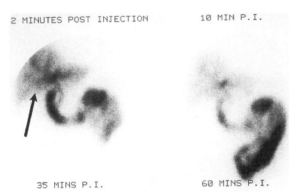

Fig. 12.4 Failure of uptake of tracer into the gall bladder in a patient with acute right subcostal pain. The arrow points to the site of the gall bladder.

stances a radionuclide (HIDA) scan may help (cholescintigraphy) (Fig. 12.4).

Although CT is less sensitive in the detection of gallstones, it can detect biliary ductal dilatation, pericholecystic fluid and any other pathology. Thickening of the gall bladder wall is a non-specific finding and can occur in other settings, in which case it is not diagnostic of acute cholecystitis (Box 12.3).

In most instances, patients with acute cholecystitis will undergo cholecystectomy and this can usually be undertaken in an elective or semi-elective setting. Occasionally the inflammatory process is so severe and the generalised effects of infection have made the patient so ill that urgent intervention is required. If the patient is not sufficiently fit for cholecystectomy, a per-

cutaneous cholecystostomy may be performed to drain the infected gall bladder. This is done under ultrasound control (see Chapter 9).

Acalculous cholecystitis

Acute inflammation of the gall bladder can occur in the absence of stones (acalculous cholecystitis). Acalculous cholecystitis is an uncommon condition outside of the ICU setting. Ultrasound, by definition, will not demonstrate gallstones but the gall bladder may be distended and tender on transducer pressure and there may be 'sludge' visible within the gall bladder. If the diagnosis remains in doubt, a radionuclide scan may be performed (see Fig. 12.4).

Cholangitis

This is usually due to a stone or stones obstructing the common bile duct. Whilst the sensitivity of ultrasonography for choledocholithiasis is in the region of 50%, the findings of stones in the gall bladder in a patient with cholangitis is usually sufficient to confirm the diagnosis.

After resuscitation, the next stage in the management of a patient with suppurative cholangitis is duct decompression. Preferably this is performed endoscopically by ERCP. The degree of urgency of the procedure will depend on the gravity of the patient's illness. The aim of ERCP is to visualise the biliary system, identify any filling defects and decompress the system. Decompression will involve a sphincterotomy and insertion of a stent (Fig. 12.5).

Occasionally it is not possible to decompress the bile duct endoscopically and a percutaneous transhe-

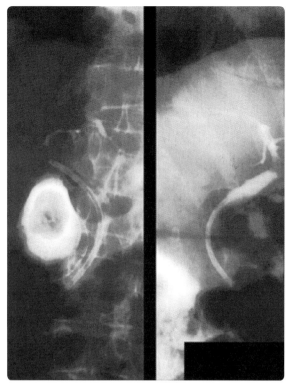

Fig. 12.5 Decompression of the common bile duct and insertion of a stent. There is a large stone in the gall bladder.

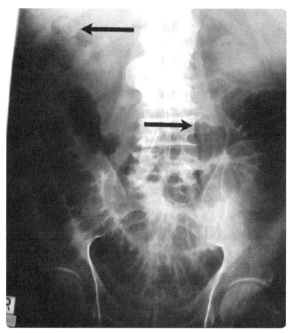

Fig. 12.6 Small bowel obstruction secondary to an impacted gallstone. There is another large stone in the gall bladder and gas in the gall bladder and biliary tree. Arrows point to the stone in the gall bladder and the stone impacted in the small bowel.

patic approach may be considered. Through a lateral approach with ultrasound or CT guidance, a fine-bore needle is introduced into the dilated intrahepatic system. A guide wire is threaded through the needle and steered into the common bile duct. When in position, a pigtailed catheter is introduced over the guide wire and left to drain the infected system (see Chapter 9).

Small bowel obstruction ('gallstone ileus')

Impaction of a gallstone in the small bowel is an uncommon cause of small bowel obstruction. Frequently the diagnosis is not made preoperatively and the patient is taken to the operating room on the basis of an unresolved obstruction.

In a patient with small bowel obstruction, the plain abdominal radiograph may give clues suggesting this unusual type of obstruction (Fig. 12.6, Box 12.4).

 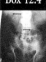

WHAT TO LOOK FOR | **Box 12.4**

on the plain X-ray gallstone ileus

- Dilated small bowel loops
- Gallstones in the gall bladder
- Gas in the biliary tree (central towards the porta hepatis)
- Gallstone in the region of the dilated loops of bowel, which may be in different positions on the erect and supine films

Extrahepatic biliary obstruction

Obstructive jaundice

The key to clinical management of obstructive jaundice is identification of the level of obstruction and the underlying aetiology.

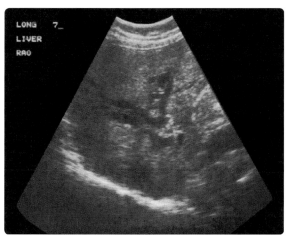

Fig. 12.7 Dilated intrahepatic ducts in a patient with jaundice. Other views taken during the examination revealed a hypoechoic mass in the head of the pancreas.

Obstructive jaundice may be due to:

- luminal obstruction, e.g. calculus
- mural obstruction, e.g. stricture, sclerosing cholangitis, cholangiocarcinoma
- extramural obstruction, e.g. pancreatitis, tumour, lymphadenopathy.

The important surgical causes of jaundice are:

- carcinoma of the head of the pancreas
- stones in the common bile duct
- metastatic disease in the porta hepatis
- cholangiocarcinoma
- metastatic disease in the liver.

In suspected obstructive jaundice, an ultrasound examination of the upper abdomen is the first line investigation (Fig. 12.7, Box 12.5).

Bile duct strictures

Bile duct strictures may affect the intrahepatic and/or the extrahepatic biliary tree. Management of the stricture will depend on its site and aetiology (Box 12.6).

Biliary strictures can be classified as:

- Benign:
  - Trauma, e.g. postcholecystectomy (Fig. 12.8)
  - Inflammatory, e.g. sclerosing cholangitis
  - Infective, e.g. liver flukes

WHAT TO LOOK FOR | Box 12.5

on the ultrasound and CT of extrahepatic biliary obstruction

- Duct dilatation, particularly intrahepatic duct dilatation
- The liver parenchyma (cirrhosis, metastatic deposits)
- Presence of gallstones, especially stones in the extrahepatic biliary tree
- Size of the gall bladder and thickness of the gall bladder wall
- Enlargement of lymph nodes in the porta hepatis
- Any masses in the head of the pancreas
- Enlargement of the pancreas with surrounding inflammatory change (pancreatitis)

- Malignant:
  - bile duct tumour
  - pancreatic tumour (Fig. 12.9)
  - gall bladder cancer
  - other extrinsic tumour, e.g. lymphoma at porta hepatis.

Pancreatic pathology

Acute pancreatitis

Most cases of acute pancreatitis will be related either to the presence of gallstones or consumption of alcohol.

In suspected or confirmed acute pancreatitis the first imaging investigation is usually an ultrasound examination of the upper abdomen. Gaseous distension and ileus reduce the accuracy of ultrasound in the early phase of pancreatitis and the gall bladder is only visualised in 70–80%. Even if there is good visualisation, the pancreas often appears normal on ultrasound and its main use is to determine the presence or absence of gallstones (Box 12.7). The ultrasound should be repeated at 6 weeks if the initial scan is negative for stones, and alcohol is not thought to be the precipitating cause.

WHAT TO LOOK FOR | Box 12.6

on the CT and ERCP/MRCP in extrahepatic biliary obstruction

CT

- Level of ductal dilatation
- Pancreatic mass or enlargement with surrounding inflammatory change (pancreatitis)
- Liver parenchyma (intrahepatic mass, cirrhosis, metastatic deposits)
- Benign or malignant process involving porta hepatis, pancreas or gall bladder
- Presence of distant disease

ERCP/MRCP

- Determine level of stricture
- Nature and length of strictured segment
- 'Beading' of ducts +/− segmental pathology typical of sclerosing cholangitis
- 'Double duct sign' suggestive of pancreatic/ampullary cancer
- Pancreatic mass on MRI

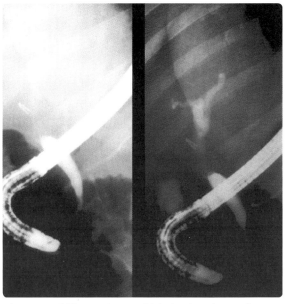

Fig. 12.8 A biliary stricture which developed several months after a laparoscopic cholecystectomy. It is probably ischaemic in origin.

WHAT TO LOOK FOR | Box 12.7

on ultrasound in pancreatitis

- The presence of gallstones
- Stones in the common bile duct
- An oedematous pancreas (enlarged and hypoechoic)

Indications for computed tomography scanning in pancreatitis

CT scanning is not indicated in all patients with pancreatitis, but may be used for initial diagnostic purposes and the assessment of potential complications (Box 12.8). In established pancreatitis it should be performed between day 3 and 5 in patients with prognostically severe pancreatitis as it is the most reliable determinant of pancreatic necrosis.

First 48 hours Diagnostic uncertainty

Days 3–5 All patients with prognostically severe pancreatitis (e.g. using the Atlanta, Glasgow scoring systems).

Delayed scanning Follow-up of pancreatic necrosis (Fig. 12.10).

Complications of pancreatitis

- pancreatic necrosis
- pancreatic abscess
- pseudocyst
- splenic vein thrombosis (Fig. 12.11).

In mild pancreatitis the pancreas and surrounding tissues appear oedematous, often with few other signs. Hallmark features of severe pancreatitis include necrosis, peripancreatic fluid collections, and areas of patchy enhancement. Complications of pancreatitis such as pseudoaneurysms, thrombosis and fluid collections

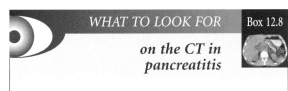

WHAT TO LOOK FOR Box 12.8

on the CT in pancreatitis

- Enlarged low density pancreas consistent with oedema
- Stranding of the peripancreatic fat
- Fluid collections within the peripancreatic region or elsewhere in the abdomen
- Loss of pancreatic enhancement following IV contrast consistent with necrosis
- Ascites
- Gallstones
- Intra-/extrahepatic biliary dilatation
- Duodenal obstruction
- Splenic vein thrombosis

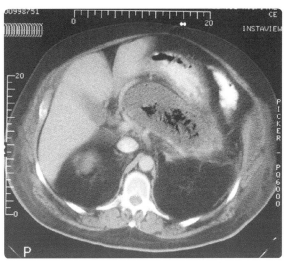

Fig. 12.10 Necrotising pancreatitis. The CT scan shows gas bubbles in the infarcted pancreas.

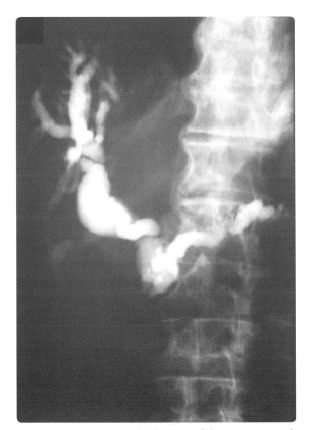

Fig. 12.9 Obstruction and dilatation of the pancreatic and bile ducts in carcinoma of the head of the pancreas.

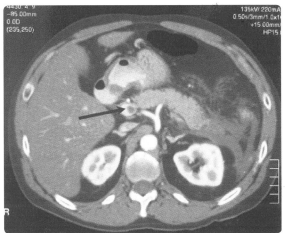

Fig. 12.11 Acute pancreatitis, with mild inflammatory changes around the tail of the gland, with stranding in the peripancreatic fat. There is a filling defect in the portal vein (arrow). Other slices showed thrombosis of the splenic vein and this cut shows the clot extending into the portal vein.

can be readily assessed with CT. Recently there has been some concern that iodinated contrast may aggravate severe pancreatitis, and in this setting MRI may be a safer alternative.

The role of ERCP in gallstone-related pancreatitis is controversial. In patients with severe pancreatitis due to gallstones, early ERCP is advocated and has been demonstrated to reduce mortality. ERCP may also be required in the delayed management of patients with gallstone related pancreatitis, for example if they are unfit to undergo cholecystectomy.

The aim of ERCP is to:

- visualise the common bile duct
- overcome any obstruction
  - sphincterotomy
  - removal of stone
  - insertion of a stent if the stone cannot be removed.

Pancreatic necrosis In a small percentage of patients with acute pancreatitis, the disease will be complicated by pancreatic necrosis and/or abscess formation. In high-risk patients or those in whom deterioration has occurred, further visualisation of the pancreas with CT scanning is recommended. The morphological changes observed in complicated pancreatitis (necrosis, abscess formation), are unlikely to be detected until several days have elapsed.

Whilst it is the clinical condition of the patient that will determine the need for any surgical intervention, the CT will help in the decision-making. A contrast enhanced CT with fine slices through the pancreas is the best method to detect pancreatic and peripancreatic necrosis, which appear as areas of patchy contrast enhancement, define its severity and plan any proposed surgery.

Pancreatic abscess A pancreatic abscess should be treated as soon as it is diagnosed. It should be suspected in any patient whose condition deteriorates several weeks after an episode of severe pancreatitis. Abscess formation is best confirmed with contrast enhanced CT scan. A key to diagnosis of infection is the presence of gas in the collection. If small, a percutaneous approach (under ultrasound or CT guidance) may allow satisfactory drainage.

There are limitations to radiological drainage, principally:

- multiloculated collections
- access considerations
- multiple collections
- non-liquified infective material.

Pancreatic pseudocyst The development of a pancreatic pseudocyst can be confirmed by CT or ultrasound (Fig. 12.12). A small pseudocyst should be left to resolve of its own accord, but cysts greater than 5 cm diameter will probably require some form of drainage. This may be open, laparoscopic or radiological (see Chapter 9). The cyst should be left several weeks to allow the wall to 'mature' and thicken before any drainage procedure is attempted. This allows a controlled puncture and drainage rather than collapse of the cyst and risk of pancreatic ascites.

Indications for drainage of peripancreatic collections are:

- suspected infection
- symptomatic
- size > 5 cm
- failure to resolve or increase in size on follow up.

Options for interventional radiological drainage include:

- aspiration
- percutaneous cyst-gastrostomy drainage.

Splenic vein thrombosis Splenic vein thrombosis is a rare complication of acute pancreatitis and may lead to the development of segmental or left-sided portal

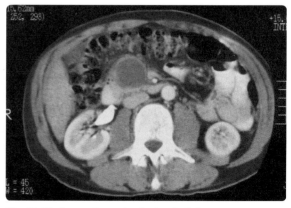

Fig. 12.12 A pseudocyst in the head of the pancreas.

hypertension. Other vascular complications of pancreatitis such as pseudoaneurysm formation may also be evident on CT (Box 12.9).

Chronic pancreatitis

Chronic pancreatitis results in diffuse atrophy of the pancreatic parenchyma and fibrosis. The changes of chronic pancreatitis are most clearly seen on CT images (see Chapter 4) (Box 12.10), although calcification of the pancreatic duct may be evident on a plain abdominal radiograph. Classical features of advanced chronic pancreatitis include dilatation of the pancreatic duct and its side branches, focal or diffuse atrophy (usually most obvious in the pancreatic head), calcification, biliary duct enlargement and changes in the peripancreatic fat. MRI is now accepted as a primary imaging modality for chronic pancreatitis and demonstrates similar changes with decreased signal intensity on T1 images due to fibrosis.

WHAT TO LOOK FOR | Box 12.9

on the CT in splenic vein thrombosis

- Failure of the splenic vein to opacify with contrast on venous phase
- Splenomegaly
- Collaterals around the greater curve of the stomach
- Absence of liver cirrhosis

WHAT TO LOOK FOR | Box 12.10

on the CT in chronic pancreatitis

- Pancreatic atrophy
- Pancreatic fibrosis, calcification
- Dilatation and irregularity of the pancreatic duct
- Calculi in the pancreatic duct

Carcinoma of the pancreas

Ductal adenocarcinoma accounts for more than 90% of malignant pancreatic tumours. Most cancers arise in the head of the pancreas and present late in the course of the disease. Periampullary carcinoma is associated with a more favourable prognosis as it presents earlier and is more likely to be resectable. Neuroendocrine tumours of the pancreas are discussed in Chapter 20.

Radiology is central to both diagnosis and treatment of pancreatic malignancy. In patients with a pancreatic mass, the aim of treatment is to:

- confirm the clinical diagnosis
- determine resectability and staging
- help plan management, e.g. surgery, stents.

Ultrasound Pancreatic carcinoma typically appears as a focal hypoechoic mass on ultrasound. Patients with advanced disease and extensive metastases may not require further investigation. Endoscopic ultrasound is also a useful investigation, especially for small peri-ampullary carcinomas which may not be evident on CT or MRI. The head of the pancreas is well visualised through the wall of the third part of the duodenum and transduodenal biopsies can be taken. Endoscopic ultrasound is also useful to anatomically define the course of the pancreatic duct.

Computed tomography Dynamic CT is the most useful imaging modality in pancreatic cancer (Box 12.11). The main role of the CT scan is to determine the resectability of the neoplasm. The accuracy of CT in predicting the resectablility of a tumour is high (>90%) (Fig. 12.13). The use of 3D CT and CT angiography improves the accuracy of CT. On dynamic CT most adenocarcinomas are hypoattenuating compared with normal pancreatic parenchyma. This facilitates detection of small lesions. Any narrowing or obliteration of adjacent blood vessels may suggest possible vascular involvement. Perivascular cuffing (increased attenuation of normal perivascular fat) also correlates with vascular invasion and suggests non-resectability.

Angiography Angiography is used in some centres as a further staging investigation in patients with potentially resectable tumours. The role of angiography has largely been replaced by MRI.

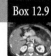

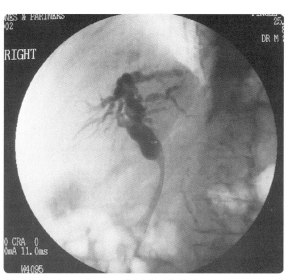

Fig. 12.14 A carcinoma of the head of the pancreas treated by decompression of the common bile duct with a metallic mesh stent. The stent has only just been inserted and is not yet fully expanded.

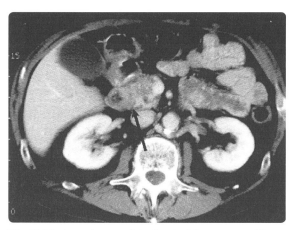

Fig. 12.13 A carcinoma of the head of the pancreas. There is invasion of the superior mesenteric vessels and the duodenum (arrow).

ERCP/MRCP MRI is of increasing importance in the diagnosis and staging of pancreatic cancer, particularly when it is used in conjunction with MRCP. Characteristic features of pancreatic head carcinoma on MRCP include encasement or obstruction of the pancreatic duct or bile duct. The 'double duct' sign is also evident on MRCP due to dilatation of both pancreatic and common bile ducts in 77% of patients. MRCP is also helpful in planning peripheral access for transhepatic drainage if required. MRI is not reliable for demonstration of small lymph nodes. Pancreatic adenocarcinoma does not take up manganese, allowing magnafodipir enhanced MRI to provide better defini-

tion of pancreatic tumour against background normal pancreatic tissue. The role of contrast enhanced MRI has still to be defined.

Controversy exists over the place of ERCP in obstructive jaundice thought due to malignancy. The protagonists argue for accuracy of diagnosis with clear visualisation of the duct systems and biopsy of the tumour. This group also argues that most cases of malignant obstruction are due to carcinoma of the head of the pancreas, and as most of these cases are inoperable at the time of presentation, a stent is good treatment. An extension of the argument is that the overall survival of carcinoma of the head of the pancreas is not much improved by pancreaticoduodenectomy, and therefore it is best to proceed straight to stenting (Fig. 12.14).

Those without such a nihilistic viewpoint argue that if a patient is thought to have a resectable lesion, ERCP should be avoided to:

- minimise the risk of sepsis
- allow the bile duct to remain dilated, thereby facilitating operative intervention.

Those who follow this latter dictum will rely on the CT scan and look for:

- size, position and local extension of the primary tumour
- relationship of the tumour to the portal vein, SMV, SMA and coeliac axis
- presence of metastatic disease.

Contrast studies have limited value in the management of pancreatic cancer and have been supplanted by endoscopy and CT scanning. However, a barium meal may show evidence of gastric outlet obstruction, duodenal narrowing or splaying of the duodenal curve (Fig. 12.15). Some centres are using MRI and MRCP for assessment of the primary tumour and ducts, but CT is still the accepted modality of choice for staging pancreatic cancer in most institutions.

Intra-hepatic cholangiocarcinomas are difficult to see on CT and often need the use of delayed postcontrast images. They may be more apparent on MRI

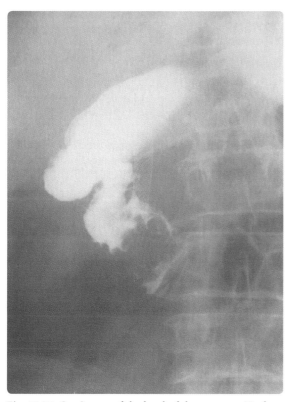

Fig. 12.15 Carcinoma of the head of the pancreas. Twelve months earlier the patient had presented with jaundice and a mesh stent (visible) had been inserted. On this occasion the patient presented with gastric outlet obstruction. The tumour is obstructing the second part of the duodenum.

(Fig. 12.16). Extrahepatic tumours and ampullary tumours are often not seen on CT.

Liver lesions

As well as their morphological appearance and that of the surrounding liver parenchyma, liver lesions are described according to their segmental distribution.

Characterisation of benign liver lesions

Benign liver lesions are relatively common and most are first noted as incidental radiological findings. Radiological investigation is the principal means of characterisation of benign liver lesions, the main purpose of which is to exclude malignancy and to identify lesions with pre-malignant potential or a high probability of complications.

The most common benign liver lesions encountered in clinical practice are:

- hepatic adenoma
- focal nodular hyperplasia
- haemangioma
- cystic lesions e.g. simple cysts, abscess, echinococcal cysts.

Careful radiological evaluation of these liver lesions gives a high degree of diagnostic certainty, often without the need for biopsy. Ultrasound and 'multiphase' CT are considered complimentary and, more recently, MRI has been added to further characterise these lesions. Hepatic angiography is only rarely required (Boxes 12.12 and 12.13).

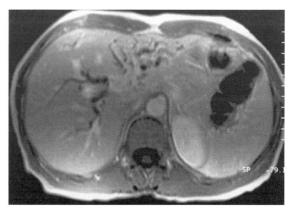

Fig. 12.16 A postcontrast MRI showing an enhancing mass at the junction of the right and left intrahepatic ducts. This is a cholangiocarcinoma.

WHAT TO LOOK FOR Box 12.12
on liver ultrasound

- Solitary or multiple lesions
- Solid or cystic structure
- Characteristics of the surrounding liver parenchyma
- Evidence of calcification
- Vascularity (Doppler enhancement)
- Features of a hydatid cyst:
  - lamellated membrane
  - fluid level with granular sand at base
  - daughter cysts within cavity

WHAT TO LOOK FOR Box 12.13
on CT of liver lesions

- Presence/absence of cirrhosis
- Solitary or multiple
- Size and position
- Stellate central 'scar' of FNH
- Enhancement pattern with contrast
- Internal haemorrhage and necrosis characteristic of adenoma
- Gradual 'disappearance' of haemangioma on delayed films

Hepatic adenoma

Hepatic adenomas are focal, well differentiated liver lesions. They are usually solitary and occur most commonly in women (thought to be related to the use of oral contraceptive pills) in an otherwise normal liver. Adenomas are characteristically well encapsulted, hypervascular lesions which are hyperdense on arterial phase CT images, but may be isodense or hypodense to liver parenchyma on venous phase scans. They have a low malignant potential but are prone to haemorrhage and necrosis, giving them a heterogenous internal appearance. The appearance alone is similar to an HCC and the lack of cirrhosis and relevant clinical history are required for differentiation.

The lesions are usually heterogenous on MRI, with mild increased signal on both T1 and T2 sequences. There is usually intense postcontrast enhancement in the arterial phase (Fig. 12.17).

Focal nodular hyperplasia

Focal nodular hyperplasia (FNH) is less common than adenoma and occurs primarily in women, although the lesions are not thought to be associated with contraceptive use. They may be multiple in up to 25% and are characterised by the presence of a central stellate 'scar' (Fig. 12.18). They are also hypervascular and enhance on arterial images, but the scar is usually hypodense in this early phase (Fig. 12.19). On delayed images the FNH is isodense to liver, but the scar demonstrates delayed enhancement. They can also be distinguished from adenomas by the use of technetium sulphur colloid scans which will demonstrate near

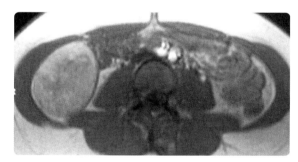

Fig. 12.17 MRI demonstrating hepatic adenoma.

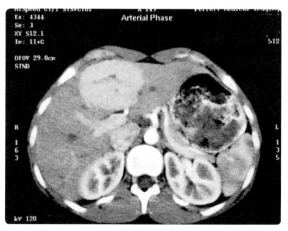

Fig. 12.18 A CT scan of focal nodular hyperplasia. This is the arterial phase scan, showing an enhancing lesion with an hypodense central stellate scar.

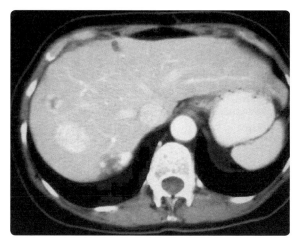

Fig. 12.19 Haemangiomas showing typical peripheral "puddling" on the arterial phase film.

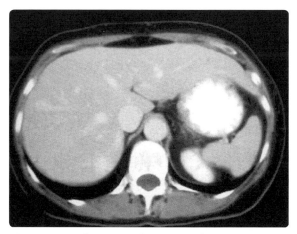

Fig. 12.20 On the venous phase image, the haemangiomas are no longer visible.

normal uptake in FNH as they usually contain Kuppfer cells, whereas the adenoma appears as a focal filling defect. Note that a hypervascular lesion with a central scar in a non-cirrhotic liver can also be a fibrolamellar variant HCC.

Haemangioma

Haemangiomas may be capillary or cavernous varieties and rarely cause clinical problems. They can be multiple and often present diagnostic difficulty and confusion with other lesions. The most characteristic radiological sign of an haemangioma is the presence of a low attenuation lesion which 'disappears' on delayed images due to progressive opacification of the lesion in a centripetal manner (Figs 12.19 and 12.20). They are classically hyperechoic on US. MRI and radionuclide imaging using tagged red blood cells may be required to confirm the diagnosis.

Simple cysts

Simple cysts are common incidental findings on CT examinations and can be difficult to distinguish from metastases. Larger lesions demonstrating fluid density with no enhancement are usually cysts, and this can be confirmed with ultrasound if it is important to clinical management. Lesions less than 1 cm are more difficult to characterise and MRI may be needed for further clarification. If a lesion has not changed in size over a 2-year period it can be safely assumed to represent a cyst.

Hydatid cysts

Hydatid disease is endemic in certain parts of the world including the southern United States, Turkey, south-eastern Australia and New Zealand. Man is an accidental intermediate host and develops cysts, most commonly in the liver. Frequently these cysts are asymptomatic but complications may occur related to enlargement of the cyst, biliary obstruction or rupture resulting in anaphylaxis.

Ultrasound is usually diagnostic, with a fluid-filled cyst containing loose material ('hydatid sand') and septa (Fig. 12.21). CT appearances are usually characteristic with a low attenuation lesion characterised by the presence of secondary cysts ('daughter cysts')

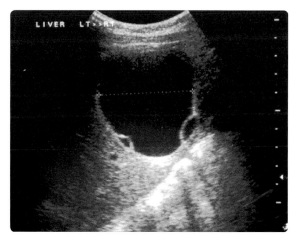

Fig. 12.21 An hydatid cyst in the liver. Several septa are visible.

within the cavity. The cyst wall may be lamellated and in longstanding cysts, contain calcium.

Further investigations of liver lesions

If the radiological patterns are not characteristic other options are:

- red cell scan for haemangioma
- sulphur colloid scan for FNH. The colloid is taken up by Kupffer cells demonstrating the absence of filling defect with FNH.

Primary hepatic malignancy

Hepatocellular carcinoma (hepatoma or HCC) is a common cancer on a world-wide basis, but usually occurs in Western society in the setting of pre-existing cirrhosis. It may present as clinical deterioration in a known cirrhotic, although many hepatomas are now detected through screening of high-risk patients.

Ultrasound Ultrasound is the first-line investigation because it is inexpensive, non-invasive, non-irradiating and has a high sensitivity for identification of a focal liver mass. Tumours as small as 1 cm in diameter can be detected. Microbubble ultrasound contrast, although not freely available, is likely to increase the use of ultrasound as a primary investigation in the future. Liver-specific microbubbles such as Levovist® can improve the sensitivity of detection of focal liver malignancies from 70% with conventional ultrasound to almost 90%. Ultrasound contrast agents have also been demonstrated to have a role in differentiating HCC from regenerating liver nodules of cirrhosis.

Dynamic computed tomography CT can be very sensitive in identification of hepatoma (Box 12.14). Typically HCC appears as a hyperdense lesion on arterial phase scans and iso- or hypodense on venous phase images. It is often heterogenous with a pseudo-capsule (Fig. 12.22). HCC is characterised by the frequency of multiple lesions and microsatellites. The main difficulty of detecting HCCs on any imaging modality is the frequent presence of background cirrhosis with multiple regenerating nodules which may demonstrate a similar appearance to an HCC.

Lipiodol computer tomography scanning Lipiodol has been used in some centres in conjunction with CT

scanning to improve the diagnosis of HCC. Lipiodol is injected into the hepatic artery and taken up by the liver cells. It is administered 2–4 weeks before scanning and is cleared by normal hepatocytes within 7 days. Lipiodol is retained and concentrated within the HCC and appears on scanning as a high density area. This technique has also been used for attachment of chemotherapeutic substances such as cisplatin and doxyrubicin. Improvements in helical scanning technology have rendered the lipiodol test all but obsolete.

Magnetic resonance imaging MRI is not used as a primary imaging modality in HCC due to its cost, although it can complement the CT findings. The

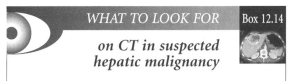

WHAT TO LOOK FOR — Box 12.14

on CT in suspected hepatic malignancy

- The lesion:
  - site
  - size
- Presence of satellite lesions
- Heterogenous appearance with early contrast enhancement
- Pseudocapsule
- Intratumoural necrosis
- Any cirrhotic change in the parenchyma
- Extrahepatic tumour spread

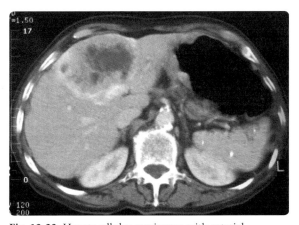

Fig. 12.22 Hepatocellular carcinoma with arterial enhancement at the pseudocapsule and necrotic foci in the centre of the lesion.

typical features of HCC are similar to those seen on CT, appearing as a hypointense lesion on T1- and as a hyperintense lesion on T2-weighted images.

Angiography With the availability of high-quality, high-resolution cross-sectional imaging, there is less need for pure angiographic imaging in problems associated with the hepatobiliary and pancreatic systems. Angiography is still occasionally required to define vascular involvement and relationships to vascular structures prior to surgical intervention. It can also be used for regional infusion of chemotherapeutic agents or embolisation prior to surgery to devascularise a bulky tumour (Fig. 12.23).

Hepatic metastases

The liver is a common site of metastatic disease, although only colorectal and neuroendocrine metastases carry a good prognosis with surgical resection.

Metastatic disease affecting the liver is most often due to primary disease of the:

- colon and rectum
- stomach
- pancreas
- lung
- breast.

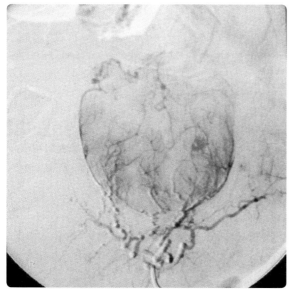

Fig. 12.23 Angiographical localisation of an hepatocellular carcinoma prior to chemotherapeutic infusion.

Dynamic computed tomography Most metastases appear as focal low attenuation lesions, although iso-dense and hyperdense lesions are encountered, which is why scanning in both arterial and venous phases is useful (Fig. 12.24, Box 12.15). Generally, only lesions >1 cm are visible on CT. The major role of imaging in metastatic liver disease is to confirm the presence and burden of metastatic disease and assess the suitability for resection or other treatment. FNA can provide a histological diagnosis if the primary site is unknown which may guide systemic treatment.

There are numerous studies into the use of MRI with liver-specific contrast agents for improved assessment of metastatic disease prior to hepatic metastasectomy (see Chapter 6). This suggests that there will be significant improvement in the sensitivity and specifi-

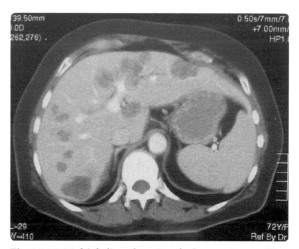

Fig. 12.24 Multiple liver deposits of adenocarcinoma. The lesions are hypodense.

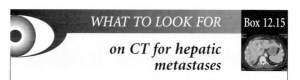

WHAT TO LOOK FOR   Box 12.15

on CT for hepatic metastases

- Size, number and distribution of lesions
- Peripheral ring enhancement
- Calcification
- Residual liver texture (cirrhosis)
- Extrahepatic nodal involvement

city of lesion detection in the future. The role of PET scanning in detection of metastatic liver disease is discussed in Chapter 8.

Further reading

Appleton GV, Bathurst NC, Virgee J et al. The value of angiography in the surgical management of pancreatic disease. Ann R Coll Surg Engl 1989; 71:92–6

Balthazar EJ, Robinson DL, Megibow AJ, Ranson JH. Acute pancreatitis: value of CT in establishing prognosis. Radiology 1990; 174:331–6

Choi BI, Park JH, Kim BH et al. Small hepatocellular carcinoma: detection with sonography, computed tomography (CT), angiography and Lipiodol-CT. Br J Surg 1989; 62:897–903

Cosgrove D, Blomley M. Liver tumours: evaluation with contrast-enhanced ultrasound. Abdom Imaging 2004; 29:446–54

Freeny PC, Traverso LW, Ryan JA. Diagnosis and staging of pancreatic adenocarcinoma with dynamic computed tomography. Am J Surg 1993; 165:600–6

Georgopoulos SK, Schwartz LH, Jarnagin WR et al. Comparison of Magnetic resonance and endoscopic retrograde cholangiopancreatography in malignant pancreaticobiliary obstruction. Arch Surg 1999; 134:1002–7

Gracie WA, Ranohoff DF. The natural history of silent gallstones: the innocent gallstone is not a myth. N Engl J Med 1982; 307:798–800

Halpert RD, Feczko PJ. Biliary system and the gall bladder. In: Gastrointestinal radiology: the requisites. Mosby, St Louis, 1999

Kalra MK, Maher MM, Sahani DV et al. Current status of imaging in pancreatic diseases. J Comput Assist Tomogr 2002; 26:661–75

Lee MG, Lee HJ, Kim MH et al. Extrahepatic biliary diseases: 3D MR cholangiopancreatography compared with endoscopic retrograde cholangiopancreatography. Radiology 1997; 202:663–9

Maniatis P, Trinatopoulou C, Sofianou E et al. Virtual CT cholangiography in patients with choledocholithiasis. Abdom Imaging 2003; 28:536–44

McKay AJ, Imrie CW, O'Neill J, Duncan JG. Is early ultrasound scan of value in acute pancreatitis? Br J Surg 1982; 69:369–72

McSherry CK, Glenn F. The incidence and causes of death following surgery for non-malignant biliary tract disease. Ann Surg 1980; 191:271–5

Motohara T, Semelk RC, Bader TR. MR chonagiopancreatography. Radiol Clin North Am 2003; 41:89–96

Neoptolemos JP, Carr-Locke DL, London NJ et al. Controlled trial of urgent endoscopic retrograde cholangiopancreatography and endoscopic sphincterotomy versus conservative treatment in patients with acute pancreatitis due to gallstones. Lancet 1988; 2:979–83

Oikarinen H, Paivansalo M, Tikkakoski T, Saarela A. Radiological findings in biliary fistula and gallstone ileus. Acta Radiol 1996; 37:917–22

Soto JA, Barish MA, Yukel EK et al. Magnetic resonance cholangiography: comparison with endoscopic retrograde cholangiopancreatography. Gastroenterology 1996; 110:589–97

Stabile Ianora AA, Memeo M, Scardapane A et al. Oral contrast-enhanced three-dimensional helical-CT cholangiography: clinical applications. Eur Radiol 2003; 13:867–73

Stockberger SM, Sherman S, Kopecky KK. Helical CT cholangiography. Abdom Imaging 1996; 21:98–104

Tanaka S, Kitamura T, Nakanishi K et al. Effectiveness of periodic checkup by ultrasonography for the early diagnosis of hepatocellular carcinoma. Cancer 1990; 66:2210–14

Xu AM, Cheng HY, Jiang WB et al. Multi-slice three-dimensional spiral CT cholangiography: a new technique for diagnosis of biliary diseases. Hepatobiliary Pancreat Dis Int 2002; 1:595–603

Zech CJ, Schoenbuerg SO, Reiser M, Helmberger T. Cross-sectional imaging of biliary tumors: current clinical status and future developments. Eur Radiol 2004; 14:1174–87

Imaging in colorectal disease

13

J.L. Sweeney

Background

As with disorders affecting the upper digestive tract, endoscopy is frequently the preferred initial diagnostic tool in the investigation of colorectal disease. Colonoscopy will always have the advantage over imaging modalities in its ability to obtain tissue diagnosis and perform therapeutic manoeuvres. Endoscopic ultrasound has proved valuable in the assessment of perianal disease, but conventional ultrasound has virtually no role in the management of colorectal disease. CT is the imaging method of choice in most colonic conditions due to its ability to accurately demonstrate mural bowel disease as well as extramural extension, pericolic soft tissues and adjacent structures. Advances in CT colonography may mean that imaging has a greater role in diagnosis and more importantly surveillance in the future. MRI has an important role in the definition of complex perianal problems such as those that may occur in Crohn's disease and rectal cancer.

RADIOLOGICAL INVESTIGATION OF COLORECTAL DISORDERS

Plain radiology

The abdominal X-ray is used in the initial assessment of the majority of colorectal and abdominal problems. It is particularly useful in the assessment of large bowel obstruction, acute problems related to inflammatory bowel disease and obstructed hernias. In the latter problem gas within bowel can occasionally be seen overlying the groin area outside the abdominal confines (see Chapter 24). The plain radiograph will help guide the clinician in determining the next most useful investigation or intervention. The supine abdominal film is often used in conjunction with the erect chest X-ray.

Contrast enemas

Double-contrast barium enema (DCBE)

Advances in endoscopic techniques and CT scanning have relegated contrast studies to a largely supportive role in the assessment of colorectal disease (Box 13.1). However the barium enema is a more cost-effective procedure than colonoscopy and does not require sedation. It is limited by only having a diagnostic role.

The technique of double-contrast barium enema is discussed in Chapter 3. Abnormalities seen on a contrast enema may be classified as to whether the lumen

---

WHAT TO LOOK FOR   Box 13.1

*on a DCBE
in colorectal investigation*

Luminal narrowing
- Spasm:
  – often associated with diverticular disease
  – smooth concentric narrowing
  – not a constant feature during observation
  – generally abolished by administration of Buscopan®
- Benign disease:
  – tapered ends
  – smooth outline
  – variable length
- Inflammatory bowel disease:
  – Crohn's strictures have predilection for ileocaecal area
  – often associated with mucosal ulceration
- Ischaemic strictures
  – usually centered between splenic flexure and sigmoid colon
- Diverticular disease:
  – look for presence of diverticula
  – may be difficult to distinguish from neoplastic lesion
  – usually in sigmoid colon
- Malignant disease:
  – shouldered edges (apple core appearance)
  – irregular lumen often with loss of mucosal detail
  – rarely >6 cm in length

- Extrinsic compression:
  – smooth with normal mucosa
  – may displace bowel from normal position
  – look for an adjacent mass/gas within an abscess

Filling defects/mucosal abnormality

- Benign disease:
  – individual polyps
  – polyposis syndromes
  – inflammatory pseudopolyps
  – diverticulae
- Malignant disease:
  – polypoidal mass with irregular surface
  – projections into wall of bowel, gives shaggy appearance to normally smooth colonic mucosal outline.
- Ulceration:
  – loss of mucosal line

Contrast outside the lumen

- Fistulae (colovesical, colovaginal, etc.)
- Anastomotic leak
- Sinus and fissures
- Perforation (barium enema contraindicated if perforation suspected)

---

is narrowed, obstructed, contains filling defects or there is extravasation of contrast outside its confines. The barium study should always be complemented by sigmoidoscopy because lesions of the rectum and rectosigmoid can be difficult to identify on enema alone.

Gastrografin® enema

Gastrografin® may be preferred as a contrast agent when it is not feasible to perform bowel preparation. The major use is in acute large bowel obstruction (LBO) as a diagnostic tool to confirm the presence of a mechanical obstruction prior to surgery or decompression. The material does not coat the mucosa as well as barium and hence mucosal detail may be lost. Other comparisons between barium and Gastrografin® are discussed in Chapter 3. Gastrografin® can be used to:

- confirm the presence, site and nature of an LBO
- diagnose 'pseudo-obstruction' by excluding mechanical LBO
- determine the integrity of left sided colonic anastomosis.

Defecating proctogram

This procedure may be performed as an adjunct to investigation of faecal incontinence, rectal prolapse, sphinter and pelvic floor disorders. It is a specialist investigation that should be used and ordered only by practitioners with a special interest in this area because it needs to be interpreted in conjunction with the clinical examination.

Endoanal ultrasound

This investigation has a role in the assessment of a number of anorectal disorders (see Chapter 5). In conjunction with anal manometery and pudendal nerve testing it can be used in the evaluation of faecal incontinence. The internal sphincter and external sphincter can easily be differentiated and the presence of sphincter tears in either can be assessed. It can be used to evaluate rectal lesions to differentiate benign from malignant, the depth of invasion and the presence of lymph node enlargement. Endoanal ultrasound is also useful in the staging of rectal carcinoma and assessment of complex anal fistulas. The small rotating probe inside a water filled balloon (rectal) or plastic cap (anal) is inserted via the anal canal. Real-time images are generated and the procedure is operator dependent.

Virtual (CT) colonoscopy or colonography

CT colonography has been advocated as a replacement for screening colonoscopy (see Chapter 23). The images obtained by CT are then computer manipulated to enable three-dimensional visualization of the colonic lumen. CT colonography can reliably detect lesions measuring 5 mm or more. Currently the patient requires a bowel preparation and rectal intubation for air insufflation and as such, it does not yet offer much advantage over conventional colonoscopy. The use of a faecal tagging substance (barium solution) taken orally to reduce the need for a rigorous bowel preparation is being evaluated. This is still combined with a low residue diet and laxative medication to reduce the faecal loading of the colon. Several reports show improved specificity for polyp differentiation and comparable sensitivity with non-statistical improvement in patient acceptance of the procedure. Virtual colonoscopy is reported to offer a sensitivity for polyps greater than 1 cm in size of between 80 and 100%, comparable to a 95% sensitivity for colonoscopy. An area of particular interest is 'flat polyps' as these are held to be associated with an increased risk of dysplasia. 'Flat polyps' are commonly found in association with hereditary non-polyposis syndrome.

Virtual colonoscopy is frequently performed using 'ultra-low dose' irradiation (e.g. as little as 3 Sv). However one of the drawbacks of this technique is the inability to characterise extracolonic lesions, reported as being 'significant' in up to 12% of patients. MR colonography is an attractive alternative as it is non-ioninsing. However, experience to date has been disappointing as MR has lower resolution than CT. MR colonography also requires the patient to retain a liquid gadolinium enema for the duration of the examination and there are difficulties with achieving adequate bowel distension.

The procedure has been advocated to replace DCBE in those patients in whom colonoscopy cannot be completed. If this can be performed on the same day it avoids the need for a second bowel preparation.

The role of colonography is yet to be established but is an evolving technique which will see an increasing role in screening in the future. Most likely it will be reserved for asymptomatic patients rather than symptomatic patients or patients positive on faecal occult blood testing. These patients would be best served by colonoscopy as the first choice because of its therapeutic potential.

Advantages of virtual colonography are:

- no sedation is required
- the risk of colonic perforation is reduced to negligible levels (rectal intubation still required)
- colonoscopy can be limited to those requiring intervention.

Current limitations of virtual colonography are:

- bowel preparation still required
- time/equipment/computing constraints.

Computed tomography

Increasing speed and resolution of CT scanners with the ability to manipulate images has seen an expansion in the use of this imaging modality in colorectal diseases in both the emergency and elective setting. CT is a particularly useful investigation in inflammatory and neoplastic colorectal disease as it provides information about colonic and extracolonic manifestations (such as abscess, fistula or metastases) that might impact on management. In some settings, CT can be used to guide percutaneous drainage of abscess collections, obviating the need for surgery.

Oral and intravenous contrast studies are usually used for abdominal imaging (see Chapter 4). If colonic disease is suspected it is important to opacify the entire colon. Therefore oral contrast may be given the night before the scan with a second dose prior to the study. If required, positive contrast agents or air can be administered via the rectum to optimize visualization of the lower colon and rectum.

In particular, CT is used (Box 13.2) to:

- help define the site and nature of large bowel obstruction
- assess patients with diverticulitis when the diagnosis is in doubt or complications such as abscess are suspected
- to stage colorectal cancer.

WHAT TO LOOK FOR Box 13.2

on the CT scan in colorectal examination

- Presence or absence of obstruction
- Presence of diverticulae
- Stranding of pericolic fat/abscess formation
- Site and extent of any primary neoplasm
- If a primary neoplasm is present:
  – locoregional lymph node involvement
  – hepatic metastases
  – ascites
  – peritoneal and/or omental deposits

Magnetic resonance imaging

MRI is most useful in the assessment of complicated perianal sepsis, staging of anorectal cancers (Figs 13.1 and 13.2) and in differentiating liver lesions identified on staging investigations for colorectal cancer. Its use in the assessment of rectal prolapse is evolving.

Indications for magnetic resonance imaging

- complicated perianal sepsis especially fistulae in Crohn's disease (Figs 13.3 and 13.4)
- staging anorectal cancers
- characterising possible liver metastases when there is diagnostic difficulty.

Radionuclide scanning

These investigations (Figs 13.5 and 13.6) form part of the management of patients with lower gastrointestinal haemorrhage and those with motility disorders (slow transit constipation) (see Chapter 7).

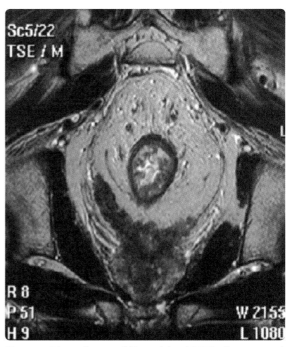

Fig. 13.1 Normal coronal T2-weighted MRI of rectum and mesorectum.

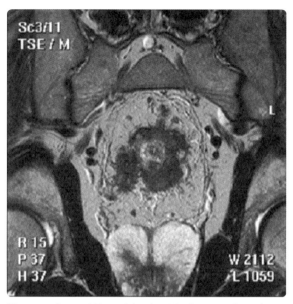

Fig. 13.2 Coronal T2-weighted MRI of a case of rectal cancer showing extension to the mesorectum and enlarged mesorectal lymph nodes.

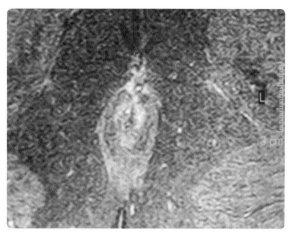

Fig. 13.4 Axial STIR MRI of same case showing fistula crossing the sphincter mechanism in the midline anteriorly (arrow).

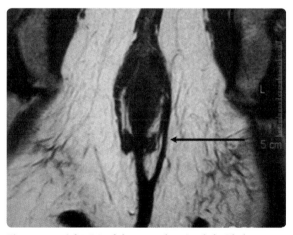

Fig. 13.3 Axial MRI of the anus showing left sided extrasphincteric fistula track (arrow).

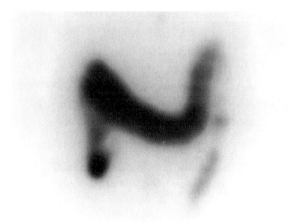

Fig. 13.5 Radionuclide scan showing delayed transit through the right colon.

Angiography

The use of angiography in colorectal disorders is mainly confined to the diagnosis and treatment (embolisation) of colonic haemorrhage (see Chapter 15).

THE CLINICAL PROBLEMS

Large bowel obstruction

Plain imaging

In patients with large bowel obstruction the initial imaging investigation will be a plain abdominal radiograph. This will help assess the:

- calibre of both small and large bowel
- distribution of gas in the colon

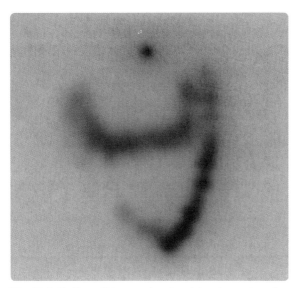

Fig. 13.6 Radionuclide scan showing delayed transit and retained tracer in the left colon.

- presence or absence of gas in the rectum (Fig. 13.7)
- degree of proximal colonic dilatation
- any associated small bowel dilatation
- presence of free gas.

Contrast studies

Generally, the further investigation of a patient with suspected large bowel obstruction will include a single-contrast enema. This study is primarily to show the site of obstruction (or lack of it, i.e. pseudo-obstruction) and the best and safest material for this is Gastrografin®. In certain circumstances a CT scan with rectal contrast may be an acceptable alternative.

Water-soluble material is best (i.e. Gastrografin®) if obstruction is suspected on the plain film (Fig. 13.8). If no obstruction is identified then the therapeutic effect of the osmolality of the gastrografin often will help with the resolution of the pseudo-obstruction.

Therapeutic options

The use of colonic stenting is discussed in Chapter 9.

Inflammatory bowel disease

Traditionally, contrast studies have been used to diagnose inflammatory bowel disease. Although contrast

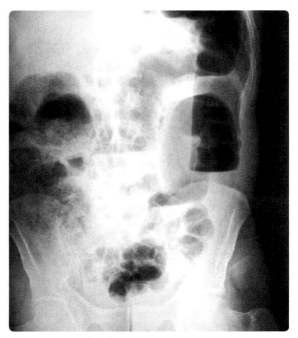

Fig. 13.7 Large bowel obstruction secondary to a stenotic lesion at the rectosigmoid junction. There is little gas in the rectum.

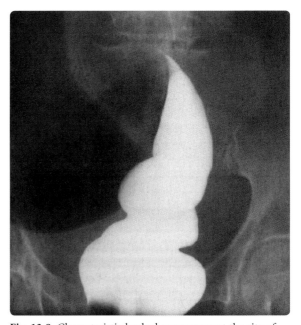

Fig. 13.8 Characteristic beaked appearance at the site of obstruction in a sigmoid volvulus. Gastrografin® is the contrast of choice as the use of barium in these circumstances makes endoscopic assessment and decompression difficult.

studies provide detailed mucosal definition they do not provide information about extraluminal disease, knowledge about which may be important for both diagnosis and management. Radiological investigation now plays a subsidiary role to endoscopic evaluation of most patients with inflammatory bowel disease except in the emergency setting. CT is used predominantly in the diagnosis and management of complications such as fistulae or abscesses. The potential problems of toxic dilatation, perforation and fistula formation are usually best managed by a combination of clinical judgement and the appropriate radiological investigation. Serial plain abdominal radiographs are used to monitor the potential development of a toxic megacolon in the setting of acute severe colitis. When the diameter of the transverse colon exceeds 8 cm there is a substantial risk of colon perforation and the patient warrants consideration of surgical intervention (Fig. 13.9).

CT scanning can also be valuable in the assessment of complicated inflammatory bowel disease. The colon can be assessed for thickening of the wall and strictures

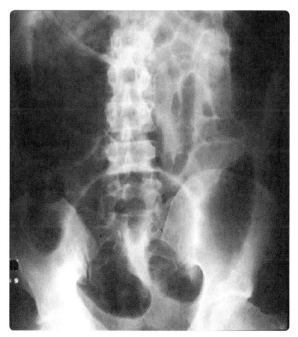

Fig. 13.9 Toxic dilatation of the colon. The diameter of the right colon exceeds 8 cm and the structure is in imminent danger of perforation.

in small and large bowel may be discernable. CT patterns of bowel thickening have been shown to correlate histologically with inflammatory activity in Crohn's disease. Layered enhancement of the bowel wall with strong mucosal enhancement and prominent low density submucosa is strongly predictive of active disease. A more homogenous pattern of bowel wall thickening is seen in quiescent disease. Abscesses and fistulae complicating Crohn's disease can also be evaluated and percutaneous drainage of any abscesses considered.

Crohn's colitis can be difficult to assess colonoscopically when there is stenosis and stricture formation. In this setting virtual colonography (by either CT or MRI) may have a role as it enables visualization above the stenotic segment. Both virtual colonography and barium enema remain inferior to colonoscopy in the assessment of ulcerated lesions.

Perianal disease

Endoscopic ultrasound (EUS) is a useful modality to evaluate perirectal and perianal complications of Crohn's disease (see Chapter 5). EUS provides more accurate anatomical information than fistulography, CT and can guide surgical intervention. Efforts to use EUS to differentiate Crohn's colitis from ulcerative colitis on the basis of transmural or superficial inflammation have so far been disappointing. EUS also has a role in monitoring perianal disease in patients treated with infliximab.

Diverticular disease

The CT scan can be used to confirm the diagnosis of diverticulitis where the clinical scenario is atypical. A presentation of left iliac fossa pain alone is common and, without the concomitant elevated temperature and white cell count, the diagnosis may be in question. In this setting, a CT can be useful in confirming or refuting a diagnosis of acute diverticulitis. A CT is not required except when the diagnosis is in doubt or there is a suspicion of complications such as an abscess.

On CT diverticulosis appears as multiple small, air-filled outpouchings, usually most prominent in the sigmoid colon. The wall of the involved segment of colon may be thickened due to muscle hypertrophy. The typical appearances of inflammation such as streaking of the mesenteric fat planes, oedema of the colon and surrounding tissues adjacent to an area of colon affected by the diverticular disease are diagnostic in the presence of diverticula (Fig. 13.10). There may be extravasation of contrast, if administered rectally (Fig. 13.11), and extracolonic gas indicating perforation. Fistula into adjacent organs, most notably bladder,

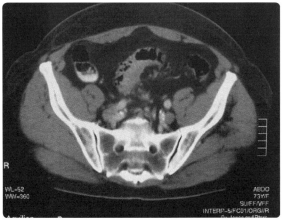

Fig. 13.10 CT scan showing a thickened sigmoid colon with oedema and fat stranding.

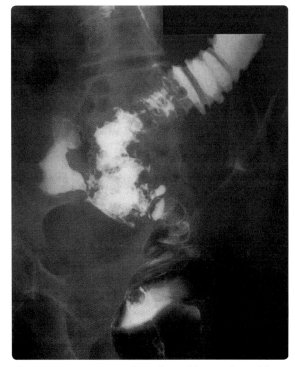

Fig. 13.11 A contrast study performed in a patient with acute diverticulitis. There is extravasation of contrast.

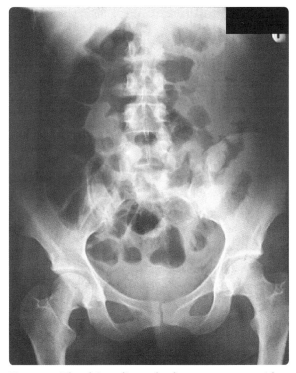

Fig. 13.12 The plain radiograph of a young woman with ischaemic colitis. The characteristic 'thumb printing' appearance of oedematous colon can be seen in the left upper quadrant.

may be identified. The features of colovesical fistula are discussed in Chapter 14.

In severe diverticular disease it may not be possible to differentiate between diverticulitis and bowel cancer on imaging features alone. The presence of lymphadenopathy in the pericolic nodes is highly suggestive of malignancy but imaging should not be considered diagnostic is this setting.

Ischaemic colitis

The characteristic imaging feature of ischaemic colitis is 'thumbprinting', which may be visible on the plain radiograph, most commonly in the region of the splenic flexure (Fig. 13.12). The presentation is generally such that colonoscopic investigation is performed without radiology but in more severe cases a CT scan may be performed.

Characteristic features on CT are circumferential, symmetric wall thickening of the affected segment of colon with enlargement of the folds. There may be evidence of intramural haemorrhage and inflammatory change in the pericolic fat. Gas may be seen within the bowel wall, mesenteric veins and portal venous system of the liver (see Chapter 10). In cases of occlusive ischaemia, thrombus may be visible in the superior mesenteric vessels. In an elderly patient with cardiovascular risk factors, ischaemic proctosigmoiditis is sometimes noted as an incidental finding on CT. This diagnosis would be suggested by isolated rectosigmoid wall thickening in association with stranding of the perirectal fat.

Colorectal cancer

Preoperative staging

Imaging is used in the preoperative staging of rectal malignancy to identify:

- the extent of local disease
- invasion into adjacent organs
- presence of lymph nodes and distant metastases.

Endorectal ultrasound is the staging tool of choice to determine the depth of rectal tumour invasion and assess nodal metastases (see Chapter 5). Accurate T staging of rectal cancer influences the treatment and allows assessment of rectal cancer with the view to patient selection for neo-adjuvant therapy. Newer surgical options, such as trans-anal endoscopic microsurgery also require accurate T staging to select patients with T0 or T1 disease. Pelvic MRI is also very useful in the assessment of rectal cancer, and can assist in surgical planning and assessment of resectability.

Preoperative staging with CT scanning is less important with colonic malignancies. Primary tumour staging with CT colonography is accurate in over 95% of patients but this procedure does not allow for biopsy and histological confirmation of malignancy. The identification of distant metastases may influence decision making in frail, elderly patients or those with suspected extensive liver metastases where resection of the primary lesion may not provide sufficient long term benefit to the patient.

Radiological surveillance/detection of metastatic disease

No proven benefit has been shown for routine scanning in follow-up of colorectal cancer. This is generally reserved for suspicion of recurrence either clinically or on blood examination (LFTs or CEA).

CT is the most widely used modality to assess patients with metastatic or recurrent colorectal cancer. The overall accuracy of CT and MRI in detecting recurrent colorectal cancer is 90–95%. The differentiation between recurrent tumour and scar tissue is problematic on CT and MRI is useful in this setting. More recently PET and PET-CT have been advocated (see Chapter 8). The role of PET has yet to be established but it may be useful in patients who have a rising CEA but indeterminate findings on imaging.

Screening

The role of imaging in screening for colorectal cancer is discussed in Chapter 23.

Faecal incontinence

Anorectal ultrasound (see Chapter 5) is the radiological investigation of choice in the assessment of the integrity of the anal sphincters (Figs 13.13 and 13.14). However, it is an operator-dependent procedure and needs to be interpreted in conjunction with the clinical findings and other appropriate investigations such as pudendal nerve terminal motor latency and anal manometry. In addition to defects in the internal and/or external sphincters, anorectal ultrasound will

Normal   Ruptured

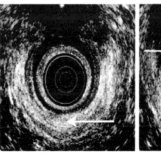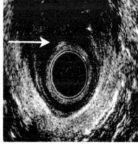

Fig. 13.13 Normal anal ultrasound (left) and the picture on the right showing disruption of external and internal sphincters anteriorly. The arrow on the left picture points to the external sphincter and the arrow on the right picture identifies the point of disruption of the internal and external sphincters.

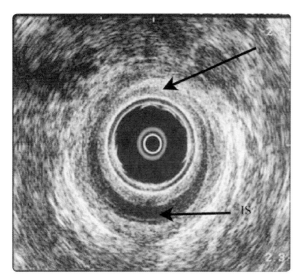

Fig. 13.14 Ultrasound showing disruption of internal sphincter (IS) after stapled haemorrhoidectomy. The upper arrow points to the damaged sphincter.

also demonstrate thinning of the perineal body, which is associated particularly with obstetric trauma.

Perianal disease

Imaging is used in perianal disease to demonstrate internal openings and complex fistula tracts which may not be evident on clinical examination (see Chapter 14). The role of imaging in the assessment of Crohn's perianal disease is discussed above.

MRI (see Chapter 6) and EUS (see Chapter 5) are useful tools in assessing complex perianal fistulae. More recently ultrasound using Levovist® contrast has been advocated. The use of Levovist® contrast significantly improves the accuracy (85%) compared with conventional ultrasound (25%). Trials are needed to compare the relative value of Levovist®, hydrogen peroxide and MRI in imaging complex perianal disease.

Further reading

Allison JE, Tekawa IS, Ransom LJ, Adrain AL. A comparison of fecal occult blood testes for colorectal cancer screening. N Engl J Med 1996; 334:155–9

Aviv RI, Shyamalan G, Watkinson A et al. Radiological palliation of malignant colonic obstruction. Clin Radiol 2002; 57(5):347–51

Blakeborough A, Sheridan MB, Chapman AH. Complications of barium enema examinations: a survey of UK consultant radiologists 1992–1994. Clin Rad 1997; 52:142

Bragg DG, Rubin P, Hricak H. Oncologic imaging, 2nd edn. WB Saunders, Philadelphia, 2002

Callstrom MR, Johnson CD, Fletcher JG et al. CT colonography without cathartic preparation: feasibility study. Radiology 2001; 219:693–8

Chaoui AS, Blake MA, Barish MA et al. Virtual colonoscopy and colorectal cancer screening. Abdominal Imaging 2000; 25:361–7

Chew SS, Yang JL, Newstead GL, Douglas PR. Anal fistula: Levovist-enhanced endoanal ultrasound: a pilot study. Dis Colon Rectum 2003; 46(3):377–84

Choi D, Jin Lee S, Ah Cho Y et al. Bowel wall thickening in patients with Crohn's disease: CT patterns and correlation with inflammatory activity. Clin Radiol 2003; 58:68–74

Dachman AH, Yoshida H. Virtual colonoscopy: past, present and future. Radiol Clin N Am 2003; 43:377–93

Dobos N, Rubesin SE. Radiologic imaging modalities in the diagnosis and management of colorectal cancer. Hematol Onocol Clin North Am 2002; 16:875–95

Fenlon HM, Nunes DP, Schroy P et al. A comparison of virtual and conventional colonoscopy for the detection of colorectal polyps. N Engl J Med 1999; 341: 496–503

Fletcher J, Johnson C, Welch T et al. Optimization of CT colonography technique: Prospective trial in 180 patients. Radiology 2000; 216:704–11

Horton KM, Corl FM, Fishman EK. CT evaluation of the colon: inflammatory disease. Radiographics 2000; 20: 399–418

Jensen J, Kewenter J, Asztely M et al. Double contrast barium enema and flexible retrosigmoidoscopy: A reliable diagnostic combination of colorectal neoplasm. Br J Surg 1990; 77:270

Keymling M. Colorectal stenting. Endoscopy 2003; 35(3): 234–8

Laghi A, Iannaccone R, Trenna S et al. Multislice spiral CT colonography in the evaluation of colorectal neoplasms. Radiol Med (Torino) 2002; 104(5–6):394–403

Lefere PA, Gryspeerdt SS, Dewyspelaere J et al. Dietary fecal tagging as a cleansing method before CT colonography: initial results polyp detection and patient acceptance. Radiology 2002; 224:393–403

Macari M, Bini EJ, Jacobs SL et al. Significance of missed polyps at CT colonography. Am J Roentgenol 2004; 183:127–34

Mendelson RM, Forbes GM. Computed tomography colonography (virtual colonoscopy): review. Aust Radiol 2002; 46:1–12

Mendelson RM, Foster NM, Edwards JT et al. Virtual colonoscopy compared with conventional colonoscopy; a developing technology. Med J Aust 2000; 173:472–5

National Health and Medical Research Council. Guidelines for the prevention, early detection and management of colorectal cancer. Available at http://www.nhmrc.gov.au/publications/pdf/cp62.pdf [accessed June 2004]

Nicholson FB, Korman MG, Stern AI. Distribution of colorectal adenomas: implications for bowel cancer screening. Med J Aust 2000; 172:428–30

Ota Y, Matsui T, Ono H et al. Value of virtual computed tomographic colonography for Crohn's colitis: comparison with endoscopy and barium enema. Abdom Imaging 2003; 28:778–83

Pappalardo G, Polettini E, Frattaroli FM et al. Magnetic resonance colonography versus conventional colonography for detection of colonic endoluminal lesions. Gastroenterology 2000; 119:300–4

Scholefield JH, Moss S, Sufi F et al. Effect of faecal occult blood screening on mortality from colorectal cancer: results from a randomised controlled trial. Gut 2002; 50:840–4

Selby JV, Friedman GD, Quesenberry CP, Weiss NS. A case control study of screening sigmoidoscopy and mortality from colorectal cancer. N Engl J Med 1992; 326:653–7

Stoker J, Rociu E, Wiersma TG, Lameris JS. Imaging of anorectal disease. Br J Surg 2000; 87(1):10–27

Thoeni RF. Colorectal cancer. Radiologic staging. Radiol Clin North Am 1997; 35(2):457–85

Tjandra JJ, Sissons GR. Magnetic resonance imaging facilitates assessment of perianal Crohn's disease. Aust N Z J Surg 1994; 64(7):470–4

Yee J. Screening CT colonography. Semin Ultrasound, CT MRI 2003; 24:12–22

Gastrointestinal fistulae

P. Rabbitt

14

Background

The role of radiology in the management of a gastrointestinal fistula is to:

- confirm the clinical suspicion of a fistula
- localise the site and level
- identify factors that may prevent spontaneous closure e.g. malignancy, distal obstruction, inflammatory bowel disease
- identify any associated pathology, e.g. mass, abscess

THE RADIOLOGICAL INVESTIGATIONS

Contrast studies

These are the traditional radiological methods for investigating gastrointestinal fistulae and involve the use of contrast media with fluoroscopic imaging. The choice of contrast material will vary according to the site, evidence of perforation and likelihood of surgery, and will be either barium or a water-soluble iodinated contrast (see Chapter 3). If surgery is planned, the patient is obstructed, or there is evidence of pneumoperitoneum, large volumes of barium should be avoided. Of high importance is clear communication between the surgeon and the radiologist of what information is required from the contrast study as there are often a number of ways of performing the procedure.

In patients with gastrointestinal fistulae, the contrast material may be administered:

- orally
- via oroenteric tube
- per rectum
- per vagina
- via the fistula ('sinogram')

While fluoroscopic studies have traditionally been the 'gold standard' and remain a valuable tool, advances in cross-sectional imaging mean they are less commonly used as a 'first line' investigation.

Computed tomography

This mode of imaging may be combined with contrast administered orally, rectally or occasionally cutaneously to demonstrate a fistula. Although CT may not always show the fistulae as well as a contrast study, it has higher sensitivity for enterovesical fistulae. It also has the advantage of providing other imaging information, such as the presence of an abscess adjacent to the suspected fistulous tract. This is particularly useful in the assessment of a suspected postoperative fistula, where the CT can be used to guide percutaneous drainage. If a CT scan is to be undertaken, it should be performed before any barium examination, as the latter contrast will cause significant artefact on CT.

Ultrasound

Endoanal ultrasound has been used to identify the presence and location of fistulous tracts in relation to the anal sphincter complex in the management of perianal sepsis. The addition of hydrogen peroxide to facilitate visualisation has been reported to improve the accuracy of detection and classification, although its use remains controversial.

Magnetic resonance imaging

MRI is increasingly used to investigate complex perianal fistulae and has been shown to have a high accuracy in determining the anatomy of a fistula (see Chapter 13). The main use of MRI in preoperative assessment is to identify unsuspected areas of sepsis and to define the relationship of the fistula to the anal sphincter complex. Areas of sepsis will appear as foci of fluid intensity and the accurate depiction of perianal anatomy enables tracts to be identified in relation to the internal and external anal sphincters and levator muscles.

THE CLINICAL PROBLEMS

Enterocutaneous fistulae

Whilst there are many causes of enterocutaneous fistulae, those of most relevance to the surgeon are Crohn's fistulae and those that develop as a complication of surgery. The higher up the digestive tract the fistula occurs, the more troublesome it is likely to prove. In dealing with a leak or fistula, the information that the surgeon requires to help management will include:

- evidence that the leak is controlled (i.e. that there is no spillage into adjacent structures)
- the volume and content of any fluid loss
- evidence of any distal obstruction
- anything that suggests prompt surgical or radiological intervention may be required (e.g. a fluid collection, septic shock).

Decisions on intervention will depend on the general state of health of the patient and the degree to which the fistula is hindering postoperative progress. In other words, a low output controlled fistula from the distal gut will usually be managed conservatively, whereas leak of duodenal contents may demand intervention. Contrast studies by themselves, or combined with CT, will usually provide the radiological answers for the surgeon.

The approach depends on the likely gastrointestinal site of fistulous formation. For assessment of a fistula following colonic resection a water-soluble contrast enema (e.g. Gastrografin®) will give the most reliable information as they are mostly related to anastomotic leakage. Oral contrast would not reach the site in sufficient concentration and pressure to reliably demonstrate the tract. A fistula related to the upper gastrointestinal tract or small bowel may be assessed by injecting contrast directly into the tract, or using oral contrast for a small bowel series. While a contrast study may provide more information regarding the level of the fistula, a CT will also demonstrate any associated abscess requiring intervention (Box 14.1).

WHAT TO LOOK FOR   Box 14.1

on a contrast study or CT of a fistula

- Confirmation of the fistula
- Site of origin of the fistula
- Any association with an anastomosis
- Flow of contrast through the remainder of the bowel lumen
- Any associated abscess collection or cavity filling with contrast

Anal fistulae

Most anal fistulae develop secondary to local sepsis and a small percentage are the result of Crohn's disease. Endoanal ultrasound is reported to give identical information to MRI with an experienced operator, but where available MRI scanning should be considered, particularly for complex fistulae (see Chapter 13). Delineation of fistulae, abscesses and secondary tracts and the anatomical relations using MRI enables pre-operative planning of surgical strategy to successfully treat recurrent, complex or Crohn's related perianal sepsis. With the recent introduction of TNF-α for the management of Crohn's fistulae, the role of radiological investigation has assumed increased importance. Accurate imaging allows patients suitable for non-operative management to be selected and their treatment response monitored (Box 14.2).

Various enhancements to MRI imaging have been advocated to increase the sensitivity of this investigation. The use of intravenous gadolinium may improve the specificity of MRI as this only highlights those tracts with granulation tissue and active inflammation rather than all areas of both current and previous inflammation. If read by an experienced radiologist, the sensitivity of MRI in detecting fistulous openings and secondary tracts is said to rival that of direct surgical exploration. However, its use in the management of simple low, cryptoglandular sepsis and fistula is superfluous to thorough examination under anaesthesia.

Internal fistulae

Although fistulae can occur between any two epithelialised surfaces, the only ones commonly encountered in the digestive tract are:

- enterocolic
- colovesical
- colovaginal
- rectovaginal.

Enterocolic fistulae

Many of these present with interesting radiological findings (e.g. Crohn's enterocolic fistulae), but are of little clinical significance. However some, such as those related to diverticular disease, present with problems that require surgical intervention. A small bowel series or contrast enema is used depending upon the level of bowel involved. In the case of an enteroenteric fistula it is necessary to perform frequent fluoroscopic assessment so as not to miss the site of the fistula. It is often very difficult to detect these fistulae on CT.

Colovesical and colovaginal fistulae

Colovesical fistulae are usually related to obstetric complications, inflammatory bowel disease or gynaecological malignancy. Clinically they are implied by recurrent urinary tract infection and pneumaturic. An unusual finding is a large volume of air in the bladder, visible on the plain radiograph (Fig. 14.1) or CT. These

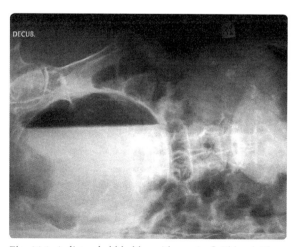

Fig. 14.1 A distended bladder with an air–fluid level. The patient had a colovesical fistula secondary to diverticular disease.

> ### WHAT TO LOOK FOR
> **Box 14.2**
>
> #### *on MRI of gastrointestinal fistulae*
>
> - Define the normal anatomy, e.g. sphincters
> - Define the tract:
>   - single or multiple
>   - the presence of any secondary tracts
>   - any traverse of the tract across the external sphincter or levator ani muscles
> - Any associated collections

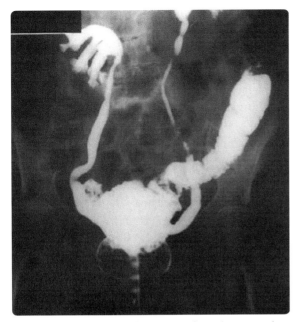

Fig. 14.2 Colovesical fistula. Contrast from the rectum has entered the bladder and refluxed up both ureters.

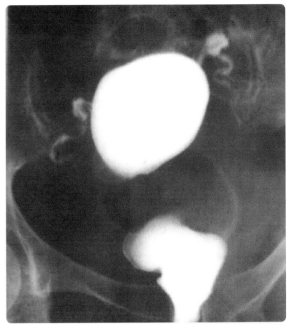

Fig. 14.3 A rectouterine fistula in a young woman with Crohn's disease. Contrast has been instilled into the rectum and has entered the uterus and salpinges.

fistulae can be difficult to positively identify on a contrast enema unless there is a large communication (Fig. 14.2). Occasionally fistulae may be seen when contrast is inserted into the vagina. Indirect signs on CT such as gas or gastrointestinal contrast within the vagina are almost diagnostic, and the underlying cause may also be demonstrated.

Colovaginal fistulae usually occur in the setting of a diverticular abscess that has decompressed via the vaginal vault in women who have had a hysterectomy. Another well-recognised but less common cause is Crohn's disease (Fig. 14.3). Conventional contrast enemas have a high false-negative rate but CT has been reported to have sensitivities as high as 90–100%, although it often relies on indirect signs. Air in the bladder in a patient who has not been catheterised and focal bladder or bowel wall thickening are highly suggestive. The use of rectal contrast increases sensitivity. Other findings such as radiation changes, contiguous pelvic mass, or adherent thickened bowel provide useful information about the aetiology of the fistula and help plan surgical repair.

NEW DEVELOPMENTS

The recent development of fibrin sealants offers new interventional radiological possibilities for the management of fistulae and sinuses, with moderate success rates for complex fistulae. The fibrin sealant can be introduced via a double lumen catheter directly into the fistula tract under radiological control.

Further reading

Brady AP, Malone DE, Deignan RW et al. Fibrin sealant in interventional radiology: a preliminary evaluation. Radiology. 1995; 196:573–8

Buchanan GN, Bartram CI, Phillips RK et al. Efficacy of fibrin sealant in the management of complex anal fistula: a prospective trial. Dis Colon Rectum 2003; 46:1167–74

Halligan S, Buchanan G. MR imaging of fistula-in-ano. Eur J Radiol 2003; 47:98–107

Henrich W, Meckies J, Friedmann W. Demonstration of a recto-vaginal fistula with the ultrasound contrast medium Echovist. Ultrasound Obstet Gynecol 2000; 15:148–9

Kuhlman JE, Fishman EK. CT evaluation of enterovaginal and vesicovaginal fistulas. J Comput Assist Tomogr 1990; 14:390–4

Maconi G, Sampietro GM, Parente F et al. Contrast radiology, computed tomography and ultrasonography in detecting internal fistulas and intra-abdominal abscesses in Crohn's disease: a prospective comparative study. Am J Gastroenterol 2003; 98:1545–55

Navarro-Luna A, Garcia-Domingo MI, Rius-Macias J, Marco-Molina C. Ultrasound study of anal fistulas with hydrogen peroxide enhancement. Dis Colon Rectum 2004; 47:108–14. Epub 2004 Jan 2005

Pickhardt PJ, Bhalla S, Balfe DM. Acquired gastrointestinal fistulas: classification, etiologies, and imaging evaluation. Radiology 2002; 224:9–23

Schwartz DA, Wiersema MJ, Dudiak KM et al. A comparison of endoscopic ultrasound, magnetic resonance imaging, and exam under anesthesia for evaluation of Crohn's perianal fistulas. Gastroenterology 2001; 121:1064–72

Sentovich SM. Fibrin glue for anal fistulas: long-term results. Dis Colon Rectum 2003; 46:498–502

Sudol-Szopinska I, Jakubowski W, Szczepkowski M. Contrast-enhanced endosonography for the diagnosis of anal and anovaginal fistulas. J Clin Ultrasound 2002; 30:145–50

Gastrointestinal bleeding

P. Worley, M. Muhlmann

15

Background

The management of patients with gastrointestinal bleeding should be multidisciplinary and involve gastroenterologists, surgeons and radiologists. Both endoscopy and radiology have had a major impact on the diagnosis and management of gastrointestinal bleeding. Therapeutic options have largely obviated the need for surgical intervention in many difficult clinical circumstances.

THE RADIOLOGICAL INVESTIGATIONS

Red cell scan

The radionuclide labeled red cell scan is a highly sensitive investigation and can detect bleeding at rates as low as 0.1 mL/min (see Chapter 7). It is non-invasive, easy to perform and patients can be scanned up to 24 hours after injection to detect intermittent bleeding (Fig. 15.1). If a scan is positive, most centres recommend angiography or endoscopy to further localise bleeding but in some cases localisation on red cell scan can lead directly to surgery (Box 15.1).

Other radionuclide studies

Radionuclide scans may also be used to look for:

- Meckel's diverticulum
- obscure anaemia (see Chapter 7).

Angiography

This can be used to localise bleeding for angiographic control or surgery (Box 15.2). It requires the patient to be actively bleeding at rates of greater than 0.5 mL/min and is often preceded by radionuclide scanning. Its reported accuracy varies between 40 and 92%. Arterial branches as small as 2 mm can be superselectively catheterised, a capability that has dramatically improved the efficacy and safety of therapeutic manoeuvres.

Vasopressin is associated with significant complications including intestinal and myocardial ischaemia and has a 50% rebleeding rate. 'Superselective' embolisation appears to have fewer ischaemic complications and a lower rebleeding rate. Angiographic intervention is used increasingly in the management of lower gastrointestinal haemorrhage and is the treatment of choice in frail or severely ill patients.

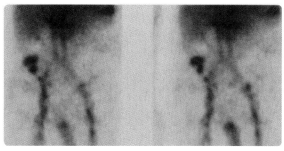

Fig. 15.1 This red cell scan, undertaken in a patient with colonic haemorrhage, shows pooling of isotope in the right side of the abdomen, consistent with a bleeding point in the right colon.

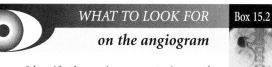

WHAT TO LOOK FOR   Box 15.1

on the red cell scan

- Focus of activity outside normal vascular pool conforming to bowel anatomy
- Increasing intensity of activity over time
- Localisation of bleeding to one side
- Anterograde and retrograde peristalsis

WHAT TO LOOK FOR   Box 15.2

on the angiogram

- Identify the major mesenteric vessels
- Is the scan selective?
- Pooling or extravasation of contrast
- A vascular tuft or early draining vein: angiodysplasia
- Contrast in a small pocket: diverticulum
- Hypervascular 'blush': tumours

Angiographic techniques to control bleeding include:

- drug-induced vasoconstriction
- embolisation.

Digital subtraction carbon dioxide ($DSA-CO_2$) angiography has also been proposed for the investigation of gastrointestinal bleeding. However, studies show that despite its potential advantage of avoiding contrast in a haemodynamically unstable patient, it is inferior to traditional iodinated contrast angiography.

Push enteroscopy

Push enteroscopy allows access to the proximal jejunum. Recent developments with video capsules (swallowed by the patient) have provided clinicians with endoscopic-like images of the small bowel. Preliminary studies have shown that this technique is able to localise 63% of small bowel lesions and that it is superior to barium studies.

CLINICAL PROBLEMS

Upper gastrointestinal haemorrhage

Radiology has a limited diagnostic role, but an important, if only occasional, therapeutic role. Most acute upper-digestive-tract bleeding problems are within range of the endoscope, which will identify the cause of the haemorrhage in more than 90% of cases. When intervention is required, some form of endoscopic manouevre (e.g. variceal banding or injection of bleeding ulcers) is usually sufficient.

The important therapeutic radiological procedures are:

- embolisation
- portosystemic decompression.

Embolisation should be considered in the following circumstances:

- bleeding lesion inaccessible to the endoscope
- bleeding despite endoscopic intervention
- patient unfit for surgical intervention.

Occasionally, patients may bleed massively from tumours and in such cases, embolisation of the feeding vessels may be more effective than an endoscopic approach to the bleeding tumour surface. Embolisation with microcoils can be effective in up to 88% of patients (see Chapter 9). Haemobilia is a rare cause of upper gastrointestinal haemorrhage and when it requires intervention, embolisation may be the only effective approach (Figs 15.2 and 15.3). Haemobilia may be secondary to trauma or aneurysm formation.

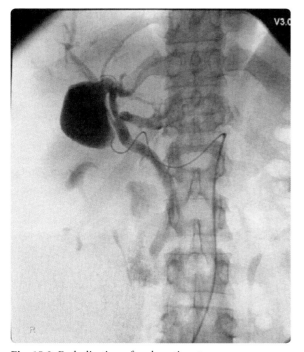

Fig. 15.2 Embolisation of an hepatic artery aneurysm. The patient presented with gastrointestinal bleeding and profuse haemobilia after a mycotic hepatic artery aneurysm had eroded into the biliary system. This image shows the aneurysm and its fistulous communication with the biliary tree. Some contrast has entered the duodenum.

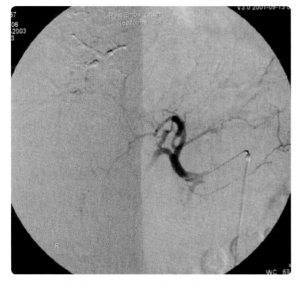

Fig. 15.3 This image was taken immediately after the feeding vessel was occluded with gelfoam. Contrast no longer enters the aneurysm.

A transjugular intrahepatic portosystemic shunt (TIPS) is a therapeutic option for massive and uncontrolled variceal haemorrhage. This radiological procedure is the treatment of choice, should the endoscopic approach fail to control bleeding (see Chapter 9). Surgical intervention in these cases is associated with mortality rates approaching 30%, but the figures associated with radiological decompression are little better. Surgery is reserved for those patients in Childs–Pugh category A or B, with good liver function and who bleed despite endoscopic efforts.

Lower gastrointestinal tract haemorrhage

Colonoscopy is usually the investigation of choice once a patient has been resuscitated, stabilised and examined with a rigid sigmoidoscope. Visualisation is often poor in the acute setting and imaging studies have a greater role here compared with the upper digestive tract. Both radionuclide scans and angiograms may be used to identify the site of bleeding and the latter investigation may also help determine the cause.

Obscure or unusual sites of gastrointestinal bleeding

There is a small group of patients who continue to bleed overtly from an unknown site despite thorough investigation of the upper and lower digestive tracts. Similarly, some patients will present with chronic iron deficiency anaemia and no gastrointestinal symptoms. In both groups, the small intestine is likely to require careful evaluation. Investigations may include:

- push enteroscopy
- video capsule
- radionuclide scanning
- angiography
- small bowel series.

Meckel's diverticulum

A Meckel's diverticulum arises from a persistent vitellointestinal duct and occurs in 2% of the population. About half of all Meckel's have ectopic gastric mucosa. This is an important cause of major gastrointestinal haemorrhage in children, but a relatively rare cause of blood loss in the adult. Bleeding may result from ulceration of the adjacent ileal mucosa secondary to acid secretion from the ectopic gastric mucosa. Intravenous

197

^{99m}technetium pertechnetate is actively absorbed by the normal gastric and any ectopic mucosa. When this is present in a Meckel's diverticulum, an area of focal radioactivity may be seen, usually in the right iliac fossa (Fig. 15.4). The scan is 90% sensitive. All that a Meckel's scan will reveal is the presence of ectopic gastric mucosa; not whether it is associated with any ulceration and bleeding – that is a clinical judgement.

Computed tomography colonography

'Virtual colonography' provides a means of accurately obtaining a full structural evaluation of the entire colon. Its place has yet to be defined in clinical use, and little is known of its role in the evaluation of haemorrhage from the lower digestive tract. It can be used to assess the colon where colonoscopy is contraindicated or unsuccessful. Currently, full bowel preparation is needed but the technique does have the advantage of the ability to detect extracolonic pathology. It is inappropriate in the emergency setting.

Other investigations in obscure gastrointestinal haemorrhage

Small bowel contrast studies have a low diagnostic yield (10–25%) but may pick up small bowel tumours or inflammatory bowel disease.

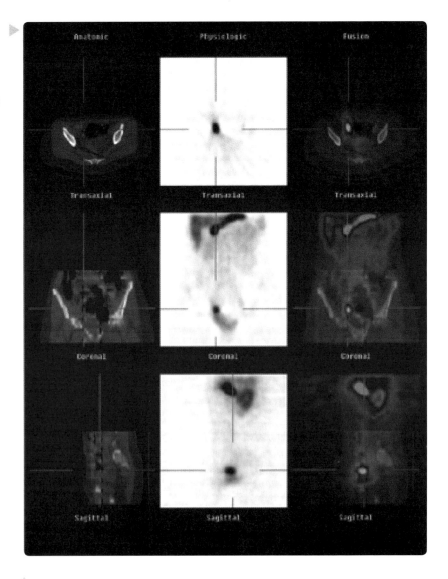

Fig. 15.4 Combined CT abdominal image 30 minutes after administration of Na ^{99m}TcO$_4$, showing uptake in a focus in the right lower quadrant consistent with gastric mucosa in Meckel's diverticulum. Note physiological uptake in stomach.

Occasionally, a CT scan will reveal an obscure cause for gastrointestinal haemorrhage, such as GIST tumours and intussusceptions of the small bowel.

The red cell scan is rarely diagnostic in low volume bleeding and is of little practical value in those patients who present with a chronic anaemia. The use of faecal excretion of ^{57}Cr autologous red cells is discussed in Chapter 7.

Angiography is only used when all other investigations have failed to reveal a site or cause and the patient continues to bleed. In this setting it is most useful in the detection of angiodysplasia, as it can do so without active bleeding.

Further reading

Ford PV, Bartold SP, Fink-Bennett DM et al. Procedure Guideline for Gastrointestinal Bleeding and Meckel's Diverticulum Scintigraphy. J Nucl Med 1999; 40:1226–32

Furaki B. Endovascular intervention for the treatment of acute arterial gastrointestinal haemorrhage. Gastroenterol Clin N Am 2002; 31:701–13

Ji H, Rolnick J, Haker S, Barrish MA. Multislice CT colonography: current status and limitations. Eur J Radiol 2003; 47:123–34

Lefkovitz Z, Cappell MS, Lookstein R et al. Radiologic diagnosis and treatment of gastrointestinal haemorrhage and ischaemia. Med Clin N Am 2002; 86:1357–99

Rosch J, Keller F. Transjugular intrahepatic portosystemic shunt: present status, comparison with endoscopic therapy and shunt surgery, and future perspectives. World J Surg 2001; 25:337–46

Royal Australasian College of Radiologists. Surgery without preoperative localisation results in more bowel resected, longer intraoperative time and greater morbidity and mortality. Imaging Guidelines, 4th edn. Royal Australasian College of Radiologists, Australia, 2001, p 118

Sandhu D, Buckenham TM, Belli AM. Using CO_2-enhanced arteriography to investigate acute gastrointestinal haemorrhage. Am J Roentol 1999; 173:1399–401

Scapa E, Jacob H, Lewkowicz S. Initial experience of wireless-capsule endoscopy for evaluating occult gastrointestinal bleeding and suspected small bowel pathology. Am J Gastroenterol 2002; 97:2776–9

The abdominal mass

16

A. Aly, M. Thomas

Background

Many abdominal masses may be managed upon clinical grounds alone, particularly those that are associated with a clear history or well defined physical signs. However, radiological imaging can be an invaluable asset in helping to determine the nature of a mass and increasing reliance is placed on this additional assessment. Abdominal masses may be classified in several ways:

- The underlying pathological process:
  - inflammation (e.g. pancreatitis)
  - infective (e.g. appendix or psoas abscess)
  - hypertrophy/hyperplasia (e.g. hepatomegaly, splenomegaly)
  - neoplastic (benign or malignant)
  - vascular (aneurysm, haematoma)
  - hernia
  - trauma (e.g. urinoma)
- The site:
  - abdominal wall
  - through the abdominal wall (i.e. hernias)
  - intraperitoneal
  - retroperitoneal
  - the organ of origin, particularly:
  - lymph nodes
    - liver
    - spleen
    - kidneys
    - bladder

THE RADIOLOGICAL INVESTIGATIONS

Plain radiology

Plain radiology is of limited value in the assessment of an abdominal mass. Occasionally a mass will show itself by:

- a poorly defined shadow (Fig. 16.1)
- alteration of gas patterns (displacement of bowel)
- obscuration of normal soft tissue outlines
- distended hollow viscus
- abnormal area of calcification (Fig. 16.2).

Ultrasound

Ultrasound is a valuable initial investigation in the assessment of the abdominal mass. The consistency of the mass as determined by ultrasound, will often give a clue to its underlying pathology. Cystic or fluid-filled masses with multiple heterogeneous internal echo

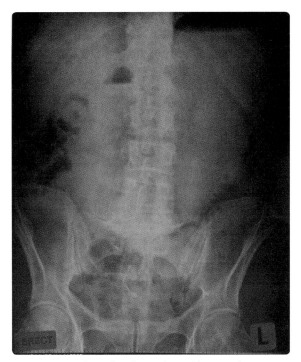

Fig. 16.1 Gastric outlet obstruction with a grossly distended stomach, full of food.

shadows may suggest necrosis, abscess formation or haematoma. Solid masses that are homogeneous and hyperechoic may well be neoplastic. Malignant masses tend to be poorly defined, with irregular or infiltrating margins. The addition of Doppler can help determine the vascularity of a mass.

The relationship of a mass to the abdominal wall and its layers is usually well defined by ultrasound since the distance from the probe is minimal. The layers of the abdominal wall are often well seen and the distinction between soft tissue masses, haematomata, abscesses and hernias is reasonably reliable. The dynamic nature of ultrasound may be helpful in confirming abdominal wall hernias by providing real time images of the hernia changing size with changes in abdominal pressure or manipulation (see Chapter 24).

Ultrasound provides good definition of masses related to the liver, spleen, kidneys, adrenals, bladder and ovaries (Fig. 16.3). It is of relatively limited value when the mass is in close proximity to a gas-filled structure, particularly when intestine intervenes between the probe and the structure to be studied (e.g. pancreas).

Laparoscopic and endoscopic ultrasound techniques have provided the surgeon with an important tool in the diagnosis and staging of intra-abdominal mass lesions. The ability to place the probe directly or very close to intra-abdominal organs and masses pro-

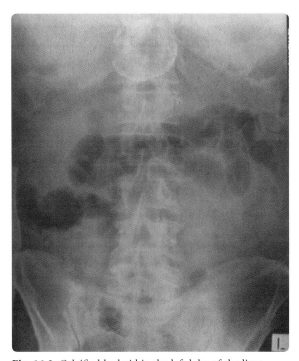

Fig. 16.2 Calcified hydatid in the left lobe of the liver.

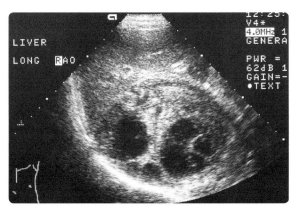

Fig. 16.3 Ultrasound examination of a mass in the liver showing a heterogenous cystic structure with a pattern characteristic of a hydatic cyst containing daughter cysts.

vides enhanced resolution images and greater diagnostic accuracy.

Ultrasound may also be used as a guide for fine-needle biopsy of an abdominal mass.

Computed tomography

Modern CT technology allows rapid acquisition of data with multiplanar and 3D reconstruction providing accurate definition of abdominal masses with regard to their:

- site
- relationship to adjacent structures
- compression
- infiltration
- morphology
- borders (well or ill-defined)
- internal structure and consistency (Fig. 16.4).

CT is far superior to ultrasound in its ability to localise and define intraperitoneal and retroperitoneal masses. The CT scan may detect changes other than those of the mass itself, which will help in the diagnosis (Fig. 16.5). These changes include local effects of the mass lesion (Box 16.1):

- Streaky changes in the surrounding fat or mesentery (inflammation)
- Luminal obstruction (e.g. colon, ureter).

Or more distant effects:

- Enlarged regional nodes (inflammation, malignancy)
- Distant disease (e.g. liver metastases)

Like ultrasound, CT is very useful in guiding needle biopsies of abdominal masses.

Magnetic resonance imaging

Where an abdominal wall mass is suspicious of a soft tissue tumour, MRI is the investigation of choice as it provides superior definition of fascial planes and distinction between adjacent structures (see Chapter 6). However, there is little evidence that MRI has any impact on outcomes (compared with CT scanning) in the management of these lesions.

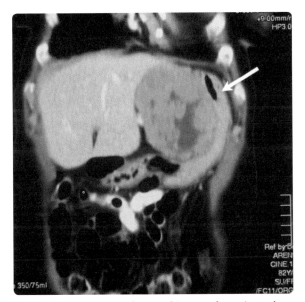

Fig. 16.4 A reconstructed coronal image of a patient who presented with anaemia and an ill-defined mass in the epigastrium. The scan shows a 10 cm heterogeneous mass adjacent to the left lobe of the liver and compressing the stomach (arrow). This is a gastrointestinal stromal tumour.

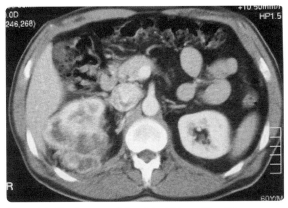

Fig. 16.5 Carcinoma of the right kidney. The CT scan shows a large irregular, lobulated mixed density mass arising from the posterior aspect of the mid and upper pole of the right kidney. The lesion shows heterogeneous contrast enhancement. It appears to be invading the perirenal fat and posteriorly, reaches the muscles of the abdominal wall. The IVC is dilated and there is a longitudinal filling defect within this vessel (confirmed on coronal reconstructions), which almost certainly represents tumour extension.

WHAT TO LOOK FOR Box 16.1

on the CT of an abdominal mass

- The distribution of oral contrast (if used)
- Intravenous contrast phases
- The mass:
  - nature, e.g. cystic/solid
  - margins
  - contrast enhancement
  - homogeneity
  - Hounsfield units (fat content)
- Site of origin:
  - intraperitoneal: viscus, mesentery, parietes or omentum
  - retroperitoneal: renal tract, adrenal, pancreas, aorta, parietes
- Relations:
  - anatomical
  - vascular, e.g. vein, aorta, IVC
- Effects:
  - obstruction, e.g. bowel, vascular, renal
  - fistula
  - ascites
- Pathological process:
  - evidence of invasion (loss of fat or fascial planes, distorted anatomy or loss of lumen)
  - inflammatory streaking
  - metastases
  - lymphadenopathy
- Free gas/fluid levels
  - abscess formation

Contrast studies

In isolation, contrast investigations now have a limited role in the management of abdominal mass lesions (see Chapter 3). A small bowel series may be helpful in elucidating the nature of a suspected Crohn's lesion, but a CT scan with oral contrast may be more useful. The latter will allow definition of structures outside the lumen of the gut.

Angiography may be used in planning treatment for an aortic aneurysm or resection of an abdominal mass, but will probably be performed in conjunction with a CT scan. Similarly, mass lesions with possible

vascular involvement or those close to major vessels will preferably be investigated with contrast-enhanced cross-sectional radiology.

Isotope scans

Isotope scans (see Chapter 7) can provide information on the nature and functionality of liver and adrenal masses (see Chapters 12 and 20).

Table 16.1 summarises the role of imaging modalities in investigation of the abdominal mass.

THE CLINICAL PROBLEMS

Abdominal wall masses

In general, these should be diagnosed on clinical grounds without the need for imaging. If required, ultrasound and/or CT scanning will define most lesions and provide sufficient information for management. Soft tissue tumours may warrant further investigation with MRI. Abdominal wall lesions to be considered include:

- skin lesions (sebaceous cyst, dermoid cysts, etc.)
- abscesses (consider fistulae from intra abdominal organs)
- soft tissue tumours (benign or malignant, e.g. desmoid tumours; Fig. 16.6)
- umbilical pathology (omphalitis, urachal or vitellointestinal duct remnants)
- rectus sheath haematoma (Fig. 16.7)
- subcutaneous haematoma.

The systematic examination of the scan is discussed further in Chapter 4 but should consider:

- Layers of abdominal wall
- Site of mass and the layer involved
- Relationships to:
  - umbilicus
  - underlying intraperitoneal organs (possible fistula)
- The mass itself:
  - encapsulated/well defined/smooth
  - poorly defined/irregular/invasive/destructive
  - CT density of muscle, fat or water (may help distinguish stromal tumours)
  - liquid component (haematoma, abscess)
  - calcification (scar, haematoma)

Modality	Good for	Limitations	Look for
Plain AXR	Faecal masses Gaseous distension Bowel obstruction	Poor anatomical precision	Bowel gas patterns Bowel displacement Calcification Soft tissue shadows
Ultrasound	Abdominal wall Gall bladder/liver Spleen/kidneys Ovaries	Body habitus Intervening bowel gas Retroperitoneal masses	Solid/cystic Site/organ of origin Organ relations Vascular relations
CT scan	Excellent anatomical and vascular relationships May define pathology Staging Abdominal wall Intraperitoneal Retroperitonium	Radiation dose	Site/organ of origin Oral contrast distribution (if given) Relations (anatomical and vascular: contrast phases) Lesion enhancement (triple phase) Loss of fat planes Invasion of adjacent structures Bowel obstruction Lymphadenopathy Liver metastases
MRI scan	As for CT Enhanced definition of fat, fascial and serosal planes	Expensive	As for CT T1/T2 distinction

◀ **Table 16.1** Imaging modalities for investigation of an abdominal mass

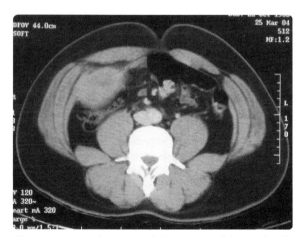

Fig. 16.6 Desmoid tumour of the anterior abdominal wall.

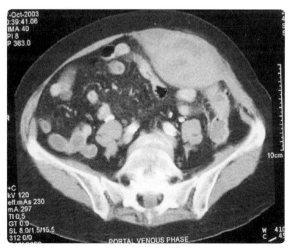

Fig. 16.7 Rectus sheath haematoma. The bleed is confined to the left rectus sheath.

Hernias

This topic is covered in Chapter 17.

Intraperitoneal masses

Multi-phase CT is the imaging modality of choice with the capacity to define the anatomical and vascular relationships of the mass within the abdomen as well as provide important clues to its likely pathology and help plan resection if appropriate. Oral and intravenous contrast should be used whenever possible. At times, ultrasound may provide complementary information, for example in outlining biliary disease or cystic disease of the liver, kidneys, ovaries or pancreas.

Causes that should be considered in the differential of an intraperitoneal mass include:

- gastric tumours/gastrointestinal stromal tumours (Fig. 16.8).
- hepatomegaly/splenomegaly/distended gall bladder/urinary bladder
- liver tumours/metastases/cysts
- small bowel tumours/inflammatory masses
- colonic tumours/diverticular phlegmon or abscess
- ovarian cysts
- mesenteric cysts/tumours
- omental cake
- faecal loading.

Common mass lesions are discussed in the relevant clinical chapters. Mesenteric lesions are discussed in Chapter 4.

Retroperitoneal masses

CT scanning is the most useful initial investigation and may provide all the information required. From a management point of view it is important to determine the relationship of the mass to other organs particularly the kidneys, ureters, pancreas, aorta and its branches and the IVC and major tributaries. Loss of fat planes or frank invasion may be demonstrated in malignant processes. Liver, lung or lymph node metastases may be evident.

MRI may provide added information particularly with respect to involvement of the spine or other neural structures and breach of fascial or serosal planes. MRI may be superior to CT in the demonstration of vessel involvement. Angiography may be important

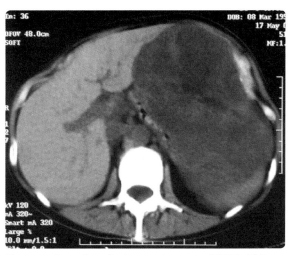

Fig. 16.8 Gastrointestinal stromal tumour (GIST). This patient was treated successfully with imatinib with a 50% reduction in tumour volume prior to surgery. This image shows the characteristic features of these large (>10 cm) tumours with well-defined but irregular margins, a heterogeneous rim of soft tissue and central fluid attenuation.

when planning resection of a retroperitoneal tumour to accurately map vascular relationships, though modern spiral CT scanning with intravenous contrast often provides a sufficient vascular 'road map.'

Retroperitoneal masses may be classified as follows:

- pancreatic neoplasms (Fig. 16.9)
- renal tumours or cysts
- retroperitoneal lymph node enlargement, lymphoma (see below)
- retroperitoneal soft tissue tumours or cysts
- retroperitoneal abscess or haematomata
- aortic or iliac artery aneurysms
- inflammatory, e.g. retroperitoneal fibrosis
- miscellaneous, e.g. urinoma

Retroperitonal neoplasms

Malignant tumours comprise 85% of retroperitoneal neoplasms. Certain of these tumours have characteristic appearances, allowing a measure of diagnostic confidence on CT imaging without biopsy. Biopsy should be considered if the tumour is unresectable, the

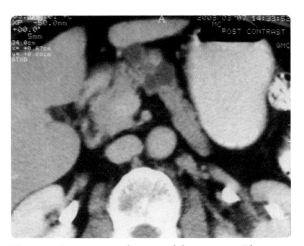

Fig. 16.9 A serous cystadenoma of the pancreas. The mass is well defined and has solid and cystic components. The margins are mostly well defined, except on the edge closest to the head of the pancreas where infiltration is occurring.

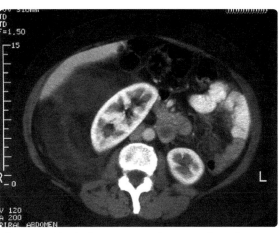

Fig. 16.10 Classical appearance of a retroperitoneal liposarcoma. Note the rotation of the kidney and the heterogeneous composition of the tumour.

diagnosis is unclear or if a chemosensitive tumour (e.g. lymphoma or germ cell tumour) is suspected.

Sarcomas are classically heterogeneous due to areas of liquefaction. Attenuation varies according to cell type and may give a clue to subtype. Biopsy is avoided, because the risk of tumour implantation may prejudice resection. Retroperitoneal liposarcomas usually arise from the perinephric fat and have a characteristic appearance on CT. The kidney, typically lies at the periphery of the mass and is encased by tumour. The kidney is rotated or displaced but still maintains its normal internal architecture with intravenous contrast (Fig. 16.10). There may be associated pelviureteric obstruction depending on the tumour size and the degree of displacement. Enhancement may occur with intravenous contrast on CT. Structures are displaced and obstructed with anterior rotation of the kidneys typical. Local infiltration and breach of planes suggests malignancy. Calcification is more typical of neurological tumours.

The CT scan can often help with the grading of these tumours, with the heterogeneity of a lesion giving an indication of its likely grade. Low-grade tumours tend to be relatively homogeneous with a characteristic fatty radiolucent appearance. Tumours of intermediate grade are usually relatively radiolucent

and have septa traversing the lesion. High-grade liposarcomas are most often dense, heterogenous and enhance with intravenous contrast.

Other retroperitoneal malignancies may also have characteristic CT findings. For example, testicular germ cell tumours may present with a retroperitoneal mass in the absence of any palpable testicular abnormality. Left-sided germ cell tumours are typically associated with para-aortic or preaortic lymphadenopathy, whereas right-sided tumours are associated with paracaval lymphadenopathy. Serum tumour markers are an important component of assessment of the obscure retroperitoneal mass.

Lymphomas characteristically show as an area of homogeneous enhancement and/or lymph node enlargement. The border of the mass is usually irregular and the mass may expand between the aorta and the IVC (Fig. 16.11).

Although MRI has an undisputed superiority to CT in the definition of soft tumours of the limbs, the apparent advantages in definition of tumours in the abdominal cavity is more controversial. Several studies have suggested an advantage with MRI, however, this view is not conclusively supported by evidence, and findings may have been superseded by current CT technology. The Radiology Diagnostic Oncology Group

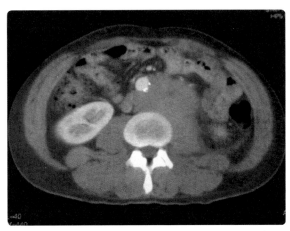

Fig. 16.11 Retroperitoneal lymphoma. Note the irregular border and the relatively anterior position of the aorta.

found, in a large well constructed trial, no significant difference in ability to assess site, size and relationship to surrounding structure and that a combination of both investigations did not increase accuracy.

Other retroperitoneal masses

Retroperitoneal haematomas are usually associated with trauma or anticoagulation. Attenuation of haemorrhage on imaging will depend on how long a haematoma has been present. Early haemorrhage is of increased density on non-contrast images. This high density will decrease over days. A diagnosis of retroperitoneal haematoma is suggested by the history (trauma, anticoagulation).

An inflammatory process will usually be localised to the primary site and be poorly demarcated. Heterogeneity and gas suggests infection. A drainable collection should be noted. Diffuse retroperitoneal fibrosis rarely presents as a clinical abdominal mass, but should be considered in the differential of a retroperitoneal mass on CT. A perirenal mass of water density (between fat and solid) is suggestive of an urinoma. Enhancement occurs only early following a leak.

Abdominal lymph node enlargement

As with most abdominal masses, the CT scan provides the most information on enlarged lymph nodes

---

WHAT TO LOOK FOR   Box 16.2

on CT of lymphadenopathy

- Size: above 10 mm is considered abnormal
- Distribution/nodal groups involved:
  - look along all major vessels: retroperitoneum and pelvis, especially at bifurcations
  - hila of liver, spleen and kidneys
  - mesenteric
- Solitary or multiple
- Calcification
- Associated mass or evidence of underlying cause
- Other indicators of lymphoma
- Organomegaly or changes in splenic density indicating infiltration
- Thickening of the gastrointestinal tract: significant at >1 cm wall thickness
- Metastatic lymph node involvement tends to vary from lymphoma:
  - smaller
  - more focal
  - more nodular

(Box 16.2). Depending on the resolution of the machine, nodes from 0.5 to 1.0 cm in diameter can be detected (see Chapter 23). The scan is best performed with intravenous and oral contrast (Fig. 16.12). Visualisation of lymph nodes is improved where there is surrounding fat. In mild lymphadenopathy, major vessels may be discernable without contrast due to their thin layer of surrounding fat, however, in gross lymphadenopathy any normal anatomy is replaced by a homogenous prevertebral mass and intravenous contrast is required to delineate vessels. Mesenteric nodes are better visualised centrally and are enhanced by a fatty mesentery. Oral contrast aids differentiation of peripheral mesenteric nodes from bowel, although this is now easier with the ability to reconstruct images in multiple planes.

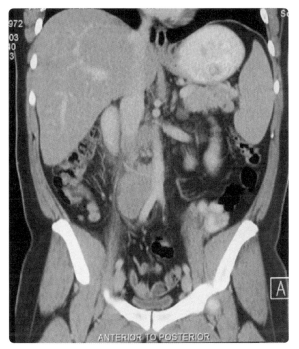

Fig. 16.12 Enlarged para-aortic lymph nodes secondary to a seminoma of the right testis. The nodes are abutting the aorta and are attached to the inferior vena cava.

Further reading

Burkill GJ, Badran M, Al-Muderis O et al. Malignant gastrointestinal stromal tumor: distribution, imaging features, and pattern of metastatic spread. Radiology 2003; 226:527–32

Feig BW, Berger DH, Fuhrman MD. The MD Anderson surgical handbook, 2nd edn. Lippincott, Williams, Wilkins, Philadelphia, 1999

Heslin MJ, Smith JK. Imaging of soft tissue sarcomas. Surg Oncol Clin N Am 1999; 8:91–107

Holm HH, Gammelgaard J, Jensen F et al. Ultrasound in the diagnosis of a palpable abdominal mass. A prospective study of 107 patients. Gastrointest Radiol 1982; 7:149–51

Hughes TM, Spillane AJ. Imaging of soft tissue tumours. Br J Surg 2000; 87:259–60

Kim Y, Cho O, Song S et al. Peritoneal lymphomatosis: CT findings. Abdom Imaging 1998; 23:87–90

Reimer P, Parize PM, Stichnoth FA. Clinical MR Imaging: a practical approach. Springer, Berlin, 1999

Spillane AJ. Retroperitoneal sarcoma: time for a change in attitude? Aust N Z J Surg 2001; 71:303–8

Tateishi U, Hasegawa T, Beppu Y et al. Primary dedifferentiated liposarcoma of the retroperitoneum: prognostic significance of computed tomography and magnetic resonance imaging features. J Comp Assist Tomogr 2003; 25:799–804

Wegener OH. Whole body computed tomography, 2nd edn. Blackwell Scientific, Oxford, 1982

Abdominal wall hernias

17

R.S. Williams

Background

Abdominal wall hernias should be diagnosed by history and physical examination in the majority of cases. Imaging is useful in the following situations:

- occult or clinically indefinite hernias
- investigation of abdominal wall pain
- preoperative evaluation of large hernias
- complications after hernia surgery.

IMAGING MODALITIES

Plain abdominal X-rays

Plain abdominal films may be useful in cases of incarcerated or strangulated hernias to check for any associated intestinal obstruction. Occasionally a hernial sac containing intestine may be visible outside the abdominal cavity outlines.

Ultrasound scanning

Ultrasound scanning of the abdominal wall is a non-invasive and dynamic assessment which is an ideal investigation for occult hernias and undiagnosed abdominal wall pain. However it is highly operator-dependent and difficult to interpret in obese patients. A high-resolution scanner with colour Doppler will give the greatest accuracy and an operator experienced in soft tissue ultrasound is essential. Examination of digital still images gives limited information. Discussion of difficult or contentious cases with the radiologist and personally viewing the study in real time can be invaluable. Surgeons may in future be performing these scans themselves.

Computed tomography

CT accurately displays the muscle and fascial layers of the abdominal wall in cross section and is particularly useful in obese patients with clinically occult hernias. Accuracy in the detection of any abdominal wall defect is increased by instructing the patient to perform the Valsalva manoeuvre during the scan. CT has an additional advantage of being able to detect other pathologies.

Magnetic resonance imaging

MRI will accurately define abdominal wall defects but can be limited by availability and costs.

Herniography

Although popular in Europe, herniography (contrast peritoneography) is not used widely elsewhere, mainly because it is invasive. It can be a useful tool in the evaluation of groin pain. A radiologist with interest and expertise in the technique is essential. Water-soluble contrast is injected into the peritoneal cavity and, with the patient in the prone and head-up position, the pelvic area is screened by fluoroscopy, looking for peritoneal bulges or evidence of contrast tracking through the inguinal canal or into the scrotum. Identification of the umbilical ligaments helps to define the anatomical site of the hernia. Complications are uncommon in experienced hands but include abdominal wall haematomas, chemical peritonitis (this usually settles spontaneously), vasovagal episodes, scrotal hydrocele formation (if a patent processus vaginalis is present) or rarely bowel injury.

CLINICAL PROBLEMS

Common hernias

Inguinal hernia

Sonography is the first-line investigation for clinically indefinite primary or recurrent inguinal hernias. Muscular, fascial and vascular landmarks are identified to allow anatomical localisation of a hernia or painful area (Box 17.1).

Experienced sonographers can identify both direct and indirect hernias and distinguish an indirect hernia from normal movement of the spermatic cord or its associated fat in the inguinal canal during straining. Changes in patient posture and repeated Valsalva manoeuvres can be necessary to complete the study (Fig. 17.1). Judgement and experience are needed to avoid overcalling equivocal cases. Comparison with the other (normal) groin should be mandatory. Scan-

ning may also identify other causes of symptoms, e.g. muscle injuries, tendoperiosteal lesions.

Herniography should be a second-line investigation (Fig. 17.2). It is particularly useful where there is pressure for early definitive diagnosis, e.g. professional sportspeople, workers' compensation cases. Patients should be aware of the small risk of a complication.

Management of a 'sonographic' inguinal hernia In this increasingly common clinical scenario, a patient with groin pain attends with an ultrasound scan reporting an inguinal hernia, but without clinical evidence of a hernia. The following points are made:

- The patient should be carefully assessed for other possible causes of groin pain before considering surgery.
- If possible, discuss the study with the reporting radiologist to assess the degree of diagnostic confidence.
- The other groin should be scanned if this has not already been done (often it will show similar appearances).
- Herniography can be ordered if clinically warranted, but a period of observation and further assessment is often wise.

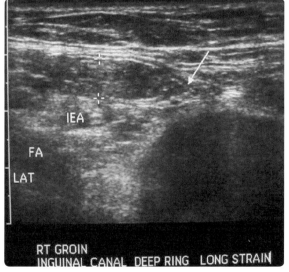

Fig. 17.1 A sonogram showing an indirect inguinal hernia (arrowed). FA, femoral artery; IEA, inferior epigastric artery; LAT, lateral.

WHAT TO LOOK FOR | Box 17.1

on the ultrasound scan of inguinal hernia

- Fascial defects
- Movement of bowel or fat through the inguinal canal
- Reducibility

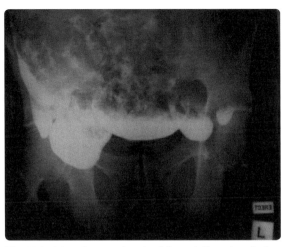

Fig. 17.2 A herniogram showing bilateral direct inguinal hernias.

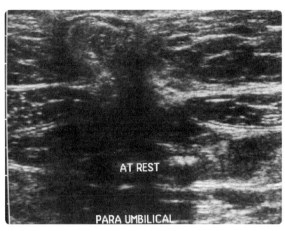

Fig. 17.3 Sonogram showing an umbilical hernia. The hernia sac can be seen bulging through the linea alba (white line).

- If surgery is undertaken in equivocal circumstances the patient should clearly understand the uncertainties.
- In footballers and other athletes it is particularly important to exclude other injuries which can present with groin pain (see below).

Femoral hernia

Femoral hernias often are irreducible and can be difficult to differentiate from enlarged groin lymph nodes. Ultrasound scanning is helpful in this situation as lymph nodes have characteristic appearances, being hypoechoic with hyperechoic centres (see Chapter 5) and are constant during dynamic examination.

Umbilical hernia

Clinical diagnosis of an umbilical hernia usually is unequivocal. Occult hernias can be identified on ultrasound scans, or on CT in obese patients (Fig. 17.3).

Epigastric (fatty) hernia

An epigastric hernia can be difficult to detect in the obese patient. The classic presentation is with epigastric pain and (often) exquisite local tenderness due to a small hernial defect with its tight neck in the linea alba. For those not clinically apparent, CT readily identifies the fascial defect and protruding fat, and generally is more useful than ultrasound scans in obese patients.

Abdominal incisional hernia

These are usually ventral in site and those not clinically evident are sometimes seen incidentally on CT scans. In cases of abdominal pain or bowel obstruction, CT can identify a previously unsuspected incarcerated hernia (Fig. 17.4). The contents of large or massive hernias can be identified on CT and can help in planning treatment, especially in relation to 'loss of domain' in the peritoneal cavity. CT readily can differentiate a true hernia from abdominal rectus divarication where the linea alba is thin but intact, or from diffuse muscle weakness.

Sportsman's hernia

Sportsman's hernia, also called athlete's groin and conjoint tendon injury, usually presents in fit young men (and occasionally women) engaged in vigorous sporting activities, most often in the football codes. These patients suffer recurrent exercise-induced pain in the inguinal region, preventing continuation of the sport and recurring after prolonged rest. There is no universal agreement about the pathogenesis of the sports hernia, but surgical repair of the posterior wall of the inguinal canal cures the condition in most cases, leading to the theory that it may represent a subclinical or incipient direct inguinal hernia. Ultrasound scanning of the groin area is useful in assessment of this condition (Box 17.2).

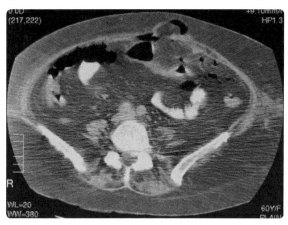

Fig. 17.4 A CT scan showing an incisional hernia and a pneumoperitoneum. In addition to the free gas under the anterior abdominal wall, there is air in the sac of the incisional hernia. This slice is taken at the level of the hernial defect. Both the pneumoperitoneum and the incisional hernia were incidental findings in a patient who had recently undergone an endoscopic examination of the stomach.

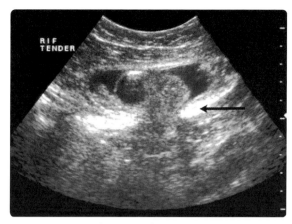

Fig. 17.5 Sonographic view of a Spigelian hernia. The sac and contents lie anterior to the rectus muscle (arrow).

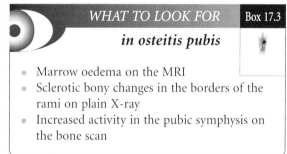

WHAT TO LOOK FOR | Box 17.3

in osteitis pubis

- Marrow oedema on the MRI
- Sclerotic bony changes in the borders of the rami on plain X-ray
- Increased activity in the pubic symphysis on the bone scan

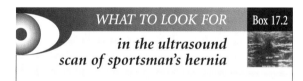

WHAT TO LOOK FOR | Box 17.2

in the ultrasound scan of sportsman's hernia

- Forward bulge of the conjoint tendon area on Valsalva
- Local tenderness to transducer pressure

Ideally, the patient should be assessed by a specialist in sports medicine to exclude other causes of chronic groin pain, such as rectus muscle/adductor tendon injuries, hip joint arthropathies and osteitis pubis.

Osteitis pubis generally causes suprapubic and bilateral groin pain. Plain X-rays can show sclerotic changes in the pubic rami, widening of the symphysis pubis or pubic instability on 'flamingo' views (patient standing on one leg). Radionuclide bone scan or MRI may be needed to diagnose early or subtle cases of osteitis pubis (Box 17.3). Bone scan typically shows increased activity in the pubic symphysis. MRI can show increased water content in the pubic bone marrow ('marrow oedema') leading to low T1 and high T2 signal intensities, the opposite of normal.

Uncommon hernias

Spigelian hernia

Spigelian hernias are interparietal hernias which protrude through the Spigelian fascia at the arcuate line of the abdominal rectus muscles, *beneath* the external oblique aponeurosis. They usually present as a lump or intermittent swelling above and medial to the inguinal canal. If the diagnosis is uncertain, sonography can be requested (Fig. 17.5). The transducer is placed over the semilunar line and the hernia usually can be demonstrated during Valsalva. In obese patients, CT is more helpful.

Lumbar hernia

Lumbar incisional hernias can occur after renal surgery. Spontaneous lumbar hernias, protruding through the superior or inferior lumbar triangles, are rare. Presentation is generally with a mass in the flank area. Sonography or CT usually will clarify clinically doubtful cases.

Obturator hernia

Obturator hernias almost always occur in thin elderly females. Atrophy of obturator fat can allow small bowel prolapse into the obturator foramen with incarceration, presenting usually as small bowel obstruction. Plain X-rays of the abdomen will show evidence of small bowel obstruction but the cause is usually not evident until after laparotomy. The increasing use of CT in assessment of acute abdominal problems may well identify some of these preoperatively.

Sciatic (gluteal) hernia

Sciatic hernias are rare hernias occurring through the greater or the lesser sciatic foramina, in the former case said to be associated with congenital maldevelopment or acquired atrophy of the piriformis muscle. Sciatic hernias are mostly seen in females and occasionally cause chronic pelvic pain. Most of the reported cases have been identified at laparoscopy or laparotomy. These hernias usually contain either an ovary or fallopian tube, although ureteric herniation is also described. In theory, the condition could be diagnosed on CT, but due to the rarity of sciatic hernias there is little literature on this.

Perineal hernia

Perineal hernias are most often seen after abdominoperineal excision of the rectum, and other major pelvic surgeries. Symptoms are often mild or absent and require no treatment. Spontaneous perineal hernias are rare. CT or herniography can be used to diagnose difficult cases.

Imaging for complications of hernias

Wound, testicular or scrotal swellings
Ultrasound scanning with colour Doppler is useful to assess:

- testicular perfusion
- testicular oedema
- postoperative wound or scrotal haematomas
- hernia recurrence.

Chronic pain after inguinal hernia repair
This most often is neuropathic pain, due to injury to local sensory nerves, but occult hernia recurrence needs to be excluded because it is surgically correctible. Sonography and herniography both are useful in assessing such patients.

Further reading
Ekberg O. Complications after herniography in adults. Am J Roentgenol 1983; 140:491–5

Fon LJ, Spence RA. Sportsman's hernia. Br J Surg 2000; 87: 545–52

Gullmo A. Herniography. Surg Clin N Am 1984; 64(2): 229–44

Holloway BJ, Belcher HE, Letourneau JG, Kunberger LE. Scrotal sonography; a valuable tool in the evaluation of complications following inguinal hernia repair. J Clin Ultrasound 1998; 26:341–4

Fitzgibbons RJ, Greenburg AG. Nyhus and Condon's Hernia, 5th edn. Lippincott Williams & Wilkins, Baltimore, 2001

Poobalan AS, Bruce J, King PM et al. Chronic pain and quality of life following inguinal hernia repair. Br J Surg 2001; 88:1122–6

Toms AP, Dixon AK, Mmurphy JM, Jamieson NV. Illustrated review of new imaging techniques in the diagnosis of abdominal wall hernias. Br J Surg 1999; 86:1243–9

Van den Berg JC, de Valois JC, Go PM, Rosenbusch G. Detection of groin hernias with physical examination, ultrasound and MRI compared with laparoscopic findings. Invest Radiol 1999; 34:739–43

Renal and genitourinary imaging

18

V. Marshall

Background

Although urology is a specialty in its own right and has its own radiological needs, there are often urological problems that fall within the domain of the general surgeon. There have been many changes in this discipline in recent years, for example the change from IVU to spiral CT and this illustrates the need to keep up with radiological developments. This chapter is a brief outline of the more commonly encountered urological problems.

THE RADIOLOGICAL INVESTIGATIONS

The plain abdominal radiograph

This simple investigation remains an important first-line tool in the assessment of stone disease, and is often performed as the preliminary to an IVU or CT urogram. Calcium oxalate stones are radiodense, whereas uric acid stones are radiolucent. Other causes of renal calcification are medullary nephrocalcinosis (e.g. medullary sponge kidney), or tuberculosis. Generally the plain X-ray is of limited value in the management of most other urological problems.

Intravenous urography

Until recently this investigation was the mainstay of investigation of the renal tract as it provides both anatomical and functional information (Fig. 18.1). An intravenous urogram (IVU) requires the injection of intravenous iodinated contrast and is therefore contraindicated in patients with an allergy to iodine or renal failure (see Chapter 3). Contrast is excreted rapidly by the kidneys allowing plain X-rays or tomograms to define the renal contour, collecting system, ureters and bladder. It provides an accurate assessment of renal excretion and drainage and should define the level of obstruction, although this may take many hours in cases of severe obstruction. Recently the IVU has been replaced by the CT urogram in the assessment of calculus disease in many centres, but it still has a role in the assessment of the upper tracts for malignancy and in confirming obstruction.

Fig. 18.1 Normal IVP.

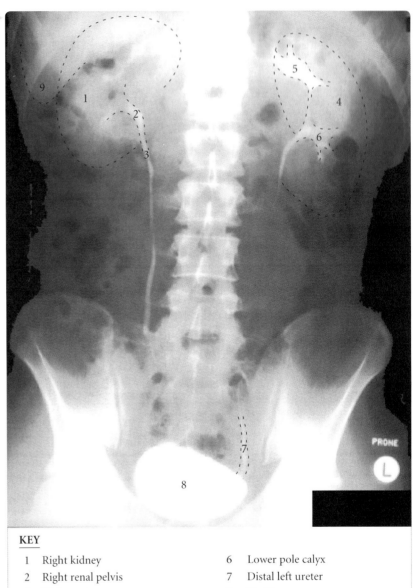

KEY

1	Right kidney	6	Lower pole calyx
2	Right renal pelvis	7	Distal left ureter
3	Right ureter	8	Bladder
4	Left kidney	9	Inferior tip of liver
5	Upper pole calyx		

Retrograde pyelography

This is performed by the urologist at the time of cystoscopy and involves catheterisation of the ureter and injection of contrast into the upper tract. A retrograde pyelogram usually provides superior distension in comparison with an IVU and is used in the assessment of urothelial tumours.

Ultrasound

Ultrasound is a very important investigation of the renal tract and usually provides detailed views of the kidneys and bladder. As at other sites, the place of ultrasound may be limited by body habitus. It is useful in the detection and assessment of mass lesions of the kidneys and bladder, detection of renal tract obstruction and calculous disease, and in the measurement of post-micturition volumes. The ureters are not usually visualised except at their most proximal and distal ends, unless they are dilated.

Computed tomography scan

The advent of the spiral CT scan has led to the virtual abandonment of intravenous urography as a diagnostic tool in suspected renal calculus disease. Low-dose non-contrast CT is used to define obstruction and the position of a calculus, while contrast enhanced CT will help characterise renal mass lesions and stage malignancies. CT angiography is also useful in defining the renal vasculature and any anomalous vessels prior to renal transplantation, having replaced conventional angiography.

Angiography

The main indication for angiography in relation to the renal tract involves the assessment of renal artery stenosis, with the ability to perform angioplasty and stent insertion. Occasionally it may be used in renal tumours if embolisation is considered.

Radionuclide imaging

Radionuclide scans provide both functional and quantitative information about the renal tract, but have limited spatial resolution. A ^{99m}Tc-DTPA scan is a dynamic scan and provides information on renal function and will demonstrate obstruction. The additional intravenous injection of frusemide 20 minutes after the radiotracer injection should promote 'washout' of the tracer. A ^{99m}Tc-DMSA scan is a static scan, with the radiotracer taken up by the renal parenchyma. The uptake of ^{99m}Tc-DMSA is a reflection of renal function, and is also used to provide information on focal scarring in children (see Chapter 7).

Magnetic resonance imaging

MRI provides good definition of the kidneys and renal tract, but the other modalities are usually sufficient to provide the information required from imaging. MRI is therefore used more as a problem solving tool for renal tumours. It has a role in the staging of prostate cancer and may also have a role in the staging of bladder cancers. MR urograms are a way of defining obstruction without ionising radiation or intravenous contrast, and may be appropriate in specific cases.

THE CLINICAL PROBLEMS

Urinary tract obstruction

Obstruction occurs frequently in the renal and genitourinary system and can occur at any level from the calyx to the urethra.

Ultrasound has become the most commonly used modality to diagnose obstruction (Fig. 18.2) (Box 18.1). Often, however, ancillary investigations are needed to establish the precise cause for the obstruction. For example, ultrasound may demonstrate a dilated collecting system and upper ureter but either a CT scan or a retrograde pyelogram may be needed to establish whether the obstruction is due to a calculus, a lesion involving the wall or lumen of the ureter, or extrinsic pressure.

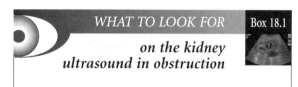

WHAT TO LOOK FOR Box 18.1

on the kidney ultrasound in obstruction

- Dilatation of calyces and upper ureter
- AP diameter of renal pelvis
- Cortical thickness of the kidney
- Presence of calculi

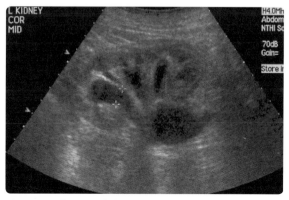

Fig. 18.2 Ultrasound showing marked dilation of the pelvicalyceal system.

The major advantage of ultrasound in the urinary tract is that no radiation is involved and it is not dependent on renal function for the urinary tract to be visualised. It can also be used to facilitate percutaneous puncture and drainage of the collecting system.

It is important to note that a dilated system does not always mean that the system is obstructed. Persisting dilatation is frequently noted after the repair of a pelviureteric obstruction and in the case of some primary megaureters. Dilatation can occur in the presence of a low pressure system and the most effective method of establishing that this is the case is to perform a DTPA (diethylenetriaminepentaacetate) scan with frusemide washout. By determining the clearance time of the isotope from the renal pelvis it is possible to establish that the system is not obstructed.

Ultrasound may on occasion demonstrate a grossly distended bladder with no associated pain which may suggest a neurogenic cause. Depending on the history and neurological examination, MRI may be necessary to establish a neurological cause for the distended bladder.

CT may also demonstrate the presence of hydronephrosis secondary to other intraabdominal pathology (Fig. 18.3).

Urinary stones

Intravenous urography, ultrasound and CT have all been used to diagnose renal, ureteric and bladder stones. Spiral CT has now become the investigation of choice to diagnose renal and ureteric stones.

Non-contrast, low-dose spiral CT can demonstrate obstruction and identify stones greater than approximately 2 mm in diameter (Fig. 18.4). The sensitivity and specificity of unenhanced helical CT in detecting ureteral calculi is >95% and is superior to both ultrasound and IVU. Features of obstruction on a CT are: demonstration of a calculus within a ureter, thickening of the ureter at the site of calculus consistent with oedema ('rim sign'), periureteric and perinephric stranding, and hydronephrosis (Box 18.2). Occasionally when there has been recent passage of a stone, ureteric dilatation and periureteric stranding will

 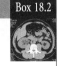

> **WHAT TO LOOK FOR** Box 18.2
> ## *on the CT urogram*
> - Presence of a calculus
> - Ureteric rim sign
> - Perinephric and periureteric stranding
> - Renal pelvic and ureteric dilatation
> - Level of calibre change

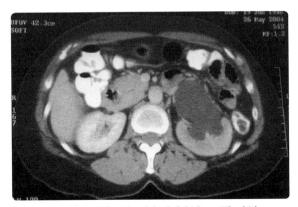

Fig. 18.3 Hydronephrosis of the left kidney. The kidney substance is well preserved, indicating that the changes are acute rather than chronic. In this patient the hydronephrosis was due to extrinsic compression of the lower ureter by a non-renal malignancy.

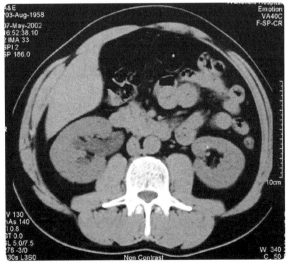

Fig. 18.4 Single axial image from a non-contrast CT scan of a patient with right sided ureteric colic. This slice shows the hydronephrotic right pelvicalyceal system. The stone was seen at the ureto-vesical junction. Note also the small stone anteriorly in the left kidney.

persist. If it is important to know whether a stone is lodged at the vessicoureteric junction or has passed into the bladder, scanning the patient prone will enable the stone to fall anteriorly if it is free. CT has the advantage of providing a rapid result compared with the delayed films often necessary with an IVU, and may demonstrate a different cause for the patient's abdominal pain.

Although the CT is the most sensitive investigation, it is not specific for stone composition, as both calcium oxalate (radio-opaque) and uric acid (radiolucent) calculi are dense on a CT. To determine the nature of a stone it is necessary to perform an AXR, which will fail to show a uric acid stone. Indinavir stones (nephrolithiasis associated with the anti-HIV protease inhibitor) are the only calculi which are not dense on CT, and diagnosis relies on the supporting signs of obstruction, with an appropriate clinical history.

Urinary tract malignancies

There has been a significant change in the radiological investigations used to diagnose urological malignancies. In the past an IVU was the most commonly used investigation but it has now been relegated to assist in the diagnosis of transitional cell carcinomas of the renal pelvis or ureter. For mass lesions of the kidney and bladder, ultrasound is the most commonly used initial investigation.

CT is extensively used to confirm the nature of mass lesions of the kidney and to stage most urological malignancies (Box 18.3).

In a renal cell carcinoma, CT can be of assistance in detecting renal vein and vena cava involvement, demonstrating penetration of Gerota's fascia and para-aortic lymph nodes (Fig. 18.5). Incidentally discovered cystic lesions of the kidney can be assessed according to the Bosniak classification (Table 18.1), which provides an indication of the likelihood of the lesion being benign or malignant. True assessment requires pre-

---

WHAT TO LOOK FOR Box 18.3

on CT of the kidney

- Focal mass within the kidney
- Homogeneous or heterogeneous
- Margins and local extension to Gerota's fascia
- Extension into renal vein or IVC on venous phase images
- Para-aortic lymphadenopathy
- If a cystic lesion:
  - homogeneity and attenuation
  - nodular or septal enhancement
  - calcification

◀ **Table 18.1** Bosniak classification of cystic renal lesions on CT

Bosniak classification	Appearances	Risk of malignancy
I	Well-defined simple cyst Homogeneous water attenuation	0
II	<3 cm diameter One or two fine septations (≤ 1 mm thick) Fine mural or septal calcification (≤ 1 mm) Homogeneous hyperdensity (>30 HU) Non-enhancement	0 (minimally complicated cysts are nominated IIF and are followed up)
III	Wall thickening or nodularity Thick or irregular calcification Multiloculated/heterogeneous Multiple enhancing septae	Indeterminate Approximately 50% malignant
IV	Irregular enhancing thick-walled cysts Large enhancing solid nodules	100% malignant

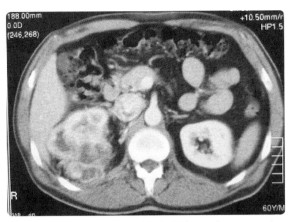

Fig. 18.5 A carcinoma of the right kidney. The tumour is extending posteriorly into Gerota's fascia.

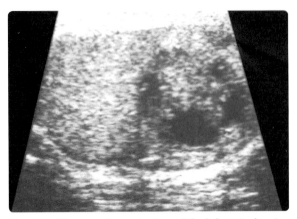

Fig. 18.7 Ultrasound examination of the left testis showing a well circumscribed cystic neoplasm. This has the characteristics of a non-seminomatous tumour.

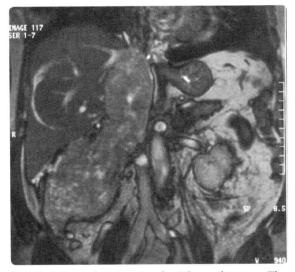

Fig. 18.6 Coronal MRI image of a right renal tumour. The image shows a large mass of tumour extending into the inferior vena cava, reaching to the level of the diaphragm.

and postcontrast scanning with fine slice thicknesses. In the case of bladder tumours CT can provide information on local extension in more advanced tumours, but is not particularly helpful in detecting lymph node involvement.

MRI is mainly used as a problem solving tool in renal cancer. It provides good definition of extension of tumour into the IVC, when CT is indeterminate (Fig. 18.6) and may occasionally be used in the further assessment of an indeterminate renal mass, particularly if iodinated intravenous contrast is contra-indicated. MRI is used to stage bladder cancers in some centres, but its role in clinical staging is still under investigation.

CT urograms following intravenous contrast have been used in the assessment of transitional cell carcinoma of the upper tracts, with coronal reconstructions in the delayed phase mimicking the appearance of an IVU. Occasionally, neither an IVU nor CT urogram will be able to identify a small transitional cell carcinoma of the renal pelvis or ureter and either a retrograde pyelogram or ureteroscopy will be necessary.

Scrotal and testicular abnormalities

Ultrasound is the most appropriate way to investigate scrotal masses. The ultrasound can differentiate cystic lesions and is now routinely used to diagnose testicular tumours (Fig. 18.7). Staging of testicular tumours involves chest and abdominal CT. Ultrasound is also useful in detecting undescended testes, particularly in the inguinal canal.

Doppler US is used to assist in the diagnosis of testicular torsion and has a sensitivity and specificity reported to range from 75 to 100%. It has a high negative predictive value and may demonstrate another cause for the patient's pain, but questions have been raised into the appropriateness of delaying surgical exploration when time is a significant factor in achieving a successful outcome. Diagnosis of torsion relies on the demonstration of decreased vascularity within the testis on colour Doppler ultrasound, but this may also be seen in severe cases of epididymo-orchitis.

Ultrasound in cases of epididymo-orchitis will usually demonstrate enlargement of the epididymis and increased vascularity within the epididymis and testis. Echogenic fluid may be present within the scrotal sac, consistent with inflammation.

Ultrasound is also valuable in the assessment of testicular trauma, and can identify whether there has been disruption of the testis and hence the need for exploration and repair.

Renal and urinary tract trauma

The standard investigation for upper urinary tract trauma is a CT with contrast if there is no evidence of significantly impaired renal function. A CT will determine the extent of the renal injury, whether there is significant urinary extravasation or devascularisation of part of the kidney (Fig. 18.8) and provides some indication as to the presence of a pedicle injury. It can also provide valuable information about other associated intra-abdominal injuries (see Chapter 25). Occasionally in pedicle or major arterial injuries renal angiography can be used to determine the precise nature of the vascular injury and severe bleeding can be stopped by the introduction of coils or other thrombotic agents.

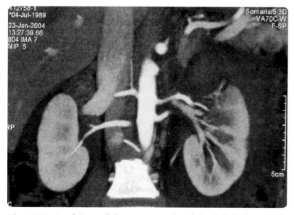

Fig. 18.8 Avulsion of the upper pole of the left kidney as the result of an injury sustained by a girl falling off a motorcycle. The upper pole is avascular.

If there is extravasation of contrast in the area of the renal pelvis but no obvious damage to the renal parenchyma this may suggest disruption of the pelvic-ureteric junction. This can be confirmed by a retrograde pyelogram.

Lower urinary tract trauma is best investigated with retrograde urethrocystogram which may be performed in the emergency department. This is covered in more detail in Chapter 25.

Transrectal ultrasound of the prostate

TRUS was originally developed in the belief that it could be used to diagnose prostate cancer. Unfortunately, although both hyper- and hypodense areas can be identified in the prostate, these areas do not correlate with cancerous changes.

TRUS is now used to assist needle biopsies to ensure samples are obtained from both the peripheral and transitional zones. The technique can also be used to facilitate the placement of radioactive seeds or wires to treat prostate cancer.

Further reading

Baker LA, Sigman D, Mathews RI et al. An analysis of clinical outcomes using color doppler testicular ultrasound for testicular torsion. Pediatrics 2000; 105:604–7

Brown JM, Taylor KJW, Alderman JL et al. Contrast enhanced ultrasonographic visualization of gonadal torsion J Ultrasound Med 1997; 16:309

Chen MY, Zagoria RJ, Saunders HS, Dyer RB. Trends in the use of unenhanced helical CT for acute urinary colic. AJR 1999; 173:1447–50

Curry NS, Cochran ST, Bissada NK. Cystic renal masses: accurate Bosniak classification requires adequate renal CT. AJR 2000; 175:339–42

Dunne PJ, O'Loughlin BS. Testicular torsion: time is the enemy. Aust N Z J Surg 2000; 70:441–2

Fedele M. Renal trauma. In: Pollack HM, McClennan BL (eds) Clinical urography, 2nd edn. WB Saunders, Philadelphia, 2000, p 1772

Heneghan JP, McGuire KA, Leder RA et al. Helical CT for nephrolithiasis and ureterolithiasis: comparison of conventional and reduced radiation-dose techniques. Radiology 2003; 229:575–80

Kravchick S, Cytron S, Leibovici O et al. Color Doppler sonography: its real role in the evaluation of children with highly suspected testicular torsion. Eur Radiol 2001; 11:1000–5

Nunez D Jr, Becerra JL, Fuentes D, Pagson S. Traumatic occlusion of the renal artery: helical CT diagnosis. AJR 1996; 167:777

Pollack HM, Wein AJ. Imaging of renal trauma. Radiology 1989; 172:297

Sheafor DH, Hertzberg BS, Freed KS et al. Nonenhanced helical CT and US in the emergency evaluation of patients with renal colic: prospective comparison. Radiology 2000; 217:792–7

Smith RC, Verga M, McCarthy S, Rosenfield AT. Diagnosis of acute flank pain: value of unenhanced helical CT. AJR 1996; 166:97

Weber DM, Rosslein R, Fliegel C. Color Doppler sonography in the diagnosis of acute scrotum in boys. Eur J Pediatr Surg 2000; 10:235–41

Wong SK, Ng LG, Tan BS et al. Acute renal colic: value of unenhanced spiral computed tomography compared with intravenous urography. Ann Acad Med Singapore 2001; 30:568–72

Breast disease and imaging 19

D. Walsh, M. Lea

Background

Breast imaging is crucial in the diagnosis and management of breast disease. A key issue in breast disease is the discrimination between benign and malignant lesions. Radiological imaging of the breast has two distinct roles in clinical practice: diagnosis and screening.

Diagnosis

In the diagnostic setting, imaging forms part of the assessment of a breast abnormality. This assessment is often referred to as the 'triple test'. The triple test involves the combination of:

1. clinical history and examination
2. fine-needle aspiration cytology
3. imaging of the breast, in an attempt to exclude or prove the presence of malignancy.

The two modalities of breast imaging employed in this setting are mammography and ultrasound, which provide complementary information regarding a breast lesion. When each component of the triple test is negative, or clear of any suspicion of malignancy, then the patient has a very small probability of breast cancer (0.5–1%). Conversely, when each component is positive for malignancy, the patient can move on to definitive management of their breast cancer. If there is discordance between components of the triple test, it is necessary to proceed with further investigations, usually core biopsy or open surgical biopsy.

Screening

Population based screening mammography is well established in many countries, with the aim of early detection, reduction of mortality and cost of treatment associated with breast cancer. Over the last decade, this use of breast imaging has greatly influenced the detection of breast malignancy in the community and has had significant impact on mortality associated with breast cancer (see Chapter 23).

THE RADIOLOGICAL INVESTIGATIONS

In the routine setting there are two modalities used in breast imaging – mammography and ultrasound. Interventional procedures based on these two techniques are often employed in the diagnosis (image-guided biopsies) and treatment (image-guided localisation) of breast lesions.

Mammography

The mammogram is the workhorse of breast imaging. Modern mammography involves minimal exposure to ionising radiation and is capable of producing consistent, high-quality images. Mammography is indicated in the assessment of a specific breast symptom, or the screening of asymptomatic women, as well as for long term follow-up of women already treated for breast cancer. In general, due to high breast density, mammography has a limited sensitivity in women below the age of 35 years and should be used selectively in this age group. Ultrasound is the preferred imaging modality in younger women. A clinical abnormality highly suspicious of malignancy should be submitted to both mammography and ultrasound regardless of age.

Standard mammogram imaging

Standard imaging includes two views, mediolateral oblique (MLO) and craniocaudal (CC) of both breasts. For the MLO projection the breast is compressed from supero-medial to infero-lateral (Fig. 19.1). The nipple should be in profile, the axillary tail included, the pectoralis major muscle visible posteriorly to the level of the nipple and the inframammary fold visible inferiorly. In CC views the breast is compressed vertically. Conventional labelling places any markers on the lateral aspect of the CC film (Fig. 19.2).

Additional projections are sometimes employed to further assess possible lesions. An 'extended CC' view may include more lateral or medial tissue to identify a lesion seen on the MLO, but not the conventional CC view. A 'true lateral' view compresses the breast horizontally, and lesions placed medially within the breast will move superiorly in relation to their position on the MLO.

Compression of the breast tissue during imaging disperses the normal tissue density and allows better appreciation of pathological lesions and their specific mammographic characteristics (Box 19.1). A perceived abnormality should be examined using a focal compression view to further help clarify the nature of the lesion, with or without magnification to assess calcifications (Figs 19.3 and 19.4). It is now routine practice to perform an ultrasound assessment of a focal abnormality detected on mammography.

Mammographic mass lesions

Several important characteristics should be considered when a mass lesion is discovered on a mammogram. Comparison with previous films is vital as a new or enlarging lesion must be viewed with considerable suspicion. A longstanding, stable mass is more likely to be benign. Differences between the mammographic appearance of both breasts, or within differing views of the same breast, will add to the perception and assessment of breast masses. Areas of clinical concern must be identified on both mammographic views and assessed specifically with increased suspicion. A skin marker can be placed during mammography to aid this process.

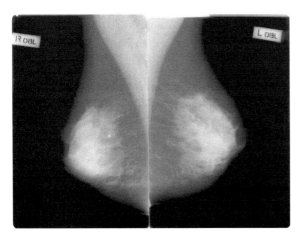

Fig. 19.1 A pair of MLO radiographs. Images are usually viewed together as a right/left pair in routine reporting and clinical review situations, allowing comparison between sides. Note triangular bands of dense tissue representing pectoral muscles.

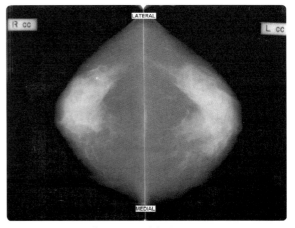

Fig. 19.2 A pair of craniocaudal view mammograms. By convention the lateral aspect of the breast is displayed at the top of the image and the medial aspect at the bottom. The nipple is displayed in profile in both projections if possible.

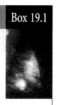
When a mass lesion is perceived on a mammogram, certain characteristics should be noted with the aim of determining the likely presence of malignancy (Table 19.1). The location of the mass should be determined and this should be expressed with reference to identifiable positions in the breast. It may be appropriate to refer to a general area such as a quadrant of the breast, but often the description of the position of a lesion considering the breast as a clock face is most accurate and clinically useful. Both breasts are considered as individual clock faces facing the examiner, so a lesion at 3 o'clock in the left breast will be lateral, whereas 3 o'clock in the right breast is medial. It is also useful to describe the distance from the nipple, usually in millimetres.

Fig. 19.3 Focal compression views showing microcalcifications in magnification view (ductal carcinoma in situ).

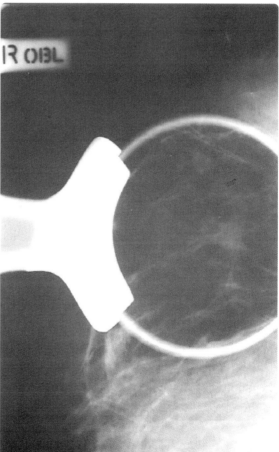

Fig. 19.4 Small stellate lesion seen with coned compression (carcinoma).

Table 19.1 Characteristics of benign and malignant lesions on mammography

Characteristics of MMG mass	Benign lesion	Malignant lesion
Prior MMG	Present Stable	New Enlarging Changing appearance
Shape	Round (Figs 19.5 and 19.6) Oval	Stellate (Fig. 19.7) Irregular Obscured
Margin	Circumscribed	Indistinct Lobulated (Fig. 19.8)
Density	Low	High
Associated microcalifications	Benign type	Malignant type
Architectural distorsion	Absent	Present
Secondary signs	Absent	Skin retraction/thickening Nipple retraction Enlarged axillary lymph nodes
Common examples	Cyst Fibroadenoma Lipoma Hamartoma Fat necrosis Haematoma Surgical scar Radial scar	Ductal carcinoma in situ (DCIS) Invasive ductal carcinoma Invasive lobular carcinoma Special type carcinomas Secondary breast malignancies (e.g. lymphoma, ovarian, melanoma, lung, sarcoma)

The size of the lesion is also expressed in millimeters. The size on mammography and ultrasound may differ, but ultrasound usually provides the more accurate measurement. The shape of the lesion should be considered. Common descriptions include a round, oval, lobulated or irregular mass. The margin of a mass is important as a clue to the diagnosis. It generally should be considered as circumscribed, obscured, ill-defined or spiculated. The density of a mass lesion can be characterised as low or high.

It is worth noting whether there is a solitary lesion or multiple masses. It is often important to decide whether the lesions are multifocal throughout a particular area such as the quadrant of the breast or truly multicentric, occurring over multiple regions of the breast. Often with mass lesions, associated calcifications and changes to the soft tissues such as the skin and nipple will be the key in the diagnosis.

Microcalcifications

Calcification is the deposition of calcium salts within tissues. This is usually in the form of calcium hydroyapatite or tricalcium phosphate. The high density of calcium salts means that their presence is relatively easy to detect and perceive on a mammogram. In mammographic screening programs up to 40–50% of women recalled will be for the further assessment of calcifications. Calcifications themselves are by-products representative of an underlying cellular pathology in the breast tissues. Once detected on a mammogram the key issue is to determine whether the underlying process is benign or malignant in nature.

Mammographic calcifications are divided into two groups on the basis of size. Fragments of calcium larger than 1 mm are termed macro-calcifications

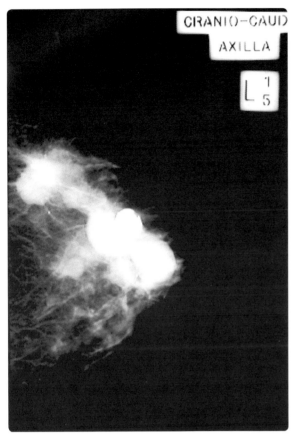

Fig. 19.5 Craniocaudal view demonstrating rounded masses with smooth margins (cysts), a calcified rounded mass (probably cyst or oil cyst from fat necrosis) and a large mass with spiculated margins (carcinoma).

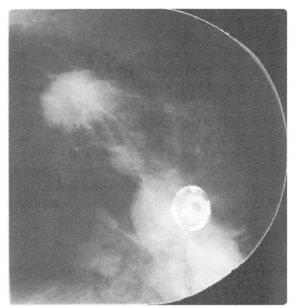

Fig. 19.6 Coned compression view better characterizing the lesions seen in Fig. 19.5.

and are generally benign, those smaller than 1 mm are referred as microcalcifications and this is the group most likely to represent a malignant process. In general, calcifications are assessed mammographically, usually by employing compression and magnified views. Although ultrasound often fails to detect or display calcifications, it has a role in their assessment. A mass lesion or soft tissue abnormality associated with calcifications often indicates malignancy.

Radiological assessment of calcifications involves classification into one of three categories:

- benign (commonest, require no further action)
- indeterminate (biopsy and follow-up required)
- malignant (biopsy and definitive management required).

As for the assessment of mass lesions, calcifications should be classified on the basis of the single most suspicious mammographic characteristic (Table 19.2). The scattered distribution of many calcifications means that a satisfactory biopsy will usually mean a core or excisional technique is required.

Ultrasound

Breast ultrasound is a technique of increasing importance in the diagnosis of breast disease. It has a major role in the assessment of a specific abnormality in the breast, discovered during clinical examination or via the use of mammography. Ultrasound is helpful in determining the characteristics of a focal abnormality, and when combined with mammography, increases the diagnostic specificity. Put simply, mammography detects lesions and ultrasound provides an interpretation of the nature of the lesion (Table 19.3). Ultrasound is the imaging modality of choice in younger women. It has a limited role in the screening of asymptomatic women, except in the assessment of mammographically detected lesions. It may be used as part of a strategy of assessment for women at higher risk of breast cancer.

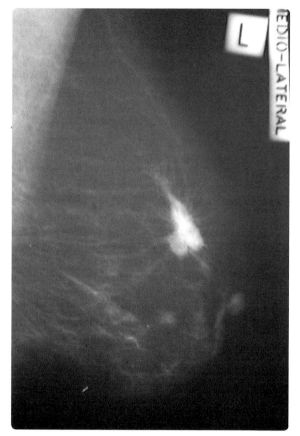

Fig. 19.7 Large stellate mass (carcinoma): note dense central body and long radiating dense strands – both features relate to the abundant collagenous fibrous tissue induced by the tumour cells.

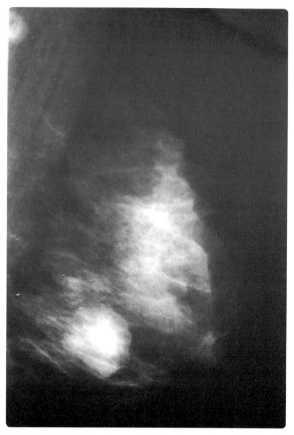

Fig. 19.8 MLO view demonstrating large, dense, lobulated mass (high grade carcinoma). High grade carcinomas are often cellular and grow rapidly with pushing margins and little fibrous response – hence the better definition and lack of stellate features. These lesions may mimic benign entities.

Table 19.2 Mammographic characteristics of calcifications

Benign	Indeterminate	Malignant
Skin location	Amorphous	Pleomorphic (Figs 19.11 and 19.12)
Vascular	Indistinct	Heterogeneous
Large rods (Fig. 19.9)		Fine
Eggshell		Linear
Milk of calcium		Branching
Layering		Casting
Diffuse		Extending to nipple
Scattered (Fig. 19.10)		

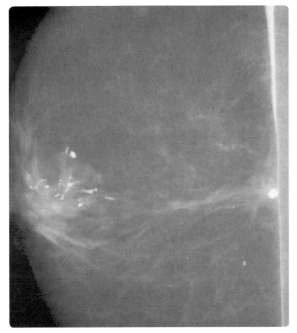

Fig. 19.9 Macrocalcification. In this postoperative breast the dense, rodlike ductal calcification is suggestive of plasma cell mastitis. The rounded density at the posterior margin of the breast suggests calcified fat necrosis within scar tissue.

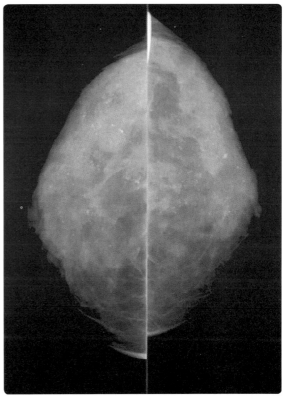

Fig. 19.10 Benign microcalcification. Abundant fine calcifications scattered throughout both breasts, in florid fibrocystic change. A few subtle rounded masses are also seen, suggesting cysts.

Table 19.3 Ultrasonographic characteristics of benign and malignant lesions

Ultrasound characteristic	Benign lesion	Malignant lesion
Cystic/solid	Simple cyst (Fig. 19.13) Anechoic	Partial cystic change Solid
Shape	Flat (width > height) Round	Tall (height > width) Irregular
Margins	Circumscribed (Fig. 19.14)	Ill defined Microlobulated
Echogenicity	Homogeneous	Heterogeneous
Acoustic properties	Enhancement	Shadowing
Doppler/vascular signal	Absent	Present
Axillary lymph nodes	Normal	Abnormal

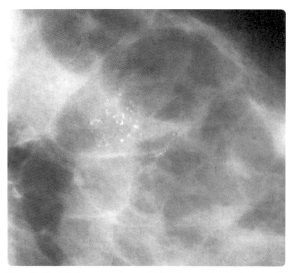

Fig. 19.11 Malignant microcalcification. A focal cluster of pleomorphic calcification (variable in size, shape and density), typical of that seen in high grade DCIS. Note the occasional linear formations due to the intraductal location of the calcification, which forms in necrotic malignant duct lining cells.

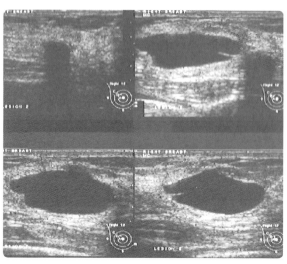

Fig. 19.13 A cyst on ultrasound. The lesion is ovoid, well defined anechoic lesion with acoustic shadowing. Placement of cursors at lesion margins allows accurate measurement of well defined lesions (measurements not shown). NB: top left frame shows a small benign calcified lesion: note acoustic shadowing due to calcium.

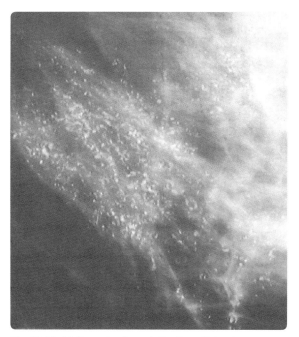

Fig. 19.12 Malignant microcalcification. Extensive pleomorphic calcification in high grade DCIS.

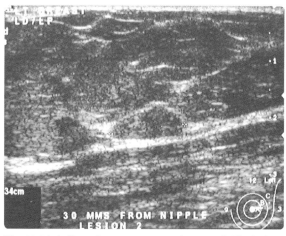

Fig. 19.14 A fibroadenoma seen on ultrasound. The lesion is ovoid, well defined, homogeneous and a solid mass. Note the echogenic (bright) needle entering the lesion for fine needle aspiration cytology.

Indications for breast ultrasound include:

- assessment of clinical breast mass
- assessment of mammographic abnormality
- age <35 years
- pregnancy
- follow-up 'benign' lesions
- guided FNAB, core biopsy, preoperative hookwire or carbon track, SLN lymphoscintography
- management of cyst, abscesses, haematoma
- biopsy in the presence of a breast implant
- surgical specimen examination.

Good ultrasound breast imaging requires both appropriate equipment (usually a 10-Hz probe) and a well-trained examiner (traditionally a radiographer/ sonographer but increasingly a radiolologist or surgeon). Real-time scanning and interpretation are vital, as the photographed images are best considered as documentation of the study rather than diagnostic images (Box 19.2). The simplicity of use, flexibility of image, portability of equipment and lack of ionising radiation give ultrasound several roles in breast imaging.

The ultrasonographic characteristics of breast carcinomas can be quite variable. Low-to-intermediate tumours often show shadowing, and tend to be heterogenous lesions with an abundant fibrous component (Fig. 19.15). Breast cancers tend to have an irregular outline (Fig. 19.16). An ultrasound appearance which

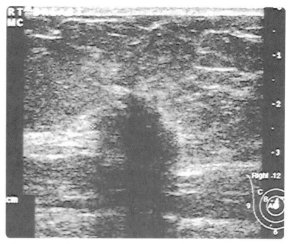

Fig. 19.15 Ultrasound appearances of a low grade carcinoma.

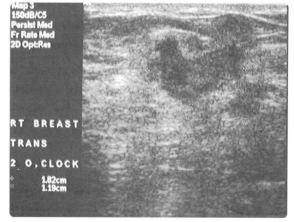

Fig. 19.16 The ultrasound appearances of a breast cancer, showing a solid, cellular lesion with irregular margins and acoustic enhancement.

shows a well-defined lesion that, homogeneous, has a cellular mass with strong acoustic enhancement is more typically a rapidly growing, high grade carcinoma (Fig. 19.17). This appearance overlaps with benign lesions such as fibroadenoma. Calcification may be present (Fig. 19.18).

Interventional techniques

The key to breast disease is establishing a tissue diagnosis. Increasingly, this is done without resort to open

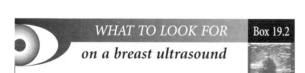

WHAT TO LOOK FOR | Box 19.2

on a breast ultrasound

- Compare with prior examinations
- Correlate with clinical and mammographic abnormalities
- Breast lesion present:
  - location
  - size
  - cystic or solid
  - shape
  - margins
  - internal echoes
  - external echoes/shadowing
  - Doppler/vascular signal
  - check axillary lymph nodes

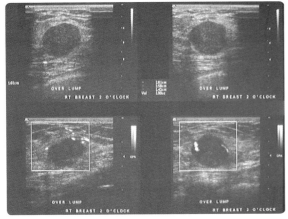

Fig. 19.17 Ultrasound of a high grade carcinoma. Note the prominent associated vessels and interruption of tissues planes.

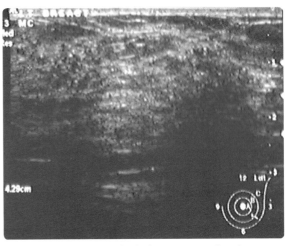

Fig. 19.18 An ultrasound of a breast cancer showing abundant calcification (punctuate bright foci) in an area of DCIS with associated invasive carcinoma.

Table 19.4 Comparison of procedures available for breast biopsy

Imaging modality	Biopsy method	Ease of use	Cost	Role
Palpation	FNAB Core	Basic	Minimal	Palpable masses
Ultrasound	FNAB Core	Moderate	Low	Masses Abundant califications
Upright stereotactic MMG	FNAB	Skilled	Moderate	Masses Calcifications
Prone table digital MMG	FNA Core Vacuum/ large core	Skilled	High	Masses Calcifications
MRI	FNAB Core	Difficult Limited availability Experimental	High	Lesions not seen on US/ MMG

surgical biopsy for abnormalities that are impalpable and are demonstrable only on imaging. Imaging-guided interventional biopsy techniques are therefore vital in breast abnormality assessment. Both mammogram and ultrasound can be used for these techniques. In general, the simplest method that will obtain an accurate diagnosis is employed (Table 19.4). This means that ultrasound is usually preferred over more complex mammographic or stereotactic-based procedures. It also means that fine-needle aspiration biopsy is used in preference to core or guided excision biopsy. The nature of the lesion being assessed is also important. Masses are generally well suited to ultrasound fine-needle aspiration, whereas microcalcifications often require a stereotactic core biopsy for satisfactory sampling.

The other important task in interventional breast radiology involves the localisation of lesions for formal surgical excision. This aspect is dealt with later in the chapter.

Use of magnetic resonance imaging

The use of magnetic resonance imaging is currently limited, but may expand in the future. In general, whilst a very sensitive technique, MRI adds little to the diagnosis of known breast abnormalities, over ultrasound and mammography. MRI is too expensive and complex for use in standard population screening programmes. When combined with appropriate gadolinium enhancement, MRI appears to be useful in both the detection of recurrence in the previously treated and scarred breast, or in assessing potential multifocal or extensive lesions detected by routine breast imaging (see Chapter 6). Likewise it may have a limited role in the screening of high-risk women known to carry a genetic mutation for breast cancer (e.g. BRCA1 or 2). The lack of a practical biopsy system based on MRI technology is a major problem for the diagnosis of MRI detected lesions.

The potential advantages of MRI breast imaging include:

- no radiation
- no breast density limitations
- determination of malignancy
- multifocal/extensive disease
- post treatment breast
- high sensitivity.

The current disadvantages of MRI breast imaging are:

- cost
- calcifications unassessable
- localised biopsy difficult
- lack of standard MR protocols
- claustrophobia/foreign metallic bodies
- low specificity.

THE CLINICAL PROBLEMS

Diagnosis of a palpable lesion

The presentation of a patient with a palpable breast lump is a common surgical problem. A benign lesion such as a simple cyst can be easily diagnosed on ultrasound and other than aspiration, no further action

taken. Any clinical abnormality which is highly suspicious of malignancy should have both mammography and ultrasound to aid the clinical diagnosis (triple test). If imaging features suggest a malignant lesion the patient should proceed to biopsy, which may be done by palpation or under imaging guidance. Surgical excision can often be performed without prior localisation.

Investigation/localisation of an impalpable lesion

The increasing use of screening mammography means that the surgeon now frequently faces the problem of the impalpable breast lesion that requires excision. The excision may be for diagnostic biopsy or for definitive management of an already diagnosed lesion. In these circumstances accurate preoperative localisation is vital to a successful procedure. As described previously, ultrasound is the easiest technique and provided the lesion is discernable by ultrasound, it is preferred to mammographic stereotactic methods. The two commonly employed localisation techniques are:

- placement of a fine wire with a barbed tip prior to the operative excision (hookwire) (Fig. 19.19)
- placement of a particulate carbon suspension (carbon track).

Hookwire

Hookwires are the most widely employed method for localised surgical excisions. It is vital for a surgeon undertaking a localised breast excision to have access

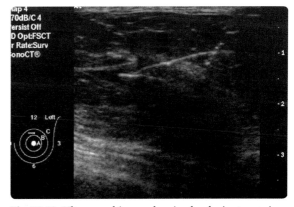

Fig. 19.19 Ultrasound image showing hookwire traversing a small, ill-defined, impalpable, stellate carcinoma.

to the patients mammograms in the operating room during the procedure. Ideally, after insertion of a hookwire, CC and 'true lateral' postinsertion mammogram views (orthogonal planes) should be obtained to ensure the lesion has been correctly localised (Figs 19.20 and 19.21). It should be noted if the wire is in fact within the lesion or lying nearby so that this can be allowed for during the excision of the lesion. Prior to commencing the procedure the surgeon should use the mammograms to map out and visualise the position of the lesion in the breast as the patient is in position for the procedure. The CC mammogram view will give the horizontal position; the vertical position can be established from the true lateral mammogram view. The position of the hookwire insertion relative to the lesion in the breast is important, particularly when planning the surgical incision. The surgical incision is usually placed over the site of the hookwire insertion, but if this approach is likely to produce a cosmetically or oncologically poor incision, the wire can be intercepted via a remotely sited incision and the lesion excised successfully.

Carbon track

An alternative approach to hookwire localisation is to place a track consisting of a carbon particle suspension. The carbon track is injected along a line from the lesion to a small tattoo on the skin surface. At operation the surgeon excises the track down to the lesion. Put simply, if all of the carbon is excised the lesion will be in the specimen. The major advantage of carbon over hookwire localisation, is that the carbon track can be placed some time prior to the day of surgery (often at the time of initial biopsy and assessment), making the logistics of surgical excision simpler. Carbon tracking generally requires an experienced radiologist and surgeon, as the track is not visible by postprocedure imaging to confirm the accuracy of placement.

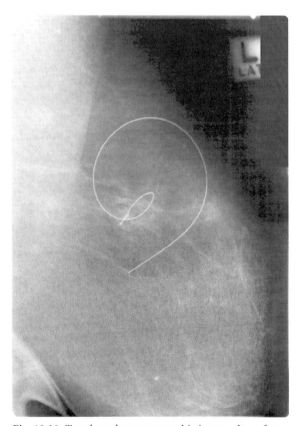

Fig. 19.20 True lateral mammographic image taken after hookwire placement to aid in surgical orientation.

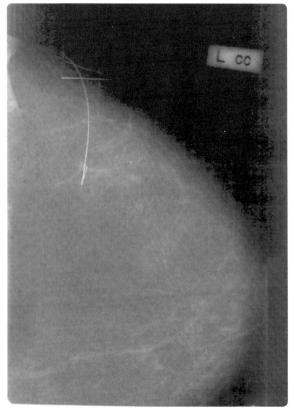

Fig. 19.21 Craniocaudal mammographic image taken after hookwire placement to aid in surgical orientation.

A number of pitfalls and potential problems exist with either localisation technique. These include:

- poor patient tolerance of hookwire/carbon insertion under local anaesthesia
- lesion altered in appearance/excised by prior biopsy
- lesions close to chest wall, immediately under nipple, extremely lateral and medial placed are the most difficult to localise
- hookwire displaced prior to surgical excision
- carbon track not continuous to lesion
- postinsertion mammography omitted
- specimen radiology not available during excision
- identification of small lesions in specimen by pathologist
- lesion not identified in specimen X-ray
- poor correlation between pre excision biopsy and specimen pathology
- omission of a 3-month post-excision mammogram to establish new mammographic baseline and to confirm lesion excision.

With either localisation technique, it is essential to confirm excision of the target lesion by performing a specimen X-ray (Box 19.3). Generally, this image is performed during the procedure so that the surgeon can consider immediate re-excision if the lesion is not present or the margins of normal breast tissue around a malignant lesion are inadequate. It is good practice to localise the specimen for accurate pathological assessment. If this orientation (usually superior, medial and lateral margins are identified) is performed using metallic surgical clips, then the specimen X-ray can be orientated for the benefit of both the operating surgeon and pathologist (Fig. 19.22). The process of localised breast lesion excision requires close coordination and communication between radiologist, surgeon and pathologist.

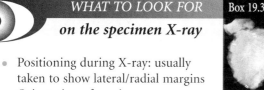

WHAT TO LOOK FOR — Box 19.3

on the specimen X-ray

- Positioning during X-ray: usually taken to show lateral/radial margins
- Orientation of specimen
- Presence of lesion: compare with preoperative MMG
- Extra lesions or changes, e.g. microcalcifications
- Margins: if malignant lesion for definitive excision
- Consider changing X-ray exposure if difficulties in interpretation (or use ultrasound)
- If re-excision performed: consider repeating specimen X-ray

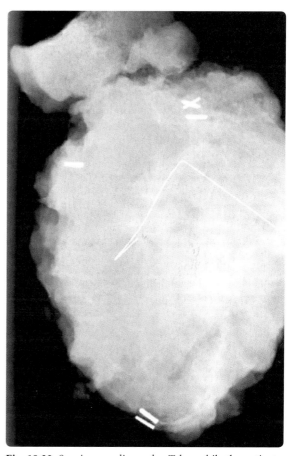

Fig. 19.22 Specimen radiography. Taken while the patient is still on the table, confirming the removal of the lesion (note hookwire). Note the surgical haemostasis clips used to mark the superior (one clip), medial (two clips) and lateral (three clips) margins of the specimen. This is important for the pathologist to identify which, if any margins are inadequately cleared of tumour.

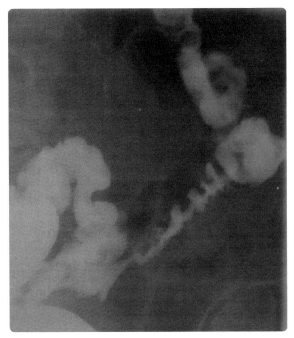

Fig. 19.23 A barium enema showing extrinsic compression of the sigmoid colon by metastatic tumour from a previously treated breast cancer.

Metastatic breast cancer

Imaging in metastatic breast cancer has several roles:

- staging prior to initial therapy
- diagnosis of recurrence in previously treated breast cancer
- monitoring of progression of disease or response to therapy.

Staging investigations include a plain chest radiograph. If there is clinical suspicion of disseminated disease (e.g. abnormal liver function tests), then further imaging is likely to include ultrasound or CT scanning of the liver. The whole body bone scan has limited value in the early stage of breast cancer (see Chapter 7), but is of more use when bone deposits are suspected (bone pain or abnormal serum biochemistry).

The initial diagnostic imaging investigations will depend on the symptoms and may involve plain radi-

ology of the chest, CT scanning of the abdomen or even contrast studies (Fig. 19.23). Monitoring of disease in response to therapy may involve either radiological or nuclear imaging (see Chapter 7).

Further reading

Baker LH. Breast cancer detection demonstration project: five-year summary report. Cancer J Clin 1982; 32:196–225

BreastScreen Australia. National Accreditation Standards. BreastScreen Australia Quality Improvement Program. BreastScreen Australia, Canberra, 2002

Ernst MF, Roukema JA. Diagnosis of non-palpable breast cancer: a review. Breast 2002; 11:13–22

Gill PG, Farshid G, Luke CG, Roder DM. Detection by screening mammography is a powerful independent predictor of survival in women diagnosed with breast cancer. Breast 2004; 13:15–22

Hata T, Takahashi H, Watanabe K et al. Magnetic resonance imaging for preoperative evaluation of breast cancer: a comparative study with mammography and ultrasound. J Am Coll Surg 2004; 198:190–7

Houssami N, Irwig L, Simpson JM et al. The contribution of work-up or additional views to the accuracy of diagnostic mammography. Breast 2003; 12(4):270–5

Irwig L, Houssami N, van Vliet C. New technologies in screening for breast cancer: a systematic review of their accuracy. Br J Cancer 2004; 90(11):2118–22

Kuhl CK. High-risk screening: multi-modality surveillance of women at high risk for breast cancer (proven or suspected carriers of a breast cancer susceptibility gene). J Exp Clin Cancer Res 2002; 21(3 Suppl):103–6

Lee JM, Orel SG, Czerniecki BJ et al. MRI before reexcision surgery in patients with breast cancer. AJR 2004; 182:473–80

Mehta TS. Current uses of ultrasound in the evaluation of the breast. Radiol Clin North Am 2003; 41:841–56

National Breast Cancer Centre/Royal Australian and New Zealand College of Radiologists. Breast imaging: a guide for clinical practice. National Breast Cancer Centre/Royal Australian and New Zealand College of Radiologists 2002. Online. Available: http://www.nbcc.org.au [accessed May 2004]

National Breast Cancer Centre/Royal Australian College of General Practitioners. Investigation of a new breast symptom. National Breast Cancer Centre/Royal Australian College of General Practitioners, 1997. Online. Available: http://www.nbcc.org.au [accessed May 2004]

Rose A, Collins JP, Neerhut P et al. Carbon localisation of impalpable breast lesions. Breast 2003; 12:264–9

Tabar L, Gad A. Screening for breast cancer: the Swedish trial. Radiology 1981; 138:219–22

Zorbas HM Breast cancer screening. MJA 2003; 178:651–2

Imaging in endocrine disease

20

P. Malycha, J. Morgan

Background

Imaging has become increasingly important in the assessment and management of endocrine disorders. Imaging investigations have a role in diagnosis, operative localisation and can be used therapeutically for some thyroid and adrenal abnormalities.

THE RADIOLOGICAL INVESTIGATIONS

Ultrasound

This is an important modality in the identification and localisation of mass lesions affecting the endocrine organs, although it is less precise in the assessment of lesions within the pancreas and adrenal glands.

Radionuclide scanning

In addition to their role in the assessment of gland function, radioisotopic studies are important in the detection and localisation of metastatic endocrine disease and ectopic glandular tissue. Radiopharmaceuticals can be used to have a direct therapeutic role or can be tagged with cytotoxic agents and used to deliver targeted chemotherapy.

Computed tomography scanning

CT characteristics have been defined that help differentiate benign from malignant lesions, particularly for adrenal lesions. With the increased sensitivity of high-resolution scanners, CT is taking over from scintigraphy in the initial investigation of adrenal disease and it is the preferred investigation to look for mass lesions within the abdominal cavity. CT scanning of the neck and chest will give excellent images of the neck and mediastinum and provide information not available from ultrasound. CT also produces an anatomical image that is more easily understood than ultrasound by most surgeons.

Magnetic resonance imaging and positron emission tomography scanning

These imaging modalities are usually second-line investigations in endocrine disease. MRI can help determine the likely content of adrenal masses and PET scanning provides information on the likelihood of such masses being malignant.

THE CLINICAL PROBLEMS

Thyroid

- Anatomy, embryology and imaging of the thyroid
- clinical problems in thyroid disease:
  - the solitary thyroid nodule

– thyroid malignancies
– benign thyroid disease.

Anatomy, embryology and imaging of the thyroid

The thyroid is not only easily palpated but also readily imaged by a variety of techniques. However the easiest and cheapest examination is real-time ultrasound (US) performed at the initial consultation. Most lesions can be adequately assessed by sonography and US-guided fine-needle aspiration cytology (FNAC). A 7.5- to 10-MHz high-resolution linear array transducer will provide an accurate measurement of cross-sectional and sagittal size of the thyroid gland and provide an immediate assessment of the physical features. The normal thyroid lobe measures approximately 20 mm wide, 30 mm deep and 40 mm in length. Ultrasonographic software will provide a read out of lobar volume which is normally between 18 and 20 mL, with females having slightly greater thyroid volume than males.

To assess the thyroid an appreciation of embryology is needed. The tongue and thyroid arise from the first and second branchial arches and are pulled down to the trachea by the developing heart and aortic sac, attracting cellular elements from the lower arches. Thus, the resulting thyroglossal tract extends from the foramen caecum of the tongue to the anterior mediastinum. The thyroid also obtains cells from the lateral ectoderm which become the tubercles of Zuckerkandl and are the origin of the calcitonin-secreting cells.

The sonographic anatomy of the thyroid is quite constant, with the carotid artery, jugular vein and larynx as stable landmarks. Saggital views clearly identify the upper pole, which is limited superiorly by the attachment of the sternothyroid muscle to the oblique line of the thyroid cartilage. Inferiorly the lower pole leads to the thyrothymic ligament and inferior thyroid vessels, which can be traced into the anterior mediastinum. Enlarged lymph nodes in the cervical chain and suprasternal area can be clearly defined with US. The surgeon's knowledge of the operative anatomy enhances clinical or image assessment of the thyroid and should be performed with potential surgical exploration in mind.

Nuclear scanning remains a favoured investigation for physicians but its value to surgeons is limited. Scintigraphy is useful for determining whether a nodule is 'hot' (lower incidence of cancer) or 'cold' (higher incidence of cancer) and while it will assess thyroid function it provides limited anatomical information other than an appreciation of gland size and retrosternal extension (see Chapter 7).

CT is ideal for the assessment of retrosternal extension and tracheal deviation or compression by a multi nodular goitre or growing tumour. It will reliably show gland size and any difference in the lobes.

MRI suffers from movement artifact and offers little more than CT. PET is not routinely used in the diagnosis of a primary thyroid cancer, however it role in metastatic thyroid cancer is under investigation.

The solitary thyroid nodule

On palpation alone, up to 7% of the population will have a thyroid nodule. On screening with ultrasound, thyroid nodules are evident in 19–46% of the population, but most are impalpable, small and insignificant. CT and MRI studies have identified thyroid incidentaloma in 15% of adult patients. With any solitary thyroid nodule, the main objective is to determine whether the lesion is benign or malignant. Most apparently solitary nodules are part of a multinodular goitre with a dominant nodule being clinically evident. US-guided fine-needle aspiration cytology remains an important investigation of a suspicious (usually solid) nodule. The needle should sample cells from a solid portion of the nodule under US guidance, ensuring that the cytology specimen is representative of the lesion. Although FNAC is highly specific if 'malignant', it has a low sensitivity. Cytology of follicular lesions is notoriously unreliable and thyroidectomy remains a diagnostic operation.

Malignancies of the thyroid

Papillary carcinoma Papillary carcinoma typically presents as a solitary nodule but is often part of a multifocal and multicentric disease process, and second or third lesions should be sought. Sonography of papillary cancers reveals a solid lesion with irregular or fuzzy margins and an absent 'halo' sign (thin low echogenicity surrounding ring) (Fig. 20.1). US may demonstrate fine punctate microcalcification associated with Psammoma bodies (Box 20.1). Such lesions are hypo- or hyperechoic with a posterior acoustic shadow and are highly vascular on Doppler. Involved

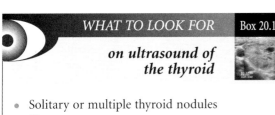

on ultrasound of the thyroid

- Solitary or multiple thyroid nodules
- Size
- Solid, cystic or complex
- Margins: 'halo' sign
- Microcalcifications
- Cervical lymphadenopathy

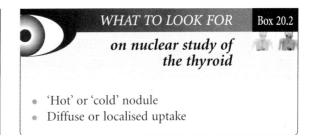

on nuclear study of the thyroid

- 'Hot' or 'cold' nodule
- Diffuse or localised uptake

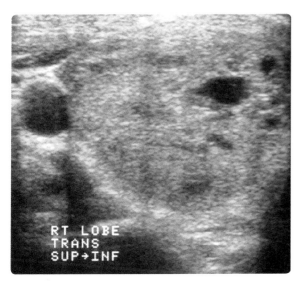

Fig. 20.1 Ultrasound appearance of a papillary carcinoma of the thyroid. The margins of the lesion are blurred.

lymph nodes are often heterogeneous, due to cystic or degenerative changes, and sometimes show microcalcifications. Despite these typical features, imaging cannot determine pathology and US-guided FNA is required. In the operating room, US is useful for directing functional neck dissections.

When a diagnosis of papillary carcinoma has been made a pre-operative US CT of the neck is necessary to assess the cervical and mediastinal lymph nodes before the tissue planes are disrupted by total thyroidectomy and functional neck dissection. Papillary carcinoma of the thyroid is usually hypodense but with variable densities and on occasion, microcalcifications can be seen within it. The radiological features do not suggest the hard sclerotic lesions often encountered at operation. When nodes are extensively involved by tumour they appear heterogeneous, often with cystic necrotic change, and with a well-defined periphery.

Nuclear scanning using radioiodine should demonstrate a cold nodule, but is non-specific (Box 20.2).

MRI does not offer more than CT and suffers from movement artefact. FDG-PET is of limited use in thyroid cancer but may play a role in establishing the source of recurrence in treated patients who develop elevated thyroglobulin levels without radioactive iodine uptake. With the increasing availability of PET for staging oncological patients, up to 3% will have incidental thyroid lesions with a high incidence of primary thyroid cancer. Most of these lesions are sclerosing occult papillary carcinomas and clinical judgement must be used in deciding which require surgery. Caution must be exercised as diffuse uptake occurs with thyroiditis, and tense neck muscles may utilise available glucose and mimic cervical nodal metastases.

Postoperative iodine-131 scanning should be performed after surgery when the TSH level is elevated to assess residual thyroid tissue and metastatic disease which can then be treated with a therapeutic dose (see Chapter 7). A preoperative contrast CT may delay radioactive iodine therapy but its value as a baseline study in recurrent disease may outweigh the risk of delay. The bioavailability of free inorganic iodide varies considerably between brands of contrast media. A study of euthyroid volunteers showed that 30 mg of iodide markedly suppressed thyroid uptake of radioactive iodine. Gadolinium enhanced MRI is an alternative to CT without the inherent problems of iodine load.

Follicular carcinoma Ultrasonographic findings are usually unhelpful in differentiating follicular cancer from other benign nodules. Follicular carcinoma is usually solitary. The diagnosis of follicular carcinoma is made by histological assessment of the capsule for vascular invasion and to a lesser extent capsular invasion. Hemithyroidectomy with paraffin section is needed for diagnosis. However sonographic signs of malignancy include irregular margins, non-encapsulation with evidence of invasion and thickening of the margin (Fig. 20.2). There may be an irregular halo effect and Doppler findings are variable. While features of a long developing cancer may be defined by these parameters, the smaller follicular cancers, minimally invasive follicular carcinoma or papillary variant of follicular carcinoma cannot be distinguished from an adenoma.

Contrast enhanced CT will not add significant information but could be considered to assess the neck and mediastinum after the diagnosis is made and before a (completion) total thyroidectomy. However it should be appreciated that follicular cancers do not usually involve cervical nodes.

Medullary carcinoma This lesion is usually unicentric and on US has similar features to papillary cancer. Amyloid is a distinguishing feature, and if present, appears as bright foci within the tumour and nodal or liver metastases. Contrast enhanced CT of neck, chest and liver are needed to assess metastatic involvement. More recently PET scanning has a role in detecting tumour metastases. Various radiolabelled ligands have been tested including 18F-FDG and 6-(^{18}F)-fluorodopamine, the latter more specific for chromaffin-rich tumours.

Anaplastic carcinoma These rapidly growing hard malignancies show US evidence of diffuse changes throughout. They are aggressive and often invade or compress the trachea, oesophagus, internal jugular vein and carotid artery. Tumour size and evidence of vascular invasion on Doppler should lead the surgeon to the diagnosis. CT will give the best assessment of its size while gadolinium enhanced MRI will identify vascular invasion of the major vessels in the upper chest.

Lymphoma Like anaplastic cancers, lymphomas grow rapidly often causing compressive symptoms. Always non-Hodgkin's in type, they can be differentiated from anaplastic cancer by their homogeneity and non-invasion of vascular structures. US, contrast CT and open biopsy to obtain fresh tissue for pathological diagnosis are required.

Metastases and rare malignancies Squamous cell carcinoma arises rarely in the thyroid or in thyroid remnants along the thyroglosssal tract. Diagnosis is by cytology and biopsy. There are no special features for these tumours on imaging. Teratomas should be considered in infants and children.

The thyroid has a large blood supply for its size and can be the site of metastases mostly from renal cell carcinoma and melanoma. Cytology and histopathology are required for diagnosis and thyroid imaging is as for other thyroid lesions. Multiple malignancies in the gland should raise the question of metastatic disease.

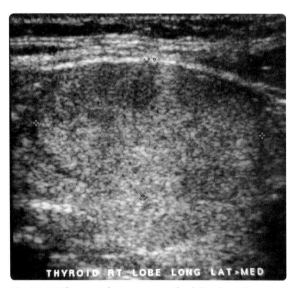

Fig. 20.2 Ultrasound appearance of a follicular cell carcinoma of the thyroid. There is increased risk of cancer when the lesion is solitary, when there is increased vascularity throughout the lesion and when it is more than 40 mm in diameter. Lesions between 10 and 40 mm are in the 'grey zone'. Follicular cancers tends to be low grade and time is often an important modality in assessment. Ultrasound is invaluable in the temporal assessment of such lesions.

Thymic lesions occur in the thymus below the thyroid in the thyrothymic ligament and into the mediastinum. These are usually found as incidental lesions on a chest radiograph or CT scan.

Benign conditions of the thyroid

Follicular adenoma The features may be the same as for follicular carcinoma and no investigation can distinguish between them. Solitary long standing thyroid lesions from 3 to 4 cm compress the surrounding gland and on US show a solid dense capsule with a peripheral hypoechoic halo. The capsule should be regular and smooth. The centre of the adenoma can undergo cystic degeneration, appearing as a dark hypoechoic mass with brighter isoechoic material particularly at the periphery of the nodule.

Nodular goitre US, CT, MRI and nuclear scanning cannot distinguish between benign and malignant nodules. Once again, US is the most helpful initial investigation. The hyperplastic nodules of nodular or adenomatous goitre are usually isoechoic when compared with the normal thyroid but will often reveal a vague capsular halo. The margins of the nodule(s) may be indistinct and the number and size of lesions can be hard to determine. However other multinodular goitres will have well defined dense nodules with a prominent halo. Cystic degeneration is common in involutionary nodules where the solid and liquid interface is easily identified. Old haemorrhage into nodules produces cysts that are sonolucent (dark), have irregular borders and show septation associated with the underlying degenerative and inflammatory response. True cysts may not exist or at least are uncommon. They are probably degenerative and part of the multinodular goitre spectrum. They can be multiple and the surgeon must remember that cancer may coexist with degenerative or other nodules in this disease.

A plain chest X-ray will give a good evaluation of the trachea and upper mediastinum, but a CT scan will best demonstrate the size of the goitre, compression or displacement of the trachea and oesophagus and retrosternal extension (Fig. 20.3). Whilst administration of iodine containing contrast may cause the Jod Basedow phenomenon, the diagnostic information obtained from contrast enhanced CT is very useful for

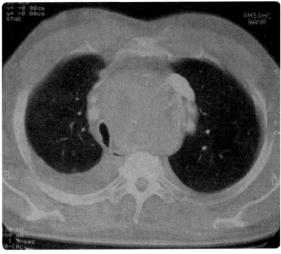

Fig. 20.3 A large retrosternal goitre with compression and deviation of the trachea and oesophagus to the right. There are areas of calcification within the gland.

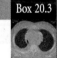

WHAT TO LOOK FOR Box 20.3

on CT of the thyroid

- Size of goitre and lobe size differences
- Neck anatomy
- Retrosternal extension
- Tracheal deviation
- Tracheal stenosis
- Oesophageal compression: tubercle of Zuckerkandl
- Calcification
- Paratracheal, centrocervical and mediastinal lymph nodes

the assessment and review of large retrosternal glands (Box 20.3). Calcification in degenerate areas within a multinodular gland are common.

Synthetic activity of the thyroid can be characterized by a [131]iodine nuclear scan. About 80% of nodules are non-functional and 'cold', and only one-fifth of these are cancerous. For this reason FNAC is more clinically relevant than nuclear scanning. Hyperthyroidism usually occurs in the diffuse goitre of Grave's disease but less commonly is due to a hyperfunctioning solitary 'hot' nodule. Less than 1% of 'hot' nodules are malignant. High uptake of thallium-201 has been investigated as an indicator of thyroid malignancy in 'cold' solitary nodules but its role in clinical practice is not yet established.

MRI has a limited role in the evaluation of a thyroid nodule. It has some advantages over CT in that more detailed anatomy is obtained. Nodules can be characterized using gadolinium enhanced scans, which do not interfere with scintigraphy and remnant ablation. However, the sensitivity of MRI remains under evaluation.

Diffuse enlargement of the thyroid can be physiological or part of Grave's disease or thyroiditis, particularly Hashimoto's. These conditions may show diffuse and varied echogenicity on US. Nuclear scanning is useful for evaluating uptake and function (see Chapter 7).

Thyroglossal remnant Cystic or solid thyroid lesions can occur along the whole tract but over half will be inferior to the thyroid. US will delineate these lesions and can be useful to monitor size and perform FNAC. Nuclear scanning has been recommended to diagnose a lingual thyroid, but US of the thyroid will tell whether it is absent from its normal position.

Parathyroid

Parathyroid localization

Relevance for considering localizing investigations
Before the enthusiasm for minimally invasive parathyroidectomy, endocrine surgeons saw no real advantage in pre-operative imaging as an experienced endocrine surgeon offered the patient a 98% chance of successful removal of the adenoma(s) without any radiological investigation.

Identification of solitary parathyroid adenomas using ^{99m}technetium sestamibi methoxyisobutylisonitrile (MIBI) has given nuclear scanning a new role (see Chapter 7). In conjunction with high-resolution ultrasound, MIBI has allowed minimally invasive parathyroidectomy (MIP) to develop and be adopted as first line surgery in selected cases. MIBI has a reported sensitivity of 75 to 100% and specificity of 75 to 90%.

About half of patients with primary hyperparathyroidism have an identifiable parathyroid adenoma and

can be treated by MIP. However bilateral cervical exploration is always indicated for undetectable adenomas and multiple hyperplastic parathyroid glands as no contemporary imaging technique will reveal them (Table 20.1).

Preoperative imaging is of little value in secondary hyperparathyroidism and multiple endocrine neoplasia (MEN). Carcinoma is rare, representing less than 1% of surgical cases in most series and is rarely diagnosed preoperatively.

Anatomy and embryology An understanding of the anatomical variations of the parathyroid glands is essential to correctly interpret any radiological investigations. The upper parathyroid comes from the fourth branchial arch and is associated with the developing thyroid, which descends to reach the trachea at 11 weeks. It travels a relatively short distance and its position near the thyroid is more constant than the lower gland.

An undescended superior gland may be found in the pharyngeal and vascular derivatives of the fourth arch from above the carotid bifurcation down to the thyroid gland. The superior gland is more constant in its position than the lower with over 90% found above and lateral to the intersection of the recurrent laryngeal nerve and inferior thyroid artery.

The lower parathyroid comes from the third branchial arch and is thus closely related to the embryological parathymus. Its position is less anatomically constant and may be found associated with the third arch derivatives from the carotid sheath, thyrothymic ligament, anterior mediastinum and occasionally the aortopulmonary window.

The average combined weight of the four glands is around 120 mg with individual glands weighing from 30 to 70 mg. An average gland measures $6 \times 5 \times 2$ mm and may be multilobular. Parathyroid glands increase in size until the fourth decade and have an increasing fat content with age. Autopsy studies show that 3% of population will have only three glands, and 13% will have supernumerary glands. Superior glands are symmetrical in about 80% cases and inferior glands 70%.

Ultrasound

High resolution US using a 7.5- to 15-MHz real-time small parts scanner is normally used. An assessment of thyroid nodularity can be performed by the surgeon

Table 20.1 Location of the parathyroid glands

Location of superior parathyroid glands

80%	Just above and lateral to intersection of the RLN and ITA
14%	Behind the superior pole thyroid gland
4%	Adjacent to ITA, behind lobe of Zuckerkandl
1%	Retropharyngeal or retro-oesophageal
0.8%	Above superior pole of thyroid
0.2%	Intrathyroid

Location of inferior parathyroid glands

46%	Behind inferior thyroid pole
26 %	Thyrothymic ligament
17%	Antero-lateral to inferior thyroid pole
6%	Just below intersection of RLN and ITA
2.8%	Above intersection of RLN and ITA
2%	Posterior mediastinum in aortopulmonary window
2%	Intrathymic
0.2%	Infrathymic

ITA, inferior thyroid artery; RLN, recurrent laryngeal nerve.

or radiologist and if multiple thyroid nodules are found there is little point in proceeding with MIBI localisation (see Chapter 7). When minimal thyroid pathology is present an adenomatous parathyroid will usually be seen with ultrasound.

Parathyroid adenomas are typically extrathyroidal, well-defined, homogenous, hypoechoic masses with a vascular pedicle arising cranially. Their shape may be round in transverse section but appear elongated in sagittal view. Using Doppler US, vascular flow can be confirmed and the relationship of the blood vessels can distinguish an adenoma from a lymph node that has hilar vessels. In addition, lymph nodes are usually multiple and will not compress or wobble. Adenomas greater than 1 cm are usually well visualised in the neck. Deep-sited small adenomas may be revealed with graded compression of the adenoma against the longus colli prevertebral muscle. Angulation of the probe behind the clavicle may allow visualisation to the level of the brachiocephalic vein but ectopic locations within the mediastinum are not visible with US.

Surgeons must understand the relations of the adenoma to anatomical and operative landmarks such as the thyroid capsule, thyrothymic ligament, carotid artery and trachea. Size and depth are also useful and simple measurements. Correlation with scintigraphy is essential and US should be repeated after scintigraphy to plan the operation. Both procedures should be undertaken as part of the formal localisation of a parathyroid adenoma. The sensitivity of US is up to 93% but is subjective and operator dependent. US is a very useful tool particularly when performed by, or in the presence of, an experienced endocrine surgeon. In addition, ultrasound is portable and can be used in the operating theatre.

Scintigraphy

Subtraction scintigraphy using thallium-201 and ^{99m}technetium pertechnetate (Tl-Tc) was used before the introduction of MIBI and had a sensitivity of up to 86%. Thyroid and parathyroid tissue take up thallium, but only thyroid takes up pertechnetate. Digital subtraction of the two isotopes then reveals a parathyroid image. This technique requires the patient to remain still and works best when the adenoma is some distance from the thyroid gland. Anterior–posterior and lateral views are especially useful when an adenoma is in the mediastinum.

Over the last decade, ^{99m}technetium hexakis-2-methoxyisobutylisonitrile or MIBI has become the scan of choice for localizing parathyroid glands. ^{99m}Technetium tetrofosmin also has its proponents. MIBI has reported sensitivities of 75 to 100% and specificities of 75–90% for detecting parathyroid adenoma at first presentation (Fig. 20.4). The principal factor that influences uptake by MIBI is gland size or more accurately gland volume with other factors such as cell type and mitochondrial content being less important. It is the mitochondria that take up MIBI that on haematoxylin and eosin staining appear pink. However, clear cell adenomas that are less mitochondria rich than oxyphil adenomas seem to take up MIBI equally. Lymph glands do not show up on MIBI.

Subtraction or dual phase protocols of nuclear scanning, single photon emission computed tomography (SPECT) and collimation add to the sensitivity of nuclear scanning. Improved diagnostic and spatial accuracy are seen with SPECT, best applied to the patient with an ectopic or multiple adenoma.

CT and MRI

Neither CT nor MRI have a role in the initial management of primary or secondary hyperparathyroidism. Sensitivities for CT are generally poor, ranging between 43 and 92%; MRI is no better, with sensitivities between 50 and 93%. In patients scheduled for reoperation for recurrent or persistent hyperparathyroidism, preoperative detection of parathyroid adenomas is necessary to reduce the extent of surgery and increase the chance of success. CT and MRI will provide detailed anatomical information that can be interpreted with greater ease by the surgeon and add strength to the MIBI and US findings.

Fine cuts on modern fast CT scanners after rapid contrast infusion are required to capture a small tumour. CT- or US-guided aspiration cytology and parathyroid hormone assay can add diagnostic certainty and, when the lesion is localised with a carbon track, the surgeon can perform the operation via a minimally invasive approach. Gadolinium-enhanced MRI can detect adenomas as bright lesions on T2-weighted images, does not irradiate the patient and does not require iodine-based intravenous contrast. However, respiration movements and carotid pulsation may compromise MR images.

The various technologies may be combined to give even greater definition of parathyroid tumours. The coregistered CT and SPECT imaging is particularly useful for identifying tumours at distant sites or where there has been previous failed surgical exploration of the neck (Fig. 20.5).

Neuroendocrine tumours of the pancreas

Neuroendocrine pancreatic tumours are derived from neuroectodermal tissue and classified by the peptide hormones they secrete. Although most occur within the islet cells of the pancreas, they are also found elsewhere in the gut. The most common types are insulinomas and gastrinomas. Other extremely rare neuroendocrine pancreatic tumours include vasoactive intestinal peptide (VIP) -omas, glucagonomas and somatostatinomas. Carcinoid tumours are of similar origin and share some features of pancreatic neuroendocrine tumours, but are distributed in the foregut (stomach, lung), mid-gut (small bowel and appendix) and hindgut (rectum).

Most of these rare tumours are slow growing and behave in an indolent fashion, even in the presence of metastatic disease. In the latter instance, therapy can be difficult and techniques have been developed to target radio and chemotherapeutic agents to the tumours. These depend on the ability of CT to identify the lesions and a scintiscan to see if agents will be taken up (Fig. 20.6).

Insulinoma

Excessive beta islet cell secretion of insulin causes life-threatening hypoglycaemia. The annual incidence

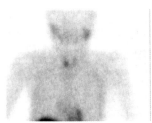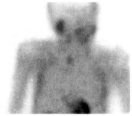

Fig. 20.4 Early and late images showing persistent uptake in a right lower parathyroid adenoma after administration of ^{99m}Tc-MIBI.

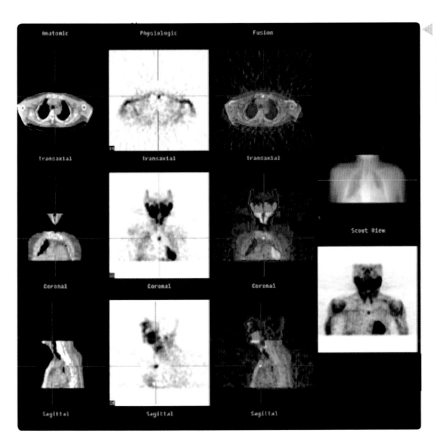

is one person per million. Diagnosis relies on clinician awareness and biochemical confirmation of inappropiate hypoglycaemia and hyperinsulinaemia. Surgical enucleation offers cure in 90% of insulinomas which are benign and solitary. Between 5 and 10% of patients with insulinomas will have MEN-1 and this group in particular have multiple insulinomas. The tumours are distributed throughout the endocrine organ, in the uncinate process, head, body and tail and due to their typical small size (6–20 mm), preoperative identification using US, CT, MRI and scintigraphy may fail. Endoscopic and intraoperative imaging of the pancreas using US has enhanced the detection of these occult lesions. By contrast, malignant insulinomas are large (>4 cm), metastasise to lymph nodes and liver, and are readily picked up on conventional imaging.

Transabdominal US is a non-invasive cheap test but will fail to identify most insulinomas. Sonography of this retroperitoneal organ is limited by body habitus, overlying bowel gas and the small size of insulinoma. Fine-slice multiphase abdominal CT dedicated to the pancreas has an improved sensitivity of up to 60%; detection rates are greater with increased tumour size. Oral contrast will outline the duodenum and bowel. Tumours are hypervascular and a contrast blush can reveal an insulinoma. MRI has similar sensitivity to CT. Tumours appear bright on T2-weighted images.

Less than half of insulinomas express somatostatin receptors and therefore scintigraphy using radiolabelled octreotide (a somatostatin analogue) may be worthless. If receptors are expressed, scintigraphy will indicate which part of the gland harbors the tumour or indeed show multiple lesions or metastases.

Endoscopic ultrasound with a 5- to 10-MHz transducer images the pancreas through the wall of the stomach and duodenum. High resolution enables the detection of the smallest of tumours at 2–3 mm. Insulinomas appear round and hypoechoic. The head of the pancreas is imaged well via the stomach, duodenal cap

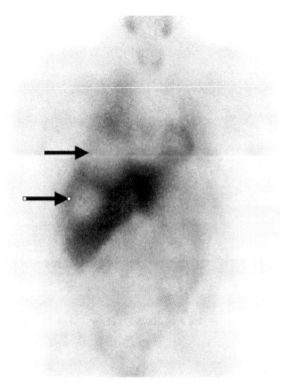

Fig. 20.6 ^{123}I-MIBG scan to determine if neuroendocrine tumour related liver masses (arrowed) were MIBG avid prior to potential therapy – they were not avid.

and from the third part of the duodenum. However, the body and tail can only be seen through the posterior wall of the stomach. The uncinate process is visualised from the third part of the duodenum.

Intraoperative US (IOUS) may be used as an adjunct to the digital palpation of the mobilised pancreas and can confirm precisely the tumour location. This will facilitate local treatment (enucleation) of the tumour. In addition, IOUS also plays a key role in identifying and protecting the pancreatic duct and vessels from damage during enucleation (see Chapter 5).

Although endoscopic and intraoperative sonography are not readily available in most centres, these tests are far superior to conventional imaging and may obviate the need for regional localisation using calcium arteriography and portal venous sampling.

Octreotide derivatives labelled with ^{111}In, ^{90}Y or other radionuclides have shown some effectiveness in the therapy of avid tumours.

Adrenal masses

The paired retroperitoneal adrenal glands are normally 30–50 mm in length and 5 mm thick. The right side is typically pyramidal in shape and lies over the right crus of the hemidiaphragm approximately at the level where the inferior vena cava becomes intrahepatic. The short right adrenal vein drains forwards and medially into the inferior vena cava. Of surgical importance an ectopic right adrenal vein may be present draining into an hepatic vein. Anterolaterally lies the bare area of the liver and inferiorly the right kidney. On the left side the gland is crescenteric and often slightly larger. The left adrenal is lateral to the ipsilateral crus of the hemidiaphragm, with the pancreas, splenic artery and peritoneum of the lesser sac anterior. The left renal vein lies inferior and into which the left adrenal vein drains. Both adrenals receive arterial blood from the superior suprarenal artery, a branch of the inferior phrenic, the middle suprarenal artery, a branch directly off the aorta and the inferior suprarenal artery, a branch of the renal artery. Within the gland an arterial plexus infiltrates the capsule, cortex and medulla.

Primary tumours of the adrenal gland arise from the cortex or medulla. They are functional endocrine tumours or non-functional. Primary adrenal carcinomas are rare, half are functional and secrete multiple cortical hormones. Imaging may have a straightforward role identifying a tumour when biochemical functional testing is positive. However, bilaterality, malignancy and ectopic sites need to be considered. Reconstructed images showing vascular anatomy may assist surgical planning.

Autopsy studies show that adrenal tumours are more prevalent with age, such that 7% of those over 70 years will have an adrenal mass. Up to 9% of those undergoing CT will have an incidental finding of an adrenal tumour (see Chapter 22). In this situation, further characterisation may be necessary and exclusion of function must be sought. If an adrenal mass is >4 cm in diameter then metastases or primary adrenal carcinoma should be suspected; 14% of adrenal carcinomas are <5 cm. Although these are common features of benign tumours, smooth margin and uniform texture are occasionally present in adrenal malignancy. Serial scanning of adenomas will show only a slow increase in size. Rapid growth, irregular outline, and heterogeneity are typical features of a malignant adrenal lesion. If considered benign and non-functional, repeat imaging with US or non-contrast CT can monitor change. With repeated measurement of adrenal lesions it is important to compare at the same cross sectional level.

Investigations

Ultrasound Ultrasound is a cheap, non-invasive and readily available investigation. If the mass is large enough to be visualised the adrenal size, texture and margins can be assessed but qualitative information is limited. It has a role in the follow up of benign lesions monitoring change, in particular growth.

Computed tomography Intracellular lipid is abundant in many adrenal cortical adenomas and helps differentiate the benign from malignant lesion (Fig. 20.7). Non-contrast CT of a lipid-rich adenoma shows low attenuation and a carcinoma has high attenuation. This is expressed in Hounsfield units (HU). An adrenal mass with less than 10 HU attenuation has a 43–71% sensitivity that it is benign but it is highly specific at 98–100%. In other words, if it is <10 HU it is almost certainly an adenoma, but approximately half of adrenal adenomas will have attenuation on non-contrast CT greater than 10 HU attributable to the lack of fat. By raising the threshold attenuation value

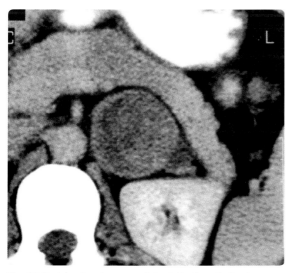

Fig. 20.7 A benign tumour of the left adrenal gland.

more adenomas are identified at the cost of reduced specificity.

Intravenous contrast CT demonstrates perfusion characteristics of adrenal lesions. Adenomas not only enhance rapidly, but they wash out contrast quickly. Carcinomas have similar vascular enhancement but retain contrast medium minutes later. The rate of washout can be assessed by measuring the attenuation in HU in the dynamic phase (60 seconds after contrast injection) and compare this with the attenuation in the delayed films (at 10 minutes). If the attenuation remains greater than 50% on delayed images then malignancy or an atypical adenoma is likely. Loss of 50% or more attenuation is specific for an adenoma and malignancy can virtually be excluded. Similarly, if the attenuation drops to 30 HU or less at 10 minutes after contrast injection malignancy is rare.

Magnetic resonance imaging As with CT, the lipid content of adrenal tumours is exploited by MRI. Chemical shift imaging has a high sensitivity and specificity differentiating adenomas from carcinoma. It relies on various resonance frequencies of protons within different tissues. Protons contained in fat have a different resonance frequency than protons in water. When fat and water protons are close together (i.e. in the same voxel) and they are made to precess in-phase, their signals are additive. If they precess out-of-phase they cancel each other out, leading to a decrease in signal. Lipid-rich adenomas therefore appear darker on out-of-phase images than in-phase images. Adrenal masses devoid of lipid (e.g. carcinomas) show no significant chemical shift with similar signal intensities for each phase. Signal intensities should be compared to the spleen rather than the liver, as the latter is often affected by disease (steatosis, cirrhosis or haemachromatosis).

Scintigraphy Iodine-131-metaiodobenzylguanidine (MIBG) is an analogue of noradrenaline and accumulates in the neurosecretory granules of the adrenal medulla. It is used to identify phaeochromocytomas. An alternative radiopharmaceutical is indium-111-diethylene triamine penta-acetic acid (DTPA)-octreotide, a somatostatin analogue. Octreotide scans identify neuroendocrine tumours which express somatostatin receptors including phaechromocytomas but also carcinoids and medullary thyroid cancers.

Noriodocholesterol (NP-59) is a cholesterol analogue and binds to low density lipoprotein receptors of the adrenal cortex. It is taken up readily by cortical functional adenomas and is useful in determining bilateral disease.

FDG-PET Malignant adrenal masses are metabolically active and utilise glucose. PET using fluorine-18 fluorodeoxyglucose (FDG) is highly sensitive in determining malignancy. Inflammatory lesions are also glucose avid, however adenomas show no increased FDG uptake (see Chapter 6).

Functional adrenal medulla tumours

Phaeochromocytoma This catecholamine secreting tumour is derived from the neuroectodermal tissue of the adrenal medulla. Extra-adrenal phaeochromocytomas known as paragangliomas occur in 10% and are found in the head, neck, and chest, adjacent to the abdominal aorta, and in the pelvis within autonomic neural plexi. Adrenal phaeochromocytomas are usually unilateral and benign, however 10% are bilateral and 10% malignant. Malignancy cannot be distinguished histologically and is diagnosed when metastases are evident. Episodic symptoms of hypertension, headache and palpations are common symptoms. Biochemical testing of raised urinary catecholamines is diagnostic, thereafter imaging is necessary to localize

the tumour, identify bilaterality or an extra-adrenal location.

Fine-slice non-contrast CT is non-invasive, should demonstrate the lesion and is unlikely to precipitate a catecholamine crisis. Whereas it was traditionally believed that CT contrast may precipitate a crisis, the only study since the introduction of non-ionic contrast showed no significant relationship between the injection of contrast media and raised catecholamine levels, and it is probably safe to use contrast if necessary. The presence of an adrenal mass confirms the diagnosis, however bilaterality should be excluded. They are usually >2 cm and 'eggshell' calcifications are occasionally seen encircling the lesion. Phaeochromocytomas have high attenuation values typically >50 HU. CT can underestimate the true size of a phaeochromocytoma by about 18%. In the absence of an adrenal lesion, a paraganglioma should be sought in the paraspinal area and around the organ of Zuckerkandl near the aortic bifurcation.

MRI is an alternative to CT and is warranted if CT fails to identify the tumour, typically in the case of paraganglioma or recurrence after surgical resection, sometimes due to malignancy. Phaeochromocytoma appear hyperintense (white) on T2-weighted images.

Scintigraphy using MIBG has a preoperative role confirming that the lesion is single or multiple (Fig. 20.8). It is also utilised in the setting of recurrence

Fig. 20.8 Intense uptake in a right adrenal phaeochromocytoma of ^{123}I-MIBG in a patient with severe hypertension.

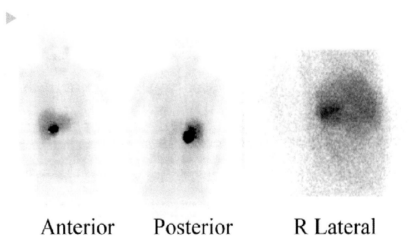

Anterior   Posterior   R Lateral

or residual disease post surgery. The bladder should be emptied with a catheter so not to miss a perivesical tumour. Abdominal or whole-body imaging is performed 24–72 hours after administration of MIBG. Whole-body imaging with MIBG has a sensitivity of 80–90% and specificity of 90–100%. Alternatively, somatostatin receptor scintigraphy can be performed. Octreotide is taken up by neuroendocrine tumours with somatostatin receptors including carcinoids and 75–90% of phaeochromocytomas. Whole-body imaging is performed at 4 and 24 hours after injection. Up to 50% of phaeochromocytomas will be identified by both MIBG and octreotide scans, the remainder will be seen on one scinitgraphy scan only. Phaeochromocytomas, particulary metastatic disease, can be treated with ^{131}I-MIBG.

Neuroblastomas This tumour is the commonest solid tumour of infancy. It arises from the developing neuroectodermal tissue and presents in neonates and infants usually as a mass. Nearly half occur within the gland itself, the rest arise from similar embryological autonomic tissue of the paraspinal region. Urinary catecholamines are raised.

CT or MRI confirms the diagnosis of a mass lesion. MIBG scan demonstrates metastases to the liver, lungs, bones and subcutaneous tissues and ^{131}I-MIBG can be used to treat the primary and metastatic lesions.

Functional adrenal cortex tumours

Functional adenomas of the cortex secrete cortisol (zona fasciculata), aldosterone (zona glomerulosa) and androgens (zona reticularis) and give rise to three syndromes of Cushing's, Conn's and virilising or feminising respectively. Investigation to anatomically identify a functional tumour is prompted by clinical suspicion and positive biochemistry of the relevant syndrome.

Cushing's syndrome Only 15–25% of patients with Cushing's syndrome will have a primary adrenal neoplasm. Most cases are due to a pituitary ACTH secreting adenoma and exclusion with pituitary MRI is relevant. Other causes are malignancies (e.g. lung) producing ectopic ACTH. Pituitary ACTH adenomas can cause bilateral adrenal enlargement in nearly two-thirds of patients, and the remainder have normal sized adrenal glands. Adrenal adenomas causing Cushing's syndrome are usually solitary, have low attenuation (lipid rich) and are >2 cm. Adrenal carcinomas are rare, much larger, heterogenous with irregular margins. Norcholesterol scintigraphy has a sensitivity of 94–100% diagnosing adrenal hypercortisolism and will demonstrate bilateral, persistent or recurrent disease.

Conn's syndrome An adrenal adenoma is responsible for 80% of cases of primary hyperaldosteronism and the other 20% are due to hyperplasia. The adenoma is usually unilateral and cured by surgical excision. Hyperplasia (idiopathic hyperaldosteronism) is bilateral, micro- or macronodular and is best managed medically with spironolactone. Rarely, adrenal carcinoma causes primary hyperaldosteronism.

Aldosterone secreting adenomas can be small with 20% <1 cm in diameter. Fine slice dedicated non-contrast CT is usually diagnostic showing a low attenuation circumscribed mass. Adrenal venous sampling can lateralise an adenoma or demonstrate bilateral disease. The femoral vein is cannulated in the angiography suite and blood is sampled from both the right and left adrenal veins and inferior vena cava. Aldosterone concentrations from each site are determined. In some centres, dexamethasone suppression norcholesterol scintigraphy is practiced and can assist in determining if the lesion is unilateral or bilateral. It has a reported sensitivity of 85% in detecting primary hyperaldosteronism. The radioligand is a cholesterol analogue and binds to low density lipoprotein receptors of the adrenal cortex and has been useful in determining bilaterality.

Non-functional adrenal lesions

Nowadays, the finding of an incidental adrenal mass on CT is common. Nearly one tenth of the population will have an adrenal mass and it is of paramount importance to establish whether the lesion is benign or malignant. Clinical examination and biochemistry is necessary to exclude a phaeochromocytoma (risk of secretory crisis) or functional cortical adenoma. In a patient with a known carcinoma, the likelihood of an adrenal lesion representing a metastasis is less than 50%. The presence of an adrenal metastasis on staging CT may have major impact upon the management plan and prognosis, and therefore detailed multimodality imaging with CT, MRI and PET is justified (see description above).

Metastasis Cancers of the lung, breast, gastrointestinal tract, kidney and melanoma commonly metastasise to the adrenal gland. When small, these lesions may appear homogenous with regular margins and may be difficult to distinguish from benign lesions. With time, non-contrast CT will usually show an irregular, locally invasive, heterogeneous mass, usually >4 cm. Attenuation is increased as malignant cells are devoid of intracytoplasmic lipid, but rarely a malignant adrenal will have an attenuation of <10 HU. Masses will often demonstrate heterogeneous contrast enhancement. There may be associated lymphadenopathy.

MRI of an adrenal carcinoma is bright on T2-weighted images, with delayed washout on gadolinium enhanced MR. Norcholesterol scintigraphy differentiates benign and malignant cortical tumours and has equivalent results to non-contrast CT. With the increasing availability of PET, oncology patients are frequently being staged using FDG. Malignant adrenal lesions are metabolically active and are FDG-PET avid.

Myelolipoma These benign tumours contain mature fat and haemopoietic tissue and occasionally calcify. The identification of pure fat within the lesion on CT is diagnostic. On MRI they are hyperintense on T1-weighted in-phase images.

Cyst Adrenal cysts are rare. The most common type is an endothelial or epithelial cyst. Adrenal haemorrhage may cause a pseudocyst, and echinococcus is an example of a parasitic cause. Ultrasound may show a hypoechoic smooth walled cyst. However internal septations and debris make distinction from malignant tumour necrosis difficult. Further imaging with CT and MRI are useful. Image guided FNAC may be indicated using a narrow spinal needle.

Haemorrhage Bilateral adrenal haemorrhage occurs in neonates caused by hypoxia or trauma. In adults haemorrhage is usually unilateral, right sided and due to trauma or infection. Acute haemorrhage is hyperechoic on US and as the blood liquifies it appears hypoechoic. With time the lesion contracts and can form a pseudocyst with coarse calcifications in the wall.

Eventually the pseudocyst collapses leaving specks of calcification within the adrenal gland. Other causes of calcification include tuberculosis and Addison's disease.

Further reading

Agarwal G, Barraclough BH, Robinson BG et al. Minimally invasive parathyroidectomy using the 'focused' lateral approach. I. Results of the first 100 consecutive cases. ANZ J Surg 2002; 72:100–4

Akerstrom G, Malmaeus J, Bergstrom R. Surgical anatomy of human parathyroid glands. Surgery 1984; 95:14–21

Arici C, Cheah WK, Ituarte PH et al. Can localization studies be used to direct focused parathyroid operations? Surgery 2001; 129:720–9

Bansal R, Tierney W, Carpenter S et al. Cost effectiveness of EUS for preoperative localization of pancreatic endocrine tumors. Gastrointest Endosc 1999; 49:19–25

Bliss RD, Gauger PG, Delbridge LW. Surgeon's approach to the thyroid gland: surgical anatomy and the importance of technique. World J Surg 2000; 24:891–7

Carpentier A, Jeannotte S, Verreault J et al. Preoperative localization of parathyroid lesions in hyperparathyroidism: relationship between technetium-99m-MIBI uptake and oxyphil cell content. Nucl Med 1998; 39:1441–4

Cases JA, Surks MI. The changing role of scintigraphy in the evaluation of thyroid nodules. Semin Nucl Med 2000; 30:81–7

Chatterton BE, Wycherley AG, Muecke TS et al. Thallium-201-technetium-99m subtraction scanning: its value in 50 cases of hyperparathyroidism submitted to surgery. Aust N Z J Surg 1987; 57:289–94

Christensen CR, Glowniak JV, Brown PH, Morton KA. The effect of gadolinium contrast media on radioiodine uptake by the thyroid gland. J Nuclear Med Technol 2000; 28:41–4

Cohen MS, Arslan N, Dehdashti F et al. Risk of malignancy in thyroid incidentalomas identified by fluorodeoxyglucose-positron emission tomography. Surgery 2001; 130:941–6

Delbridge L. Total thyroidectomy: the evolution of surgical technique. Aust N Z J Surg 2003; 73:761–8

Delorme S, Hoffner S. Diagnosis of hyperparathyroidism. Radiology 2003; 43:275–83

Doherty GM, Doppman JL, Shawker TH et al. Results of a prospective strategy to diagnose, localize, and resect insulinomas. Surgery 1991; 110:989–96; discussion 996–7

Fidler JL, Fletcher JG, Reading CC. Preoperative detection of pancreatic insulinomas on multiphasic helical CT. AJR 2003; 181:775–80

Gourgiotis L, Sarlis NJ, Reynolds JC et al. Localization of medullary thyroid carcinoma metastasis in a multiple endocrine neoplasia type 2A patient by 6-[18F]-fluorodopamine positron emission tomography. J Clin Endocrinol Metab 2003; 88:637–41

Grant CS, van Heerden J, Charboneau JW et al. Insulinoma. The value of intraoperative ultrasonography. Arch Surg 1988; 123:843–8

Grumbach MM, Biller BM, Braunstein GD et al. Management of the clinically inapparent adrenal mass ('incidentaloma'). Ann Intern Med 2003; 138:424–9

Hisham AN, Aina EN. Zuckerkandl's tubercle of the thyroid gland in association with pressure symptoms: a coincidence or consequence? Aust N Z J Surg 2000; 70:251–3

Kennedy RJ, Roberts AP, Reece GJ, Malycha PL. Minimally invasive parathyroidectomy for recurrent or persistent hyperparathyroidism using carbon track localization. Aust N Z J Surg 2003; 73:853–5

Kessler A, Rappaport Y, Blank A et al. Cystic appearance of cervical lymph nodes is characteristic of metastatic papillary thyroid carcinoma. J Clin Ultrasound 2003; 31(1):21–5

Kim N, Lavertu P. Evaluation of a thyroid nodule. Otolaryngol Clin North Am 2003; 36:17–33

Kouriefs C, Mokbel K, Choy C. Is MRI more accurate than CT in estimating the real size of adrenal tumours? Eur J Surg Oncol 2001; 27:487–90

Lau H, Lo CY, Lam KY. Surgical implications of underestimation of adrenal tumour size by computed tomography. Br J Surg 1999; 86:385–7

Laurie AJ, Lyon SG, Lasser EC. Contrast material iodides: potential effects on radioactive iodine thyroid uptake. J Nucl Med 1992; 33:237–8

Lorberboym M, Minski I, Macadziob S et al. Incremental diagnostic value of preoperative 99mTc-MIBI SPECT in patients with a parathyroid adenoma. J Nucl Med 2003; 44:904–8

Lumachi F, Ermani M, Basso S et al. Localization of parathyroid tumours in the minimally invasive era: which technique should be chosen? Population-based analysis of 253 patients undergoing parathyroidectomy and factors affecting parathyroid gland detection. Endocr Relat Cancer 2001; 1:63–9

Lumachi F, Marzola MC, Zucchetta P et al. Non-invasive adrenal imaging in primary aldosteronism. Sensitivity and positive predictive value of radiocholesterol scintigraphy, CT scan and MRI. Nucl Med Commun 2003; 24:683–8

Lumachi F, Zucchetta P, Marzola MC et al. Usefulness of CT scan, MRI and radiocholesterol scintigraphy for adrenal imaging in Cushing's syndrome. Nucl Med Commun 2002; 23:469–73

Magill SB, Raff H, Shaker JL et al. Comparison of adrenal vein sampling and computed tomography in the differentiation of primary hyperaldosteronism. J Clin Endocrinol Metab 2001; 86:1066–71

Mayo-Smith WW, Boland GW, Noto RB, Lee MJ. State-of-the-art adrenal imaging. Radiographics 2001; 995–1012

McDougall IR, Davidson J, Segall GM. Positron emission tomography of the thyroid with an emphasis on thyroid cancer. Nuc Med Commun 2001; 22:485–92

Morgan JL, Serpell JW, Cheng MS. Fine-needle aspiration cytology of thyroid nodules: how useful is it? Aust N Z J Surg 2003; 73:480–3

Mukherjee JJ, Peppercorn PD, Reznek RH. Pheochromocytoma: effect of nonionic contrast medium in CT on circulating catecholamine levels. Radiology 1997; 202:227–31

Nwariaku FE, Champine J, Kim LT et al. Radiological characterization of adrenal masses: the role of computed tomography-derived attenuation values. Surgery 2001; 130:1068–71

O'Doherty MJ, Kettle AG. Parathyroid imaging: preoperative localization. Nuc Med Commun 2003; 2:125–31

Piñero A, Rodríguez JM, Martínez-Barba E et al. Tc99m-sestamibi scintigraphy and cell proliferation in primary hyperparathyroidism: a causal or casual relationship? Surgery 2003; 134:41–4

Piñero A, Rodríguez JM, Ortiz S et al. Relation of biochemical, cytologic, and morphologic parameters to the result of gammagraphy with technetium 99m sestamibi in primary hyperparathyroidism. Otolaryngol Head Neck Surg 2000; 122:851–5

Reeder SB, Desser TS, Weigel RJ, Jeffery RB. Sonography in primary hyperparathyroidism. Review with emphasis on scanning technique. J Ultrasound Med 2002; 21:539–52

Roti E, Uberti ED. Iodine excess and hyperthyroidism. Thyroid 2001; 11:493–500

Sekiyama K, Akakura K, Mikami K et al. Usefulness of diagnostic imaging in primary hyperparathyroidism. Int J Urol 2003; 10:7–11; discussion 12

Shon IH, Roach PJ, Bernard E et al. Superimposed double parathyroid adenoma on Tc-99m MIBI imaging: the value of oblique images. Clin Nucl Med 2001; 26:876–7

Sternthal E, Lipworth L, Stanley B et al. Suppression of thyroid radioiodine uptake by various doses of stable iodide. N Engl J Med 1980; 303:1083–8

Van den Bruel A, Maes A, De Potter T et al. Clinical relevance of thyroid fluorodeoxyglucose-whole body positron emission tomography incidentaloma. J Clin Endocrinol Metab 2002; 87:1517–20

Westreich RW, Brandwein M, Mechanick JI et al. Preoperative parathyroid localization: correlating false-negative technetium 99m sestamibi scans with parathyroid disease. Laryngoscope 2003; 113:567–72

Imaging in vascular disease

21

D. Roach, R. Sebben, R. Fitridge

Background

Perhaps in more than any other surgical discipline, imaging is an integral component of the diagnosis and management of vascular disorders. The advent of reliable and accurate non-invasive imaging tools has led to the redefinition of many procedures, particularly in venous disease. Venography has lost its importance and has been superseded by duplex scanning, and, whilst the dedicated contrast study still remains the gold standard in arterial disease, developments in high-definition CT and MRI may well see angiography *per se* lose its importance.

This chapter focuses on diagnostic imaging. The role of interventional radiology in vascular disease is discussed in Chapter 9.

THE RADIOLOGICAL INVESTIGATIONS

Ultrasound

Colour and pulsed Doppler imaging have assumed a prominent role for non-invasively evaluating lower-extremity arterial occlusive disease. Ultrasound imaging is used to screen for lower-extremity arterial disease, aortic disease and carotid disease. It provides not only specific information regarding location, severity, and frequency of disease, but it can also determine the optimal therapeutic approach before more invasive procedures are undertaken. Using ultrasound for graft surveillance is mandatory for identifying flow-reducing lesions that may lead to subsequent bypass failure. Ultrasound is used routinely for assessment of venous disease, including both thrombotic and chronic venous insufficiency and has now become an invaluable tool in vascular practice.

Digital subtraction angiography

Digital subtraction angiography (DSA) remains the one imaging tool which provides the detail of definition often required for diagnosis and therapeutic intervention in arterial disease, particularly of the lower limb. It provides an accurate picture of the anatomy of the vasculature and details of changes within the vessel lumen, but provides limited information of what is happening outside the lumen. Emboli may be differentiated from thrombi, but the exact dimensions of an aneurysm in the presence of sac thrombus may escape estimation.

Indications for angiography include:

- delineation of arterial luminal anatomy
- delineation of disease: emboli, thrombi, chronic atherosclerotic disease
- therapeutic intervention: angioplasty, stenting, thrombolysis, suction thrombectomy.

Emboli can be identified by a crescentic meniscus of clot and lack of developed collateral vessels

(Fig. 21.1). Thrombotic disease is more likely when there are increased collateral vessels and preservation of run-off vessels (Box 21.1).

Angiography is an invasive procedure with risks related to arterial puncture, embolisation and contrast load particularly in renally impaired patients. Heavily calcified vessels or tortuous vessels may be difficult to catheterise, increasing the complication rate. *N*-acetyl cysteine is often used as a nephron-protective agent in renally impaired patients (see Chapter 3).

Carbon dioxide angiography (CO_2-DSA) may be used in investigations for vascular disease. The advantage of carbon dioxide is the absence of nephrotoxicity and allergic reactions. However, although studies have shown good diagnostic quality images in large vessels, it is not feasible to perform interventional procedures (e.g. stenting or angioplasty) using CO_2-DSA. The quality of images below the level of the popliteal artery is poor, limiting its use for distal disease. The main role of CO_2-DSA is in high-risk patients with severe renal impairment or contrast allergy.

Computed tomography angiography

Modern computerised tomography scanners utilising 8- to 64-slice technology are able to perform multiple axial images through contrast enhanced vessels. These images can then be reformatted to give 2D or 3D images of the vascular tree in a similar fashion to conventional angiography. There can be used to:

- evaluate claudication/rest pain and ulcers (Fig. 21.18)
- check for distal vessel patency (may show more vessels than DSA)
- clarify duplex findings

Advantages of CT angiography:

- all vascular beds are assessable including cardiac
- depicts calcium/thrombus/ulcers
- can visualise other organs
- radiation exposure is less than with conventional DSA

Disadvantages of CT angiography:

- ionising radiation
- heavy calcification/metallic prostheses can be problematic
- contraindicated in patients with contrast allergy and chronic renal failure
- need modern scanner and quality software for reconstructions
- imaging only, no intervention possible unlike DSA

Magnetic resonance angiography

MRA is a rapidly developing field. Spatial resolution, signal-to-noise ratio and acquisition times are all

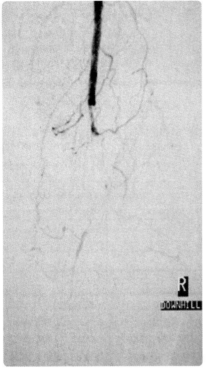

Fig. 21.1 An angiogram showing occlusion of the common femoral artery by embolus. The crescentic meniscus is clearly visible.

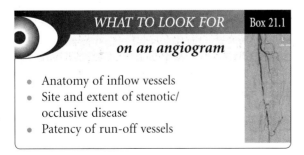

WHAT TO LOOK FOR   Box 21.1

on an angiogram

- Anatomy of inflow vessels
- Site and extent of stenotic/ occlusive disease
- Patency of run-off vessels

improving. Gadolinium can be used as an intravascular contrast medium with properties similar to iodinated intravenous contrast (see Chapter 6).

Advantages of MRA:

- good for assessing patency, particularly of small distal vessels
- no radiation
- suitable for patients with contrast allergy and chronic renal failure.

Disadvantages of MRA:

- can overestimate the level of stenosis
- lower spatial resolution than CTA
- artefacts with metal implants
- not suitable in claustrophobic patients, those with pacemakers and other ferrous metallic implantable prostheses or devices
- availability.

THE CLINICAL PROBLEMS

Venous thromboembolic disorders

Venous duplex scanning is the mainstay of diagnosis of lower extremity deep venous thrombosis (DVT). The diagnostic criteria for acute DVT on ultrasound include:

- B mode:
  - incomplete compression of vein walls with transducer (Figs 21.2 and 21.3)
  - low-level echoes within the vessel
  - venous distension seen with recent thrombosis
  - free-floating thrombus
  - collateral venous channels which enlarge rapidly during the acute phase of venous thrombosis
- Doppler spectral analysis:
  - absent or decreased venous Doppler flow proximal to thrombosed segment
  - lack of respiratory variation with continuous venous flow suggests proximal obstruction. This may be due to proximal iliac thrombosis or iliac vein compression (e.g. May–Thurner syndrome). With extrinsic compression, there is typically high-velocity continuous flow seen at area of compression
  - no augmentation or decreased augmentation with distal compression manoeuvres may indicate venous obstruction between the transducer and the level of distal compression.
- Colour Doppler:
  - incomplete or absent colour filling.

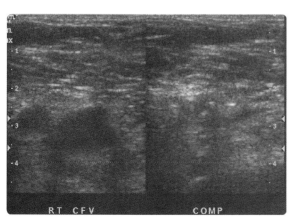

Fig. 21.2 A compressible normal femoral vein. The vein can be seen as a round structure in cross section on the left image, but is compressed and therefore not seen on the right image.

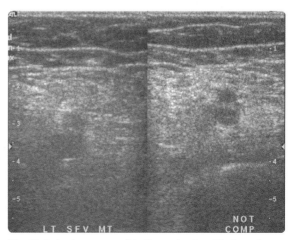

Fig. 21.3 An incompressible femoral vein with thrombus present. The vein can be seen as a round structure in both views.

An acute DVT will require treatment, whereas one that is established and chronic may not require any anticoagulation. The following points are made:

- it is often difficult to establish the age of the thrombus
- the level of echogencity increases over several days to weeks
- there is less venous distension in older thrombi
- thrombus size will reduce due to retraction and lysis
- adherence of thrombus increases with time
- there will be a reappearance of flow on colour Doppler as blood flow obstruction decreases with clot lysis
- with time, there will be thickening of valve cusps, adherence of valve cusps to vein wall and restricted cusp motion.

If there is a high index of suspicion of DVT, but the Duplex scan is negative, the patient can be rescanned within 1–3 days. Duplex scanning is associated with a false-negative rate of 0–5% and rather than submit a patient to anticoagulation on clinical grounds alone, it may be safer to wait and rescan the patient.

Varicose veins

Duplex ultrasonography is widely used in the management of patients with varicose veins (Box 21.2). Duplex scanning is more accurate than clinical assessment in determining the sites of venous incompetence causing varicose veins. Duplex assessment includes the absence or presence of clot in each vein segment as well as assessing the competency of the veins. Incompetence

is defined as reversal of flow in the vein (whilst in reverse Trendelenburg persisting for >0.5 second, although many surgeons and radiologists use 1.0 second as their cut-off).

Venography has previously been regarded as the gold standard but is rarely performed now due to invasiveness and improved overall accuracy of duplex scanning with excellent correlation between the two studies (85–90%) Although some surgeons use handheld Doppler to assess the saphenofemoral and saphenopopliteal junctions for incompetence, the technique is limited, with a sensitivity of 80–90% and a specificity of 50–90%. Many surgeons perform a duplex scan on all patients presenting with varicose veins in order to plan optimal surgical intervention or to predict the value of adjunctive percutaneous techniques such as sclerotherapy.

The common sites of incompetence are shown in Table 21.1. Venous duplex scanning is mandatory in all individuals being considered for surgery with recurrent varicose veins or venous ulceration. Of those patients with venous ulcers, only half have deep venous incompetence.

Preoperative mapping of sites of incompetence is useful in several scenarios:

- The saphenopopliteal junction is variable in position and unless its relationship to the knee

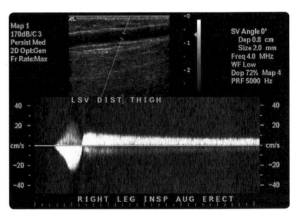

Fig. 21.4 A duplex scan showing an incompetent long saphenous vein. Augmentation is performed (flow below baseline) with calf compression which then shows reversal (above baseline) of flow in the long saphenous vein for greater than one second. Each large marker at bottom of the image represents one second.

WHAT TO LOOK FOR Box 21.2

on the duplex report

- Sites of incompetence: deep venous system or superficial venous system
- Incompetence at main stem junctions: saphenofemoral and saphenopopliteal (Fig. 21.4)
- Incompetent perforators
- Patency of the deep veins

Site of incompetence	Primary varicose veins	Recurrent varicose veins	
Saphenofemoral	53–64%	55–69%	**Table 21.1** Approximate sites of incompetence in primary and recurrent varicose veins
Saphenopopliteal	13–21%	25%	
Deep system	22%	28%	
Greater saphenous (excluding junction)	3–24%	26%	
Perforators:			
mid-thigh	5.4%	16%	
calf	31%	69%	
mid-thigh and calf	1%		
Multiple sites of reflux	6	45	

crease is known (e.g. 3 cm above), then preoperative marking should be performed.

- Incompetent perforators (mid-thigh or calf) should be marked if ligation is planned.
- Recurrent varicose veins secondary to residual long saphenous incompetence (usually following a high tie only) are best managed by marking the long saphenous vein from upper calf to the proximal extent of the vein. The vein can then be readily located just below the knee and removed from there up to its proximal extent.

Aortic disorders

Abdominal aortic aneurysms

Most abdominal aortic aneurysms (AAA) are diagnosed incidentally on abdominal ultrasound or CT performed for an unrelated indication. These aneurysms predominantly occur in males over 60 years of age. Approximately 5% of males aged between 65 and 80 years have an infrarenal aorta of >3 cm diameter. Risk factors include smoking, hypertension and hypercholesterolaemia. Diabetes mellitus in isolation is not associated with aneurysmal disease. There is a genetic predisposition to aneurysmal disease. Surgery is considered if:

- the rate of expansion is over 1 cm per year
- the aneurysm becomes tender
- the diameter exceeds 5.5 cm.

Recently, endoluminal repair has been developed as a minimally invasive technique for stenting aortic aneu-

rysms. The role of endoluminal stenting is discussed in Chapter 9.

It is important to exclude an abdominal aortic aneurysm in any patient presenting with peripheral vascular disease, particularly males over 60 years of age. Siblings or children of individuals with aneurysms should also undergo an ultrasound at approximately 50 years of age.

Ultrasound Ultrasound should be used to diagnose/exclude aneurysm disease when clinical suspicion is high and should also be used for surveillance (Fig. 21.5, Box 21.3).

Current data from randomised controlled trials show that the risk of rupture of aneurysms between 4 and 5.5 cm is approximately 1% per year and thus these patients should undergo ultrasound surveillance. Ultrasound surveillance is usually performed every 6 months depending on size of the aneurysm and the rate of expansion.

Computed tomography angiography CT angiography is usually performed when surgery is being planned. Axial and 3D reconstructions are used to define the:

- anatomy and structure of the aneurysm
- relationship of the aneurysm to the renal arteries
- anatomy of the iliac vessels.

The reconstructions also allow for the design of purpose built endoluminal stents. At least 95% of

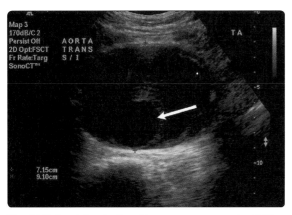

Fig. 21.5 An abdominal aortic aneurysm measuring 7.15 (anterior–posterior) by 9.1 cm (transverse) dimensions. Most of the aneurysmal sac is filled with clot, with flow in the dark circle (arrow).

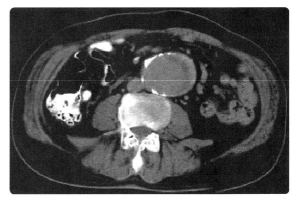

Fig. 21.6 An abdominal aortic aneurysm with a crescentic sign within the mural thrombus on the left. Note the mural calcification on this non-contrast image.

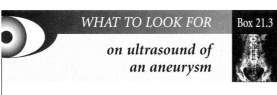

WHAT TO LOOK FOR   Box 21.3

on ultrasound of an aneurysm

- Size of aneurysm in transverse and anterior-posterior dimensions
- Site of aneurysm: aorta in relation to renal vessels, involvement of iliac vessels
- For peripheral aneurysms: the state of the runoff vessels
- Thrombus (mural or intraluminal)

aortic aneurysms are infrarenal. A hyperattentuating crescent sign seen on a CT angiogram may suggest an acute or impending rupture of an AAA. This sign consists of a crescent shaped area of hyper-attenuation within the aortic wall or mural thrombus of the aneurysm (Fig. 21.6).

CT angiography is used in inflammatory aneurysms to assess:

- involvement of surrounding structures such as the duodenum and ureters
- postoperative results in terms of maximal fibrotic-mantle thickness, both in millimetres and percentage of change.

Angiography Angiography is sometimes used when patients are being considered for endoluminal aneurysm repair or when there are concerns about distal occlusive disease. Indications for angiography include:

- defining anatomical details, e.g. aneurysm neck, sac and iliac vessels
- assessing branch vessel perfusion in aortic dissection to offer interventions such as fenestration or stenting.

Magnetic resonance angiography MRA is indicated in evaluation of aneurysms being considered for repair, especially in patients with contrast allergies or renal failure. Marked enhancement of pre-aortic tissue can be seen in inflammatory aneurysms (Fig. 21.7).

Aortic dissection

CT angiography is generally used to diagnose and assess the extent of aortic dissection (Box 21.4). Aortic dissections are differentiated into two main types depending on the proximal extent of the dissection. Type A includes all of the dissections involving the ascending aorta and Type B defines those dissections limited to the aorta distal to the left subclavian artery.

MRA is also useful in defining aortic dissections and is particularly valuable if renal impairment is present.

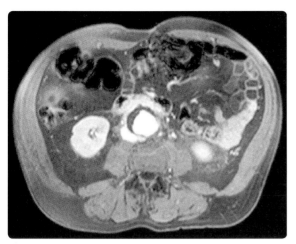

Fig. 21.7 An inflammatory aneurysm with characteristic enhancement of the preaortic tissue.

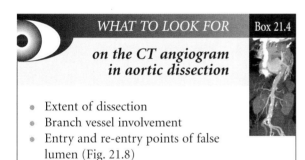

WHAT TO LOOK FOR   Box 21.4

on the CT angiogram in aortic dissection

- Extent of dissection
- Branch vessel involvement
- Entry and re-entry points of false lumen (Fig. 21.8)

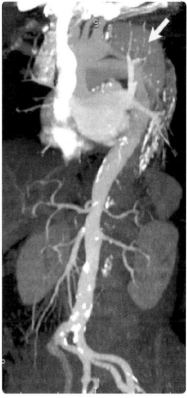

Fig. 21.8 The CT angiogram shows the false lumen on the upper outer aspect of the arch of the aorta (arrow).

Carotid artery disease

Based on the results of well-randomised controlled trials, symptomatic carotid territory lesions are considered for carotid endarterectomy when the level of stenosis reaches approximately 70%. Carotid stenting for high-risk patients is discussed in Chapter 9. Asymptomatic lesions are often considered for surgery at 60% stenosis based on trial data; however, many clinicians use higher degrees of stenosis for consideration for surgery in these patients. Asymptomatic disease is associated with a relatively low risk of stroke and hence management of these patients remains controversial at present. Many surgeons will intervene on those with 80+% stenoses especially if there is contralateral disease and/or the patient is considered at low risk for surgery.

Ultrasound Ultrasound is the first investigation and is used to investigate:

- carotid bruits
- symptomatic carotid territory cerebrovascular accidents, transient ischaemic attacks or amaurosis fugax
- other carotid pathology such as dissection, occlusion, carotid body tumours and fibromuscular disease.

Ultrasound is also used in the surveillance of:

- known carotid stenoses
- patients post-carotid endarterectomy.

The level of stenosis is established by consideration of three factors:

- peak systolic velocity of blood flow in internal carotid artery (ICA)

- end diastolic blood flow in ICA
- the peak systolic velocity ratio between ICA and common carotid artery (Fig. 21.9).

The character of the atherosclerotic plaque is also taken into consideration. The major disadvantage with carotid ultrasound is that the presence of heavy calcification in a plaque can obscure the vessel posterior to

it. This can sometimes be minimised by changing the probe insonation angle or by using another imaging modality. Another limitation is that ultrasound cannot always distinguish between a very tight stenosis (99%) and complete carotid occlusion. Very tight lesions show as a 'string sign' on angiography in which there is a collapsed distal internal carotid artery with very slow flow (Fig. 21.10, Box 21.5).

Fig. 21.9 Carotid duplex scans showing normal waveforms and velocities at the origin of the internal carotid.

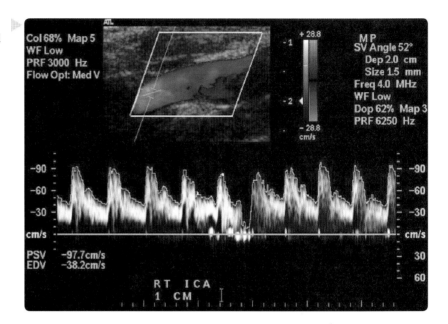

Fig. 21.10 Carotid duplex scan showing low velocity trickle flow with almost complete occlusion

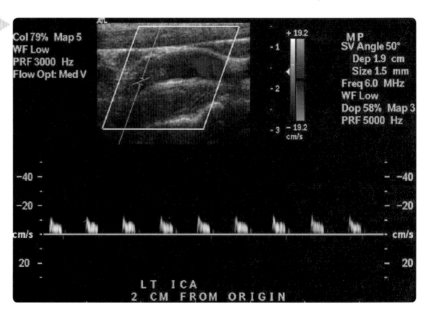

WHAT TO LOOK FOR Box 21.5

on carotid duplex

- Peak systolic velocities in the common and internal carotid arteries and the ratio between both (Fig. 21.11)
- Overall level of internal carotid artery stenosis based on above velocities/ratios
- Character of the plaque
- Direction of flow within the vertebral arteries

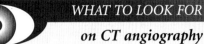 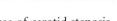 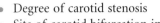

WHAT TO LOOK FOR Box 21.6

on CT angiography

- Degree of carotid stenosis
- Site of carotid bifurcation in relation to bony landmarks
- Any swallowing artefacts which might affect carotid studies
- Visualization of tandem lesions, particularly at level of carotid siphon

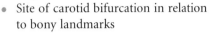

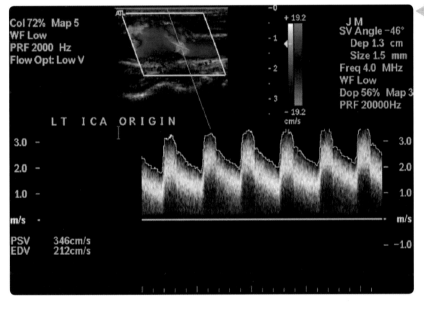

Fig. 21.11 High-grade stenosis at the origin of the internal carotid artery. High peak systolic velocity and high end-diastolic velocity.

Computed tomography angiography CT angiography is used to define the degree of stenosis of the internal carotid artery, particularly if endarterectomy is planned (Figs 21.12 and 21.13, Box 21.6). It is often used in conjunction with ultrasound. The CT angiogram will show the vascular anatomy from the arch of the aorta to the brain.

Magnetic resonance angiography MRA is a useful technique for imaging extra and intracranial carotid and vertebral disease. In the context of extracranial carotid disease, this technique has a tendency to over estimate the degree of internal artery stenosis. Once again, MRA is indicated in patients with renal failure or contrast allergy. It may also be performed if magnetic resonance imaging of the brain is required in the investigation of their cerebral symptoms.

Angiography Although the angiogram is still considered the gold standard in the assessment of carotid stenosis, it is an invasive procedure with a complication of up to 1.2% (Fig 21.14). For this reason, the non-invasive imaging modalities tend to be used in

Fig. 21.12 CT angiogram showing a high-grade stenosis at the origin of the internal carotid with calcium deposits in the plaque.

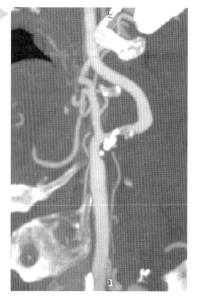
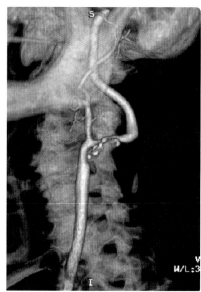

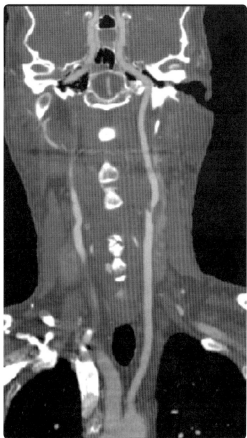

Fig. 21.13 CT angiogram showing a high-grade stenosis and anatomy from arch to brain.

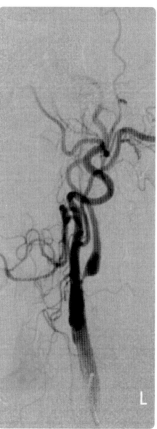

Fig. 21.14 Carotid angiogram showing a tight stenosis at the origin of the internal carotid (arrow). (The external carotid artery has multiple branches).

preference. There is still a role for carotid angiography with the following indications:

- any discrepancy of the level of a stenosis among the non-invasive imaging modalities
- difficulty with interpretation of either the ultrasound or CT, particularly in the setting of heavy calcification
- delineation of high or intracerebral vascular lesions.

Leg ischaemia

The most commonly used tool for basic screening of leg pain and ischaemia is the ankle to brachial pressure index (ABPI). This is a ratio of the blood pressure between one of the foot vessels and the brachial artery, measured using a hand-held Doppler probe and a sphygmomanometer cuff. In patients with heavily calcified and incompressible vessels, (such as in diabetes), toe pressures are often required to indicate the level of distal perfusion.

Although angiography remains the gold standard for the investigation of infrainguinal arterial disease, the other imaging modalities can be used to obtain accurate and often sufficient information to allow management decisions to be made.

Ultrasound Ultrasound is used in infrainguinal arterial disease to:

- assess disease and sites of involvement
- assess the level of stenosis/occlusion and the haemodynamic significance
- assess suitability of atherosclerotic stenotic or occlusive lesions for intervention, thus allowing directed angiography
- undertake surveillance of vein bypasses to diagnose development of graft or native vessel stenoses (Figs 21.15 and 21.16)
- assess and treat false aneurysms (Fig. 21.17)
- diagnose true aneurysms of femoral and popliteal vessels.

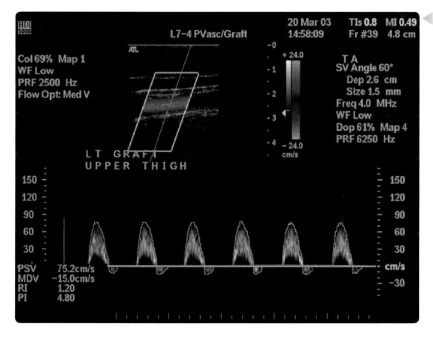

Fig. 21.15 Normal graft appearance with normal peak systolic velocity.

Specific clinical perspectives

Fig. 21.16 A view of the same graft as Fig. 21.15 but imaged in the lower section of the graft. The wave form has changed to show a high peak systolic velocity, consistent with a tight stenosis.

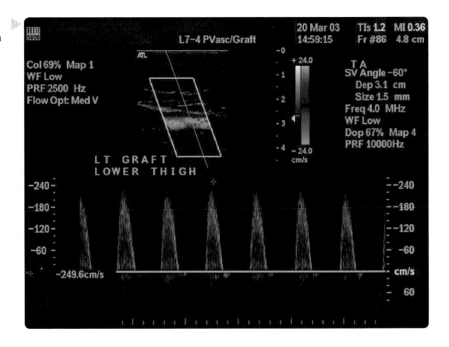

Fig. 21.17 A false aneurysm with a jet of flow through the wall of the femoral artery into the false aneurysm sac.

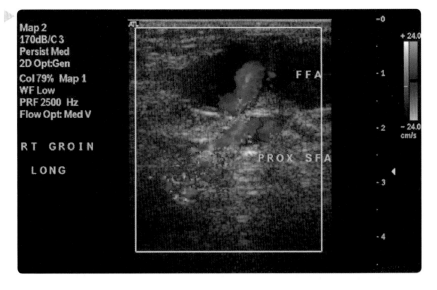

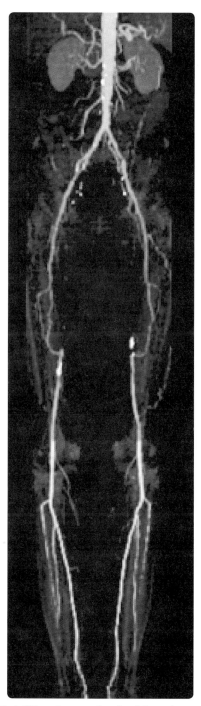

Fig. 21.18 A CT angiogram showing bilateral superficial femoral artery occlusion with collateral circulations.

Angiography Conventional angiography is considered the gold standard for investigation of infrainguinal arterial disease (Fig. 21.19). It allows both diagnosis and therapeutic intervention. Emboli are often identified by a crescentic meniscus of clot and lack of developed collateral vessels (see Fig. 21.1). Thrombotic disease is more likely when there are increased collateral vessels and preservation of runoff vessels (Fig. 21.20). As it is only the lumen that is seen on angiograms, it is not possible to define the exact dimensions of aneurysm disease in the presence of sac thrombus.

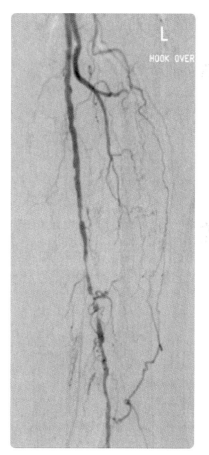

Fig. 21.19 An angiogram showing severe artherosclerotic disease of the superficial femoral artery with a collateral circulation.

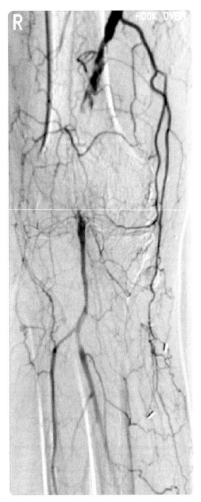

Fig. 21.20 Angiogram of thrombus occluding the superficial femoral artery. There is a good collateral circulation.

Further reading

Baldt MM, Bohler K, Zontsich T et al. Preoperative imaging of lower extremity varicose veins: color coded duplex sonography or venography. J Ultrasound Med 1996; 15:143–54

Beese RC, Bees NR, Belli AM. Renal angiography using carbon dioxide. Br J Radiol 2000; 73:3–6

Cooper DG, Hillman-Cooper CS, Barker SG, Hollingsworth SJ. Primary varicose veins: the sapheno-femoral junction, distribution of varicosities and patterns of incompetence. Eur J Vasc Endovasc Surg 2003; 25:53–9

Diaz LP, Pabon IP, Garcia JA, de la Cal Lopez MA. Assessment of CO_2 arteriography in arterial occlusive disease of the lower extremities. J Vasc Interv Radiol 2000; 11:163–9

Englund R. Duplex scanning for recurrent varicose veins. Aust N Z J Surg 1996; 66:618–20

Executive Committee for the Asymptomatic Carotid Atherosclerosis Study. Endarterectomy for asymptomatic carotid artery stenosis. JAMA 1995; 273:1421–8

Gonsalves CF. The hyperattenuating crescent sign. Radiology 1999; 211:37–8

Ho CF, Chern MA, Wu MH et al. Carbon dioxide angiography in lower limbs: a prospective comparative study with selected iodinated contrast angiography. Kaohsiung J Med Sci 2003; 19:599–607

Kristo DA, Perry ME, Kollef MH. Comparison of venography, duplex imaging and bilateral impedance plethysmography for diagnosis of lower extremity deep vein thrombosis. South Med J 1994; 87:55–60

Labropoulos N, Tassiopoulos AK, Kang SS et al. Prevalence of deep venous reflux in patients with primary superficial vein incompetence. J Vasc Surg 2000; 32:663–8

Lederle FA, Wilson SE, Johnson GR et al. Aneurysm detection and management: Veterans Affairs Cooperative Study Group. Immediate repair compared with surveillance of small abdominal aortic aneurysms. N Engl J Med 2002; 346:1437–44

Lindholt JS. Radiocontrast induced nephropathy. Eur J Vasc Endovasc Surg 2003; 25:296–304

MRC European Carotid Surgery Trial (ECST). Randomised trial of endarterectomy for recently symptomatic carotid stenosis: final results of the MRC European Carotid Surgery Trial (ECST). Lancet 1998; 351:1379–87

North American Symptomatic Carotid Endarterectomy Trial Collaborators. Beneficial effect of carotid endarterectomy in symptomatic patients with high-grade carotid stenosis. N Engl J Med 1991; 325:445–53

Pistolese GR, Ippoliti A, Mauriello A et al. Postoperative regression of retroperitoneal fibrosis in patients with inflammatory abdominal aortic aneurysms: evaluation with spiral computed tomography. Ann Vasc Surg 2002; 16:201–9

Prince MR, Narasimham DL, Stanley JC et al. Gadolinium-enhanced magnetic resonance angiography of abdominal aortic aneurysms. J Vasc Surg 1995; 21:656–69

Rubin GD, Schmidt AJ, Logan LJ, Sofilos MC. Multi-detector row CT angiography of lower extremity arterial inflow and runoff: initial experience. Radiology 2001; 221:146–58

Siegel CL, Cohan RH, Korobkin M et al. Abdominal aortic aneurysm morphology: CT features in patients with ruptured and nonruptured aneurysms. AJR Am J Roentgenol 1994; 163:1123–9

Thomsen HS, Morcos SK. Contrast media and metformin: guidelines to diminish the risk of lactic acidosis in non-insulin-dependent diabetics after administration of contrast media. ESUR Contrast Media Safety Committee. Eur Radiol 1999; 9:738–40

UK Small Aneurysm Trial Participants. Mortality results for randomised controlled trial of early elective surgery or ultrasonographic surveillance for small abdominal aortic aneurysms. Lancet, 1998; 352:1649–55

van der Heijden FH, Bruyninckx CM. Preoperative colour-coded duplex scanning in varicose veins of the lower extremity. Eur J Surg 1993; 15:329–33

Wong, JK, Duncan JL, Nichols DM. Whole-leg duplex mapping for varicose veins: observations on patterns of reflux in recurrent and primary legs, with clinical correlation. Eur J Vasc Endovasc Surg 2003; 25:267–75

Management of the asymptomatic 'incidentaloma'

22

S.J. Neuhaus

Background

The term 'incidentaloma' was originally coined to describe the unexpected finding of an adrenal tumour on abdominal imaging. It has since been extended to include other asymptomatic lesions detected during investigation for other pathology. The clinical significance of many of these lesions is unclear. As newer methods of imaging become more widespread, it is likely that the number of incidentally detected lesions will increase. This creates a significant burden for health resources, as further investigations, such as biopsy, are usually required to characterise the lesion or reassure the patient. It also increases the risk to which patients are put, who might otherwise have lived in blissful ignorance of a truly incidental 'abnormality.'

Radiological investigations are:

- CXR
- US

COMMONLY DETECTED INCIDENTAL LESIONS

Adrenal

Since the introduction of the multislice CT scanner in the 1980s, the finding of an incidental adrenal mass has increased four-fold. Reported as approximately 2% in 1982, it is now probably closer to the 9% documented in postmortem studies. Most lesions will represent a non-functioning adenoma (Fig. 22.1) but it is important to exclude unsuspected functional lesions, particularly phaeochromocytoma (Box 22.1) (see Chapter 20).

The larger the adrenal lesion, the greater the risk of malignancy. Adrenalomas and carcinomas can sometimes be distinguished by enhancement patterns on CT (see Chapter 20). Even if it is an incidental finding, a lesion bigger than 5 cm diameter should be resected. Smaller lesions should be further assessed on imaging to prove a diagnosis of adrenal adenoma or kept under regular surveillance. Even in the setting of malignancy elsewhere, an incidental adrenal lesion <2 cm is more likely to be an adenoma than a metastasis. If it will alter the patient's management a biopsy may be required.

Solitary pulmonary nodule

The major concern with an asymptomatic solitary pulmonary nodule is to exclude bronchogenic carcinoma (see Chapter 4) (Box 22.2).

WHAT TO LOOK FOR | Box 22.1

on CT of the adrenal glands

- Size of the lesion
- Adreniform or nodular shape
- Homogenous or heterogeneous internal appearance
- Presence of fat or calcification
- Unilateral or bilateral

Common causes of an adrenal mass include:

- adenoma
- hyperplasia
- phaeochromocytoma
- carcinoma
- metastasis.

Further assessment should include:

- individual or family history of an endocrine abnormality
- blood pressure measurement
- serum electrolytes
- urinary catecholamines, cortisol, VMA.

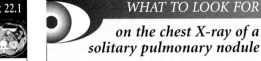

WHAT TO LOOK FOR | Box 22.2

on the chest X-ray of a solitary pulmonary nodule

- Evidence of distal collapse/consolidation
- Hilar lymphadenopathy
- Parenchymal lung disease
- Internal calcification or cavitation

Common causes of a solitary nodule include:

- bronchogenic carcinoma
- solitary metastasis
- granuloma, e.g. TB
- hamartoma.

Cavitation (Fig. 22.2) within a solitary pulmonary nodule could be associated with:

- tuberculosis
- resolving staphylococcal pneumonia
- neoplasia (primary or secondary)
- infarction.

Further assessment should include:

- history of smoking, haemoptysis, weight loss etc
- comparison with previous CXR
- sputum cytology (may require bronchoscopy or CT-guided FNA)
- CT chest to characterise lesion and ascertain any evidence of metastatic disease.

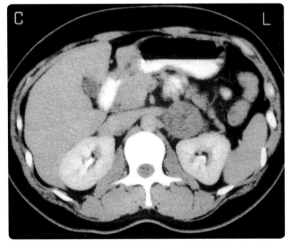

Fig. 22.1 Incidental finding of a 4 cm left sided adrenal tumour.

The PET scan may also have a role to play in the characterisation of the solitary pulmonary nodule, particularly if the patient has risk factors for malignancy (Fig. 22.3).

Gallstones

Gallstones are common. By the age of 55, 12% of men and 20% of women have gallstones. Most gallstones are asymptomatic and many are detected incidentally on a plain abdominal radiograph (as calcifications) or during upper abdominal ultrasound (see Chapter 12) (Box 22.3). The management of asymptomatic gallstones is controversial as less than 2% of these patients will develop symptoms over a year.

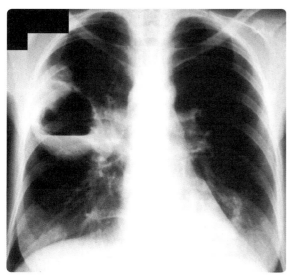

Fig. 22.2 A cavitating lung lesion found incidentally on a chest radiograph.

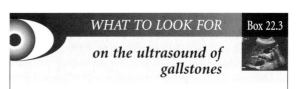

WHAT TO LOOK FOR · Box 22.3

on the ultrasound of gallstones

- Solitary or multiple stones
- Dilatation of extra or intrahepatic bile ducts (particularly CBD diameter)
- Thickening of the gall bladder wall
- Presence of adenoma or 'porcelain' gall bladder (calcification within the wall of the gallbladder) (Fig. 22.4)

Further assessment should include:

- careful history looking for biliary symptoms
- history of diabetes
- liver function tests.

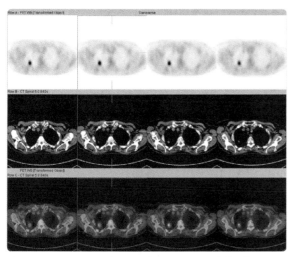

Fig. 22.3 Coregistered CT and PET image of the thorax showing a solitary FDG-avid pulmonary nodule. This proved to be a squamous cell carcinoma.

Liver lesions

Benign liver lesions are often detected incidentally on ultrasound or CT. They can be difficult to differentiate from malignant lesions and often require multiple radiological and other investigations to establish a diagnosis (see Chapter 12).

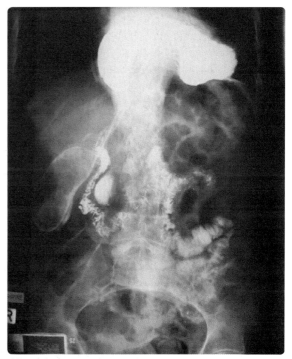

Fig. 22.4 A patient with a gastric volvulus and an incidental porcelain gall bladder.

Common and often asymptomatic solitary liver lesions include:

- fatty infiltration
- cysts (including hydatid)
- metastases
- adenoma
- focal nodular hyperplasia
- haemangioma
- hepatocellular carcinoma.

Further assessment should include:

- A detailed history inquiring about:
  - drug use (e.g. oral contraceptive pill)
  - farm exposure
  - hepatitis
  - cirrhosis
- Liver function tests
- Further imaging (see Chapter 12)
- Biopsy (this is controversial).

Abdominal aortic aneurysm

Incidental aneurysms of the abdominal aorta are most commonly detected on ultrasound or CT scans undertaken for investigation of other pathology (Box 22.4). Aneurysmal dilatation of the abdominal aorta affects 2–4% of the population and the risk of rupture is

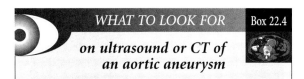

WHAT TO LOOK FOR Box 22.4

on ultrasound or CT of an aortic aneurysm

- Maximum transverse diameter of aneurysm
- Extension above renal arteries (95% are infrarenal)
- Involvement of iliac arteries
- Fusiform or saccular
- Clot within the aneurysmal sac
- Evidence of threatened leak (focal ulceration)

Further assessment should include:

- history of risk factors
- examination for other aneurysms
- referral for further radiological / vascular assessment.

directly related to the diameter of the aneurysm. Surgery or radiological intervention (stenting) is usually advised when the diameter is greater than 5.5 cm. The risk of rupture is reduced by the elective repair of an asymptomatic aneurysm (see Chapter 21).

Endoluminal metallic stenting is now performed at many centres, saving the patient from a major laparotomy. Workup for an endoluminal stent requires specialised CT angiography to assess suitability and calibrate stents (see Chapter 9).

OTHER INCIDENTALLY DETECTED LESIONS

Incidentally detected adnexal pathology

Incidental adnexal lesions on CT performed for another indication have been detected in up to 5% of patients. The majority of these (70%) are benign, even in patients known to have a malignancy elsewhere. It is important to differentiate benign ovarian pathology from metastatic disease as the latter has implications for staging and prognosis. Biopsy (often with laparoscopy) is usually required to differentiate benign from malignant pathology.

Premalignant lesions on positron emission tomography scanning

PET scanning is being increasingly utilised for the staging of malignancies (see Chapter 8). In approximately 3% of scans an abnormal and unexpected focus of hypermetabolism is identified. Of these, approximately 70% represent either a second malignancy (i.e. unrelated to the cancer for which the patient was being scanned) or a premalignant lesion. Most of the unexpected foci of hypermetabolism are colonic, due to either adenomas or asymptomatic colon cancer. Detection of asymptomatic thyroid malignancy is also reported in up to 3% of PET scans, most of these being papillary carcinoma.

Patient self-referral for 'whole-body scanning'

The use of 'whole-body' scanning in the asymptomatic patient is addressed in Chapter 1. The yield for detection of clinically significant lesions is low, but there is a significant cost due to the generation of 'follow-up' investigations.

Further reading

Agress H, Cooper BZ. Detection of clinically unexpected malignant and premalignant tumours with whole body FDG PET: Histopathologic comparison. Radiology 2004; 230:417–22

Dunnick NR, Korobkin M, Francis I. Adrenal radiology: distinguishing benign from malignant adrenal masses. AJR 1996; 167:861–7

Fenton JJ, Deyo RA. Patient self referral for radiologic screening tests: clinical and ethical concerns. J Am Board Fam Pract 2003; 16:494–501

Gracie WA, Ransahoff DF. The natural history of silent gallstones: the innocent gallstone is not a myth. N Engl J Med 1982; 307:798–800

Grumbach MM, Biller BM, Braunstein GD et al. Management of the clinically inapparent adrenal mass ('incidentaloma'). Ann Intern Med 2003; 138:424–9

Korobkin M, Francis IR, Kloos RT, Dunnick NR. The incidental adrenal mass. Radiol Clin N Am 1996; 34:1037–54

McSherry CK, Glenn F. The incidence and causes of death following surgery for non-malignant biliary tract disease. Ann Surg 1980; 191:271–5

Royal Australasian and New Zealand College of Radiologists. Imaging guidelines, 4th edn. The Royal Australasian and New Zealand College of Radiologists, Australia, 2001

Slanetz PJ, Hahn PF, Hall DA Mueller PR. The frequency and significance of adnexal lesions incidentally revealed by CT. AJR 1997; 168:647–50

UK Small Aneurysm Trial Participants. Mortality results for randomised controlled trial of early elective surgery or ultrasonographic surveillance for small abdominal aortic aneurysms. Lancet 1998; 9141:1649–55

van den Bruel A, Maes A, de Potter T et al. Clinical relevance of thyroid fluorodeoxyglucose-whole body positron emission tomography incidentaloma. J Clin Endocrinol Metab 2002; 87:1517–20

Webb WR. Radiological evaluation of the solitary pulmonary nodule. AJR 1990; 154:701–8

Wilmink ABM, Quick CRG. Epidemiology and potential for prevention of abdominal aortic aneurysm. BJS 1998; 85:155–62

Yankelevitz DF, Henschke CI. Does 2 year stability imply that pulmonary nodules are benign? AJR 1997; 168:325–8

Screening, staging and follow-up in malignancy

23

P.G. Devitt, S. Saloniklis, J. Heysen

Background

Few decisions are made in the diagnosis, investigation and treatment of solid organ malignancy without radiological input. This chapter provides an overview of the role of radiology in screening for malignant disease, staging of established disease and follow up of treated disease.

RADIOLOGICAL SCREENING FOR MALIGNANCY

Screening is the process of looking for disease in asymptomatic individuals. Screening aims to detect treatable disease at an early stage and therefore reduce mortality. Whatever screening instrument is adopted, it must have high sensitivity to minimise the chance of missing an individual with the disease. When the test is positive, it is always followed by another investiga-tion to confirm or refute the presence of the disease. This chapter examines the role of radiological screen-ing of solid organ malignancy. The issues of whole-body scanning as a screening tool are discussed elsewhere (see Chapter 1).

There are a number of diseases in which the role of screening has been clearly defined and is a viable process both in terms of cost effectiveness and improved survival. When considering the efficacy of a screening programme, there are a number of issues to be considered. These have been defined by the World Health Organization and include the definition of any at-risk groups and an understanding of the natural history of the disease to be screened. Issues of test acceptability need to be considered, together with the cost of the test to the individual and to the community.

The place and role of screening for breast cancer is well documented and is described below. This disease is relatively common in Western communities and if detected and treated early, can lead to improved sur-vival. Mammography has proven to be cost effective when applied to the groups most at risk of developing breast cancer.

There are other common conditions, such as colo-rectal cancer, where screening also has a potentially beneficial role and could lead to improved survival with earlier diagnosis, but whether or not the cost and effort of screening large populations can be justified is still debated. On one hand the major cost of screening for colorectal cancer is limited to faecal occult blood testing and is relatively cheap and easy to perform, with minimal risk to the person. On the other hand, some forms of screening for other kinds of cancers will involve imaging, with costs of personnel, equipment and radiation risks to the individual.

The case for the screening of high-risk groups is easier to make. The groups tend to be relatively small, easily defined and have a pick-up rate that justifies the screening in terms of cost effectiveness and improved survival. In colorectal cancer this particularly applies for patients with ulcerative colitis and families with familial adenomatous polyposis. Patients in such groups tend to be kept in a register and under regular surveillance. Currently, the means of surveillance is endoscopic, but arguments have been advanced to use imaging techniques, on the basis that they are fewer invasive with less potential complications.

The place of radiological investigation in the staging of malignancy is more clearly defined and its application is described in detail in the clinical sections of this book. The principles of staging are explained in this chapter.

Follow-up of established disease is one of the fundamentals of medical practice. The place of radiological investigation in follow up is not always clear-cut. As with screening, the question to be addressed is will the detection of asymptomatic disease at an early stage alter progress of the disease and be to the overall advantage of the patient both in terms of quality of life and long-term survival. The answer may be yes in such situations such as the resection of isolated metastases in the liver, lung or brain from some solid tumours (e.g. colorectal, sarcoma) but it is of no proven advantage in other malignancies such as gastric cancer.

Breast cancer

Breast cancer represents the most common malignancy in females. The clinical course is potentially alterable by treatment. The risk of breast cancer is most common over the age of 40 years and increases with age throughout life, representing the age groups where mammography is most sensitive in malignancy detection.

It is generally accepted that mammographic screening has decreased mortality from breast cancer. Several randomised controlled trials have been performed in North America and Europe assessing mortality reductions and have shown the potential effectiveness of population mammographic breast screening. Initial studies, such as the Health Insurance Plan (HIP) in North America in the 1960s, stimulated the important 1970s studies such as the Breast Cancer Detection Demonstration Project (BCDDP), also from the USA, and the widely quoted Two Counties study based in Sweden. These studies showed that 90% of cancers could be detected by mammography alone and at an earlier stage than on clinical grounds alone. This early detection appears to have translated into a reduced breast cancer mortality and morbidity. Despite recent concerns from some authors leading to a surge of new literature, mortality reductions have been validated. A meta-analysis of the most recent studies indicates a 24% reduction in mortality associated with mammographic screening. The mammogram aids in detection of multifocal disease and bilateral disease.

Although the efficacy of mammography has been demonstrated, the test does have limitations. False negatives and positives can be a result of interpretation, technical limitations, (e.g. dense breast tissue which might obscure a cancer), or quality assurance failures. There are also concerns regarding detection and over-treatment of ductal carcinoma in situ (DCIS) because not all cases are progressive.

Screening programmes

Successful screening programmes must attract the target group of women in sufficient numbers to see reduced breast cancer mortality and to be viable in terms of cost effectiveness. Strategies such as issuing personalised invitations based on the electoral register have been employed, as well as advertising campaigns through the media. Women detected as having an abnormal mammogram are generally recalled for further assessment and investigation as part of the screening service. This will include clinical examination, further specific mammography, ultrasound and often biopsy. For screening to succeed, the establishment of benchmarks and quality control measures is vital. These need to be individualised for each screening programme based on population characteristics, the breast cancer incidence and the available programme budget. Outcomes are generally recorded at all stages to assess the efficiency and quality of screening.

Typical benchmarks for screening programmes include:

- percentage of women attending screening from target population
- mammographic quality

- diversity of age, race, socioeconomic status in screened women
- percentage of women recalled for assessment after incidence screening (first MMG)
- percentage of women recalled for assessment after prevalence screening (subsequent MMGs)
- time to complete assessment of MMG abnormality
- time to treat screen-detected cancers
- number of cancers detected
- number of small/early cancers detected
- DCIS versus invasive cancers detected
- number of interval/missed cancers diagnosed between screening rounds
- influence on treatment offered (morbidity)
- influence on survival (mortality).

Current recommendations

Current Australian recommendations are that women at average risk should begin mammography at age 40 (Table 23.1).

Data from two trials have provided evidence that younger women will likely benefit more from annual screening than postmenopausal women. This is based on evidence supporting faster tumour growth rates in younger women and therefore detection of cancers at a smaller size. In women aged less than 50 years the lead time is estimated at 2 years, compared with 3–4 years in women over 50 years.

The case for screening older women is not so clear. Breast cancer mortality increases with advancing age. Diagnosis of invasive breast cancer in women aged 65 and older accounts for approximately 45% of all new breast cancer cases. Performance and effectiveness of mammography is as good and possibly better, in women aged 70 years and older compared to younger women. The potential benefit, however, of detecting breast cancers in this age group needs to be weighed up against their estimated life expectancy. Therefore the case for screening older women will need to be individualised depending on the patient's risk of dying from other causes.

Screening modalities

Mammography remains the 'gold standard' in screening for breast cancer. For women over the age of 35 the radiation risk of mammography is negligible. With typical two-view mammography (200 mrad each view) there is a 0.1% increased cancer risk. The risk will increase with increasing radiation exposure and in young women. It has been suggested that radiation sensitivity is increased in people with BRCA1 and BRCA2, which hypothetically may lead to a radiation-induced cancer. This has not been supported by current research.

Ultrasound has a limited role in screening. It is generally used for targeted examination, limiting the scanned area to the clinical or mammographic area of concern. Its major role is to guide fine needle and core biopsies, and differentiate solid from cystic masses. Ultrasound is poor at detecting microcalcification, particularly in the absence of an associated mass. The rate of false positive sonographically detected cancers is higher than in mammography. In younger women, with dense breast tissue specificity is reduced compared to older women. As a result, it is not acceptable as a sole test for detecting early breast cancer but rather as an adjunct to mammography.

Breast MRI can detect some mammographically and clinically occult breast cancers. MRI relies on the enhancement pattern of tumours after administration of a contrast agent. Unlike mammography and ultrasound, this is not typically influenced by breast density. MRI has some advantages over sonography. The prevalence of cancer at MRI screening in high-risk women is 2–7% and this is higher than sonographic screening. MRI is more sensitive than ultrasound in detecting DCIS. The positive predictive value of biopsy in studies

Country	Age	Interval	Views
USA	40–70 years	1 year	2 views
Australia	40–70 years	2 years (1 year high risk)	2 views
United Kingdom	50–70 years	3 years	1 view

Table 23.1 National screening recommendation for breast cancer

of MRI screening is 18–88%, which is greater than sonography (7–14% positive predictive value of biopsy in studies of screening sonography). Recently, it has been suggested that breast MRI screening is likely to have the highest yield in women with both a family history and personal history of breast cancer. The disadvantages of MRI relate to its expense and limited access, particularly in regard to biopsy systems. This results in a significant management problem when a lesion has been identified on MRI but is not seen on ultrasound or MMG, making localisation and biopsy problematic.

Screening in high-risk women

A number of risk factors have been identified for breast cancer, most importantly age and sex. After controlling for age, the greatest increased risk is a positive family history of breast and/or ovarian cancer. A life-time breast cancer risk of up to 85% has been calculated for women with germline mutations in either BRCA1 or BRCA2 susceptibility genes. Women at high risk may benefit from additional strategies to detect cancer at an early stage. The specificity and sensitivity of mammography in women less than 40 years is not known.

Some possibilities include initiation of mammography at 25–30 years of age, shorter screening intervals and additional modalities, for example MRI. Women who have received mantle radiation for Hodgkin's disease are also at increased risk of breast cancer and should begin annual mammographic screening 8 years after completion of radiation.

Lung cancer

Since 1980, the American Cancer Society has focused on lung cancer prevention rather than screening radiographs to detect early lung cancer. The move away from radiographic screening was influenced by the results of three large randomised trials conducted in the USA and Europe. These trials used frequent (3- to 6-monthly) 2D chest radiography as a screening tool. They found that although more cancers were resectable and there was an improved 5-year survival rate in the screened group, compared to the control groups, there was no significant reduction in disease specific mortality. These data are not universally accepted.

CT screening has been shown to be more sensitive than chest radiographs at detecting small pulmonary nodules. As a result CT is more likely to detect small, early stage cancers and potentially reduce lung cancer specific mortality. To date no trials have shown a reduction in lung cancer mortality as a result of low dose CT screening. Results of baseline screening from the Early Lung Cancer Action Project (ELCAP) study are encouraging. This study consisted of 1000 asymptomatic subjects with a moderate smoking history aged over 60. They were screened with low dose CT and conventional chest radiographs. The detection rates of non-calcified pulmonary nodules were 23.3%, while only 7% had abnormalities detected on CXR. Of the CT detected nodules 12% were eventually diagnosed with malignancy. The positive predictive value was 0.116, which is the highest reported rate from studies to date. The majority (85%) of cancers detected were stage I tumours. The data from the study however is subject to the effect of lead-time and selection bias which may erroneously lead to more favourable outcomes. Other studies are currently in progress to further evaluate CT and CXR screening for lung cancer. The cost of one study of 50 000 high-risk subjects has been estimated at US$200 million.

Colon cancer

Colorectal cancer is one of the most common cancers reported to cancer registries. In many Western communities it is the second most common cause of cancer death after lung cancer. For this reason screening for colorectal cancer is increasingly used in a bid to identify the lesions at an earlier stage and hence prevent the mortality associated with the disease. The most suitable mode of screening is not yet established.

Population-based screening for colorectal cancer starts with faecal occult blood testing. This is the appropriate method of screening low risk groups. Positive tests will be followed up with a further intervention, usually colonoscopy or double contrast barium enema. Subjects at high risk of developing colon cancer require regular screening, and this is usually performed with colonoscopy.

CT and 'virtual colonoscopy'

There is no role for routine abdominal and pelvic CT scans in screening for colorectal cancer screening. The bowel is not cleaned or inflated and the bowel lumen is not adequately visualised with this test. In addition stool and collapsed bowel can mimic tumours. However, virtual colonoscopic techniques for imaging of the colon are being developed and show promising results in terms of polyp and cancer detection rates. The improvement in both hardware and software capabilities and developments in multislice CT scanners has meant rapid scan times and reduced post-processing times. Scans are acquired in both supine and prone positions. Most use low dosage regimes and images can be acquired in one breath hold. Image reconstruction is between 1- and 2-mm intervals and this gives hundreds of images. The software then allows multiplanar reconstructions with endoluminal views from the acquired data set (Fig. 23.1). The published studies report sensitivities of 73–91% for polyps greater or equal to 10 mm and 22–82% for intermediate-sized polyps.

Unlike endoscopy, CT colonoscopy allows evaluation of the abdomen and pelvis outside of the colon, even with low-dose scans, with the possibility of detection of other asymptomatic conditions. At this stage, in terms of diagnostic accuracy, conventional colonoscopy still remains the gold standard for the detection of colonic neoplasms, particularly those less than 6 mm in diameter. Conventional colonoscopy has the

advantage that biopsy or removal of polyps can be performed at the same procedure.

MR colonoscopy

MR colonoscopy is a similar concept to CT colonoscopy except that the images are based on MR data sets. Reports show high sensitivity for detecting polyps greater or equal to 8 mm in size. Although MR has reduced spatial resolution compared with CT it has improved soft tissue resolution and does not expose the patient to ionising radiation. Extracolonic lesions can also be detected. In terms of convenience, the technique can hardly be considered a screening tool for anything other than small high-risk groups. Current CT and MR colonoscopy methods require cathartic bowel preparations. Recent interest has focused on improving techniques through faecal tagging agents. This would allow the signal of faeces imaged by MR to be modulated by adding contrast to meals.

Positron emission tomography scanning

Recently, PET scanning has been proposed for colorectal cancer screening in asymptomatic individuals. The sensitivity of PET in the detection of early colorectal cancer is high, potentially allowing resection at a curable stage. PET can demonstrate lesions larger than 0.7 cm and detect premalignant adenomas. It is unlikely however that PET will prove cost effective, except for high-risk patients.

Hepatocellular carcinoma

Screening has been advocated for hepatocellular cancer, where the aim is to detect early disease in high-risk patients. In communities such as South-east Asia where the disease has a high prevalence, screening programmes appear to be effective. High-risk groups include cirrhotics and chronic hepatitis B and C individuals. Those who are hepatitis B antigen positive have a risk 10–20 times greater than antigen negative persons. The conventional screening approach for high risk patients is a check of serum alpha-fetoprotein at 3- to 6-monthly intervals and an ultrasound examination of the liver at 6-monthly intervals. Up to two-thirds of the tumours detected are less than 2 cm diameter and potentially resectable (Fig. 23.2). Similar programmes in Western communities have not been so successful, and it is possible that the disease runs a more indolent course in Asian societies.

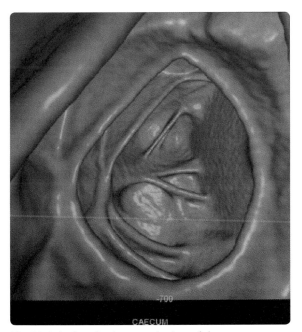

Fig. 23.1 A virtual colonoscopic view of the caecum.

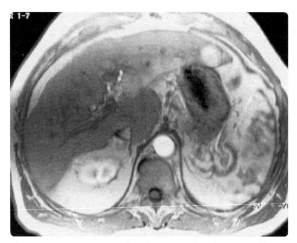

Fig. 23.2 An MRI scan showing a small and potentially resectable hepatocellular carcinoma in segment III.

The sensitivity of ultrasound for detecting focal liver lesions varies and has been reported at 79–82%. Sonography with microbubble contrast media now offers another method for identifying arterialised nodules. Detection rates decrease in people with large body habitus, hepatic steatosis and fibrosis, which will attenuate the ultrasound beam. Large tumours tend to be easy to diagnose, however the ultrasound features of small benign and malignant nodules typically overlap. This will often lead to other imaging techniques for further lesion characterisation.

STAGING OF MALIGNANCY

Radiological investigations form an integral part of the combined clinical, surgical and biochemical staging process for malignant disease. The aim of radiological staging is to accurately depict local and distant spread of malignant disease (TNM) to enable appropriate treatment planning and implementation. Neoadjuvant therapies are increasingly advocated to downstage certain tumour types prior to surgery (e.g. some oesophageal and rectal cancers), and appropriate imaging can provide a baseline measurement. This allows assessment of disease response to any treatment prior to (or instead of) surgical intervention.

The aim of staging is three-fold. It is to assess:

- local disease (i.e. structure of origin)
- locoregional disease (nodal metastases)
- distant metastases (solid organ).

The imaging tools used for staging are reliant upon knowledge of the particular disease process and its pattern of spread, along with the relative efficacy of a particular imaging modality. For example, in breast cancer a mammogram/breast US, CXR and liver US are often all that is required, whereas in pancreatic cancer a CT of the chest, abdomen and pelvis will usually be performed, perhaps together with endoscopic ultrasound. Ideally, radiological staging will be performed prior to treatment, but in some instances the primary tumour may already have been treated (e.g. resection of an acutely obstructing colorectal cancer). More recently, PET has been advocated as a cost effective means of staging malignancies, particularly when the pattern of metastasis is unpredictable (e.g. melanoma) or outside of the field of conventional imaging. There is evidence that PET may restage up to 20% of patients with lung cancer and prevent unnecessary or futile thoracotomy (Fig. 23.3)(Box 23.1).

Ideally any imaging undertaken should be non-invasive and be of high sensitivity and specificity for the presence or absence of the disease being sought. This should involve the least number of modalities as possible. Image-guided biopsy is often a part of the staging procedure. Biopsy may be required if there is diagnostic uncertainty, particularly for suspected metastatic disease or if there is an option of neoadjuvant therapy.

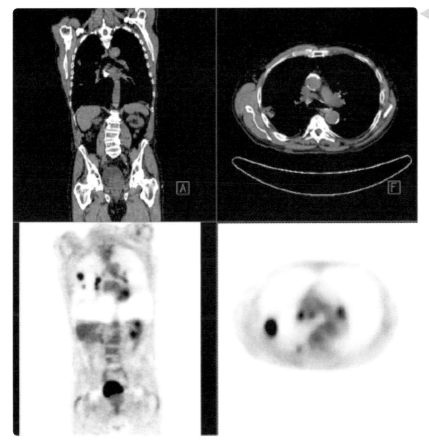

Fig. 23.3 Coregistered CT and PET image of the thorax of a patient with a carcinoma of the lung. The PET scan has picked up a lesion at the left hilum, not identified on the CT scan.

Primary tumour

Imaging of a primary tumour is important to establish T stage, particularly if neoadjuvant therapy is being considered. From a surgeon's perspective, the main role of any imaging is to help determine tumour resectability or the best approach to resection. This information might relate to the relationship of a pancreatic cancer to the portal vein (Fig. 23.4) or the size of a gastrointestinal stromal tumour being considered for laparoscopic resection.

The mainstay of staging in most solid malignancies is the CT scan. Alternative imaging is preferred for certain tumours or disease sites, especially where high-resolution, small-structure definition is required. Examples include mammogram and ultrasound for breast carcinoma, ultrasound for thyroid cancer, endorectal ultrasound/high-resolution MRI for rectal carcinoma, and high resolution MRI for tumours of the prostate and cervix. Ultrasound is often more useful in establishing the T and N status of gastrointestinal cancers however, CT may provide evidence of metastatic disease, particularly when it is unexpected. The preferred investigations for different primary tumours and their metastases are discussed in the appropriate chapters.

Lymph node assessment

Computed tomography

Radiological assessment of metastatic lymph nodes remains a diagnostic challenge, as the majority of techniques have relatively high false-positive and false-negative rates. CT remains the mainstay for nodal staging (Fig. 23.5), with other modalities used in spe-

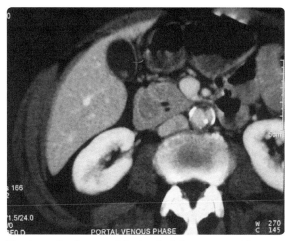

Fig. 23.4 Carcinoma of the head of the pancreas. The tumour is abutting the duodenum and is well clear of the portal vein, thus making the lesion potentially resectable.

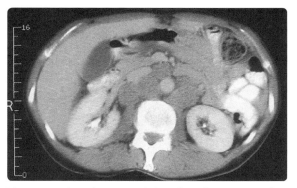

Fig. 23.5 Enlarged para-aortic lymph nodes in a case of non-Hodgkin's lymphoma.

cific circumstances (Table 23.2). CT does not usually provide information on the internal structure of a lymph node and uses an arbitrary cut-off value for size (Table 23.3) to indicate the likelihood of a node containing a metastatic deposit. Generally accepted size limits are used, although this is an area of ongoing debate. It is well documented that enlarged nodes may be reactive and smaller nodes contain metastatic foci, and there is a trade-off between sensitivity and specificity. The smaller the cut-off value, the higher the sensitivity, with an increase in the number of false positives. In the literature CT has reported sensitivities ranging from 11 to 93% and specificities of 58–100%. If a patient has a solitary suspicious node on CT imaging, further imaging for example with PET, or FNA/biopsy should be considered.

Ultrasound

Ultrasound can provide accurate nodal staging of accessible nodal basins, e.g. groin and axilla. It provides morphological information about the node and its internal architecture. Ultrasound is currently being evaluated as a surveillance and staging tool for patients with intermediate thickness melanoma. Combined with fine-needle aspirate of suspicious nodes, ultrasound has a specificity and sensitivity approaching 100% and 60%, respectively. As a non-invasive and relatively inexpensive technique, lymph node ultra-

sound may either replace sentinel node biopsy in the future or allow for more appropriate patient selection.

Positron emission tomography scan

The introduction of PET scanning has improved the ability to detect metastases within normal and enlarged nodes (see Chapter 8). It is limited by the metabolic activity of the tumour, and nodes adjacent to the primary tumour are often not seen as separate from tracer uptake within the primary due to lower spatial resolution. The more recent advent of PET-CT has provided further improvements and will have an important role in the staging of primary and recurrent malignancy in the future. The role of PET for the staging of lung cancer and head and neck cancers has now reached the stage where guidelines are being drawn up advising its use in the assessment of the patient being considered for resection.

Magnetic resonance imaging

Advances in MRI have produced improved sensitivity and specificity of metastatic lymph node detection. In pelvic cancers such as rectal and prostatic carcinoma the pre-operative identification of suspicious lymph nodes in the pelvic side-wall may alter the type of treatment, or lead the surgeon to perform an extended lymphadenectomy. The use of superparamagnetic iron oxide particles has had promising results, with detection of microscopic foci as small as 3 mm within normal sized nodes. This is still a research tool and it

◀ **Table 23.2** Use of different modalities in lymph node assessment

Modality	Advantages	Disadvantages
Ultrasound	Readily available Non ionising Assesses morphology of the node	Requires an experienced sonographer
CT	Readily available Usually part of primary imaging rather than separate investigation Mainstay of nodal assessment	Uses size criteria rather than morphology Low sensitivity for small nodes
PET	Good for metabolically active tumour in nodes at distant sites	Difficult to detect metastatic nodes adjacent to primary tumour
MRI	New contrast agents are highly sensitive and specific for small nodes	Expensive with limited availability therefore main current role is research

◀ **Table 23.3** Suggested size limits for lymph nodes on CT

Location	Upper limit for normal size
Head and neck	10 mm
Mediastinum	10 mm
Retrocrural	6 mm
Abdominal	10 mm (portahepatis 7 mm, gastrohepatic ligament 8 mm, para-aortic 9–11 mm)
Pelvic	10 mm (common iliac 9 mm, obturator 8 mm)
Inguinal	15 mm

is too early to say whether or not the technique will be of practical and clinical value.

Metastases

Depending on the symptoms produced by the primary tumour, one of the main factors that will influence management will be evidence of metastatic disease. The type and extent of imaging performed will depend on the type of primary tumour, an understanding of the natural history of the particular disease and any clinical information that might suggest spread. Investigations are usually confined to sites where metastatic spread is common. For example, staging investigations of gastrointestinal tract neoplasms tend to be confined to the abdomen and chest, as deposits in other parts of the body are uncommon. This approach is not failsafe and patients will sometimes present in the postoperative period with metastatic disease that was unsuspected on presentation and not looked for on initial workup (Fig. 23.6).

Metastatic liver disease

Many cancers and particularly those of the gut, lung, and breast commonly metastasise to the liver. Between 25 and 40% of these patients will have liver metastases at the time of their initial presentation. It should be standard practice to scan the liver of all patients with these primary cancers.

Scanning may use either ultrasound or contrast-enhanced CT. If a patient is unable to have intravenous contrast, the sensitivity of CT for detecting hepatic metastases is significantly lowered and ultrasound or MRI should be considered. The main aim of liver imaging in possible metastatic disease is the maximisa-

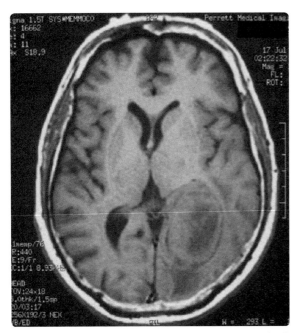

Fig. 23.6 A metastatic deposit in the left posterior cerebral hemisphere of a man who presented with a persistent headache several weeks after resection of a colon cancer. This had undoubtedly been present during initial workup.

tion of liver-to-lesion contrast, to provide maximum conspicuity of lesions. Depending on whether a lesion is hypo- or hypervascular it will have different enhancement patterns and the phase of enhancement is important (see Chapter 12).

The use of microbubble intravascular contrast agents in US also increases lesion conspicuity and helps in lesion characterisiation. Gadolinium-enhanced MRI is helpful in lesion characterisation and the use of a liver-specific contrast agent aids in lesion detection prior to hepatic metastasectomy. In many centres this has replaced CT arterial portography. Intraoperative ultrasonography allows the greatest degree of spatial resolution due to proximity of access, and in expert hands can detect lesions as small as 2 mm. Allowing for the invasive nature of the assessment, intraoperative ultrasonography is markedly superior to other forms of preoperative imaging.

Suspicious lesions identified on CT may sometimes be too small to accurately characterise as benign or malignant and too small to be accurately targeted for biopsy. In these cases management decisions may then have to be made on clinical grounds or other investigations considered. Provided the lesion is between 5 and 10 mm, ultrasound may help determine if it is cystic in nature. Multiple small lesions can be characterised on MRI if it will significantly alter the patient's management. The preferred management may be to arrange a follow-up investigation to see if there has been any change in the lesion.

Metastatic lung disease

Large autopsy series of patients with extra-thoracic malignancy reveal pulmonary metastatic disease in 20–54% of patients, and common primary tumours include breast, colon, kidney, uterus, head and neck. Less common neoplasms, but those with relatively high risk of lung dissemination include choriocarcinoma, osteosarcoma, testicular tumours, melanoma, Ewing's sarcoma, and carcinoma of the thyroid.

Whereas a plain chest radiograph may suffice for those tumours with a low risk of pulmonary metastatic spread, CT scan is now the accepted standard imaging tool. The resolution of the CT will allow detection of small nodules within the lung (Fig. 23.7), mediastinum or pleura and also detect malignant infiltration (lymphangitis).

The typical appearances of metastases on X-ray and CT are classically those of rounded or slightly lobulated nodules of soft tissue density, commonly referred to as 'coin' or 'cannon-ball' lesions. Less common, but recognised manifestations include cavitating masses, calcifying nodules, pneumothorax, and airspace consolidation. Atelectasis or segmental/lobar collapse may occur with endobronchial metastases or due to direct invasion of bronchi.

The solitary nodule detected in staging of malignancy may lead to difficulty in differentiation between a solitary secondary, a coexistent primary tumour or a benign incidental lesion (see Chapter 4). Lesions detected in this circumstance represent an isolated metastasis in between 25% (CXR detection), and 45% (CT detection) of cases. Specificity is increased if lesions are >2.5 cm and non-calcified, or multiple. Likelihood will also vary according to histological type of the primary tumour and the patient's age. Absolute differentiation between benign (e.g. sarcoid, TB), and malignant, or primary versus secondary disease may remain equivocal, and require follow up imaging or biopsy for diagnosis.

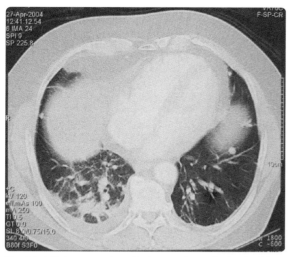

Fig. 23.7 Pulmonary deposits in a patient admitted with a gastrointestinal haemorrhage and previous treatment for an angiosarcoma of the right atrium. These were not visible on the plain chest radiograph. There is also evidence of consolidation at the base of the right lung.

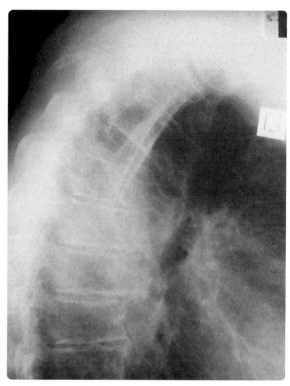

Fig. 23.8 A crush fracture of T5 in a patient with a previously treated squamous cell carcinoma of the oesophagus. The vertebral body is osteopaenic, suggesting a metastatic cause for the crush.

Skeletal metastases

Skeletal metastases occur in between 30–70% of all cancer patients. Primary tumours most commonly associated with bony metastases include breast, lung and kidney. Others include carcinoma of the rectum, pancreas, stomach, colon and ovary. Ninety percent of metastatic lesions are found in the distribution of red marrow in adults, namely the vertebra, pelvis, proximal femora and skull; 10% of lesions are solitary and up to 25–40% of asymptomatic patients with malignancy have scintigraphic evidence of skeletal metastases.

Plain X-rays are generally less sensitive than bone scintigraphy and are relatively insensitive to early metastatic disease. Lesions may be lytic, sclerotic, mixed or expansile (Figs 23.8 and 23.9). Sclerotic metastases are typically associated with breast or prostate cancer. Other bony metastases tend to have a lytic or mixed appearance. An X-ray of a specific area of concern on bone scan will help differentiate benign from malignant lesions, and may also be used to assess for a pathological fracture at a known metastatic site.

Bony metastases are usually identified on CT as an incidental finding when a patient has undergone scanning for assessment of soft tissue metastases. Occasionally CT will be used specifically in the preoperative assessment of bone texture if internal fixation is planned, or in the assessment of cord compression when MRI is contraindicated.

Radioisotope bone scanning is the mainstay of staging the bony skeleton, as it is significantly more sensitive than a plain radiograph or CT and can assess the entire skeleton in one examination. Specificity may be reduced in isolated rib or periarticular lesions, which may be mimicked by trauma or degenerative changes. These can be further assessed on plain X-ray.

MRI is highly sensitive and specific in staging the bone marrow, and is the first line of investigation in a patient with signs of acute cord compression (Fig. 23.10). The limited area of coverage and longer imaging times limit its ease of use in screening for metastases,

287

Fig. 23.9 There is increased accumulation of tracer at the fracture site identified in Fig. 23.8. In addition there are increased areas of activity in the region of T11 and in several of the ribs. These changes are highly suggestive of skeletal metastases.

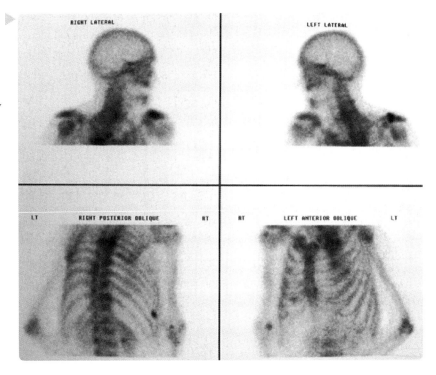

which is better provided by radionuclide scanning. It is however useful in haematological malignancies such as multiple myeloma, which may be isotope negative. MRI proves particularly useful in differentiating benign from malignant vertebral fractures.

Other sites of metastatic disease

Adrenal metastases are present in 25% of patients dying of cancer. Significant overlap in the imaging appearances of benign incidental lesions and metastatic lesions is seen, although there are some techniques to differentiate the two (see Chapter 20).

Metastases to the brain (and meninges) occur in 10–25% of autopsied patients dying of an extracranial malignancy, and 60–85% are multiple. Both contrast enhanced CT and MRI are highly sensitive and specific for detection. MRI is significantly more sensitive for meningeal and base of skull involvement (see Chapter 4).

Peritoneal (transcoelomic) dissemination is characteristic of ovarian and gastric cancer and is also seen in melanoma. Common imaging findings include ascites, increased nodularity and density in the omentum, and nodular deposits along the peritoneal surface, particularly in the pelvis and around the liver (Fig. 23.11).

The limits of resolution imposed by current imaging technology means that laparoscopy is still a more sensitive staging tool for detection of peritoneal deposits and the latter will frequently detect tumour missed by CT or ultrasound. In both pancreatic and gastric cancer, laparoscopy prior to planned surgery may avoid unnecessary operation in up to 23% of patients listed for curative resection. Until small (<6 mm) lesions can be reliably detected radiologically, some form of laparoscopic intervention will remain the preferred tool for the accurate staging of gut malignancies.

More unusual sites of metastatic dissemination include the skin, subcutaneous tissues and small intestine. Malignant melanoma is a tumour that characteristically metastasises to unusual sites and in particular the small bowel. Deposits at this site may present with haemorrhage or obstruction and a CT scan will often provide the diagnosis (see Chapter 10).

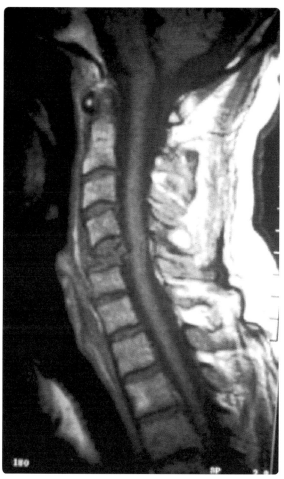

Fig. 23.10 An MRI scan showing a cervical spine metastatic deposits, with vertebral collapse and involvement of the spinal cord.

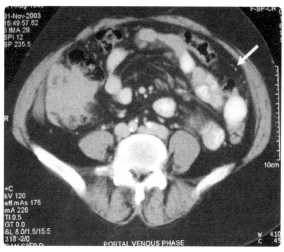

Fig. 23.11 Metastatic peritoneal deposits (arrow) from breast cancer. There is also a large tumour mass abutting the right colon.

FOLLOW UP

The aims of imaging investigations in the follow-up of a patient with previously treated malignancy are several-fold. First, if the disease has only been partially treated by surgical intervention, imaging may be required to establish a baseline of residual disease and how the disease is responding to other treatment modalities (e.g. chemotherapy). Second, the patient may develop new symptoms in the follow-up period and imaging may be required to determine the origin and cause of the symptoms to aid in their management. Third, and more difficult to be dogmatic about, is the role of investigations in the follow up of the asymptomatic patient. If it can be shown that detection and treatment of recurrent disease will increase the well-being of the patient and improve survival, then the case is easily made. If detection (and subsequent treatment) of recurrent disease is unlikely to improve the patient's outlook, then the role of routine surveillance procedures is more contentious. These issues are perhaps best illustrated by considering gastric and colorectal cancer. There is no evidence that early detection of recurrent gastric cancer and subsequent treatment does anything to improve survival. Thus there is no place in the follow up management of these patients for routine radiological investigation.

On the other hand, detection and resection of isolated hepatic metastases in colorectal cancer can be associated with improved survival. Five-year figures approaching 50% are reported following resection of isolated metastatic disease. Even the resection of several metastatic lesions from the liver can be associated with improved survival. If follow-up investigations are to be undertaken, it may be more cost-effective to screen with tumour markers and reserve imaging for cases of suspected recurrent disease.

Further reading

Albrect T, Blomley MJ, Burns PN et al. Improved detection of hepatic metastases with pulse inversion US during the liver-specific phase of SHU 508A: multicentre study. Radiology 2003; 227:361–70

American Cancer Society Surveillance Program. Estimated new cancer cases by sex and age. American Cancer Society, Atlanta, GA, 2003

Anderson I, Janzon L. Reduced breast cancer mortality in women under age 50: updated results from the Malmo mammographic screening program. J Natl Cancer Inst Monogr 1997; 22:63–7

Baker ME, Pelley R. Hepatic metastases: basic principles for radiologists. Radiology 1995; 197:329–37

Benvegnu L, Fattovich G, Noventa F et al. Concurrent hepatitis B and C virus infection and risk of hepatocellular carcinoma in cirrhosis. Cancer 1994; 74:2442–8

Bepler G, Goodridge Carney D, Djulbegovic B et al. A systematic review and lessons learned from early lung cancer detection trials using low dose computed tomography of the chest. Cancer Control 2003; 10:306–14

Blackshaw GR, Barry JD, Edwards P et al. Laparoscopy significantly improves the perceived preoperative stage of gastric cancer. Gastric Cancer 2003; 6:225–9

Brett GZ. The value of lung cancer detection by six monthly chest radiographs. Thorax 1968; 23:414–20

Burke W, Daly M, Garber J et al. Recommendations for follow up care of individuals with an inherited predisposition to cancer. II: BRRA1 and BRCA 2. JAMA 1997; 277:997–1003

Callebaut I, Mornon JP. From BRCA1 to RAP1: a widespread BRCT module closely associated with DNA repair. FEBS Lett 1997; 400:25–30

Chen YK, Kao CH, Lioa AC et al. Colorectal cancer screening in asymptomatic adults: the role of FDG PET scan. Anticancer Res 2003; 23:4357–61

Choi MY, Lee JW, Jang KJ. Distinction between benign and malignant causes of cervical, axillary, and inguinal lymphadenopathy: value of Doppler spectral waveform. AJR 1995; 165:981–4

Coffin CM, Diche T, Mahfouz A et al. Benign and malignant hepatocellular tumours: evaluation of tumoural enhancement after magnafodipir trisodium injection on MR imaging. Eur Radiol 1999; 9:444–9

Cohen CJ, Jennings TS. Screening for ovarian cancer: The role of noninvasive imaging techniques. Am J Obs Gynecol 1994; 174:1088–94

Coppage L, Shaw C, Curtis A. Metastatic disease to chest in patients with extrathoracic malignancy. J Thoracic Imaging 1987; 2:24–37

Cotton PB, Durkalski VL, Pineau BC et al. Computed tomographic colonography (virtual colonoscopy): a multicenter comparison with standard colonoscopy for detection of colorectal neoplasia. JAMA 2004; 291:1713–19

Curtin HD, Ishwaran H, Mancuso AA et al. Comparison of CT and MR imaging in staging of neck metastases. Radiology 1988; 207:123–30

Dershaw DD. Mammographic screening of the high risk woman. Am J Surg 2000; 180:288–9

Deutch SJ, Sandler MA, Alpern MB. Abdominal lymphadenopathy in benign diseases: CT detection. Radiology 1987; 163:335–8

Dorfman RE, Alpern MB, Gross BH, Sandler MA. Upper abdominal lymph nodes: criteria for normal size determined with CT. Radiology 1991; 180:319–22

Eddy DM. Screening for lung cancer. Ann Intern Med 1989; 111:232–7

Einstein DM, Singer AA, Chilcote WA, Desai RK. Abdominal lymphadenopathy: spectrum of CT findings. Radiographics 1991; 11:457–72

Fontana RS, Sanderson DR, Woolner LB et al. Lung cancer screening: the Mayo program. J Occup Med 1986; 28:746–50

Fukuya T, Honda H, Hayashi T et al. Lymph node metastases: efficacy for detection with helical CT in patients with gastric cancer. Radiology 1995; 197:705–11

Gordon PB. Ultrasound for breast cancer screening and staging. Radiol Clin North Am 2002; 40:431–41

Gross BH, Glazer GM, Ominger MB. Bronchogenic carcinoma metastatic to normal sized lymph nodes: frequency and significance. Radiology 1988; 166:71–4

Heneghan JP. Transrectal sonography in staging rectal carcinoma: role of grey scale, colour flow and Doppler imaging analysis. AJR 1997; 169:1247–52

Henschke CI, McCauley DI, Yankelevitz DF et al. Early lung cancer action project: overall design and findings from screening. Lancet 1999; 354:99–105

Henschke CI, Yankelevitz DF, Kostis WJ. CT screening for lung cancer. Semin Ultrasound, CT, MRI 2003; 24:23–32

Hilton S, Herr HW, Teitcher JB et al. CT detection of retroperitoneal lymph node metastases in patients with clinical stage I testicular nonseminomatous germ cell cancer: assessment of size and distribution criteria. AJR 1997; 169:521–5

Hopper KD, Singapuri K, Finkel A. Body CT and oncologic imaging. Radiology 2000; 215:27–40

Husband JES, Reznek RH. Imaging in oncology. ISIS Medical Media, Oxford, 1998

Ikeda K, Saitoh S, Koida I et al. A multivariate analysis of risk factors for hepatocellular carcinogenesis: a prospective observation of 795 patients with viral and alcoholic cirrhosis. Hepatology 1993; 18:47–53

Imamura H, Seyama Y, Kokudo N et al. Multiple resections of multiple hepatic metastases of colorectal origin. Surgery 2004; 135:508–17

Kodera Y, Ito S, Yamamura Y et al. Follow-up surveillance for recurrence after curative gastric cancer surgery lacks survival benefit. Ann Surg Oncol. 2003; 10:898–902

Koh DM, Brown G, Temple L et al. Rectal cancer: mesorectal lymph nodes at MR imaging with USPIO versus histopathologic findings – initial observations. Radiology 2004; 231:91–9

Kolb TM, Lichy J, Newhouse JH. Occult cancer in women with dense breasts: detection with screening US – diagnostic yield and tumour characteristics. Radiology 1998; 207:191–9

Kozuka T, Johkoh T, Hamada S et al. Detection of pulmonary metastases with multi detector row CT scans of 5mm nominal section thickness: Autopsy Lung Study. Radiology 2003; 226:231–4

Kubik A, Polak J. Lung cancer detection: results of a randomized prospective study in Czechoslovakia. Cancer 1986; 57:2427–37

Kuhl CK, Schmutzler RK, Leutner CC et al. Breast MR imaging screening in 192 women proved or suspected to be carriers of a breast cancer susceptibility gene: Preliminary results. Radiology 2000; 209:267–79

Love C, Din AS, Tomas MB et al. Radionucleide bone imaging: an illustrative review. Radiographics 2003; 23:341–58

Lowy AM, Mansfield PF, Leach SD, Ajani J. Laparoscopic staging for gastric cancer. Surgery 1996; 119:611–14

Mandel JS, Bond JH, Church TR et al. The effect of fecal occult-blood screening on the incidence of colorectal cancer. N Engl J Med 2000; 343:1603–7

McCarthy EP, Burns RB, Freund KM et al. Mammography use, breast cancer stage at diagnosis, and survival among older women. J Am Geriatr Soc 2000; 48:1226–33

Mizowaki T, Nishimura Y, Shimada Y et al. Optimal size criteria of malignant lymph nodes in the treatment planning of radiotherapy for oesophageal cancer: evaluation by computed tomography and magnetic resonance imaging. Int J Radiat Oncol Biol Phys 1996; 36:1091–8

Monig S, Zirbes TK, Schroder W et al. Staging of gastric cancer: correlation of lymph node size and metastatic infiltration. AJR 1999; 173:365–7

Morris EA. Screening for breast cancer. Semin Ultrasound, CT MRI 2003; 24:45–54

National Cancer Institute. National lung cancer screening trial. Online. Available: http://www.nci.nih.gov/NLST

Nazarian, LN, Alexander AA, Kurtz AB et al. Superficial melanoma metastases: appearances on grey scale and colour Doppler sonography. AJR 1998; 170:459–63

Nicholson FB, Korman MG, Stern AI. Distribution of colorectal adenomas: implications for bowel cancer screening. Med J Aust 2000; 172:428–30

O'Driscoll D, Warren R, MacKay J et al. Screening with breast ultrasound in a population at moderate risk due to family history. J Med Screen 2001; 8:106–9

Oka H, Tamori A, Kuroki T et al. Prospective study of alpha-fetoprotein in cirrhotic patients monitored for development of hepatocellular carcinoma. Hepatology 1994; 19:61–6

Olsen O, Gøtzsche PC. Systematic review of screening for breast cancer mammography. Online. Available: http://image.thelancet.com/lancet/extra/fullreport.pdf [accessed February 2004]

Osborne A. Diagnostic neuroradiology. Mosby, St Louis, 1994

Patz EF Jr, Goodman PC, Bepler G. Screening for lung cancer. N Engl J Med 2000; 343:1627–33

Prenzel KL, Monig SP, Sinning JM et al. Lymph node size and metastatic infiltration in non-small cell lung cancer. Chest 2003; 123:463–7

Rasanen JV, Sihvo EI, Knuuti MJ et al. Prospective analysis of accuracy of PET, computed tomography and endoscopic ultrasonography in adenocarcinoma of the esophagus and the esophago-gastric junction. Ann Surg Oncol 2003; 10:954–60

Rossi CR, Mocellin S, Scagnet B et al. The role of preoperative ultrasound scan in detecting lymph node metastasis before sentinel node biopsy in melanoma patients. J Surg Oncol 2003; 83:80–4

Rubaltelli L, Proto E, Salmaso R et al. Sonography of abnormal lymph nodes in vitro: correlation of sonographic and histological findings. AJR 1990; 155:1241–4

Rummeny EJ, Torres CG, Kurdziel JC et al. MnDPDP for MR imaging of the liver. Results of independent image evaluation of the European phase III studies. Acta Radiol 1997; 38;623–5

Selby JV, Friedman GD, Quesenberry CP, Weiss NS. A case control study of screening sigmoidoscopy and mortality from colorectal cancer. N Engl J Med 1992; 326:653–7

Seo JB, Im JG, Goo JM et al. Atypical pulmonary metastases: spectrum of radiologic findings. Radiographics 2001; 21:403–17

Sherman M, Peltekian KM, Lee C. Screening for hepatocellular carcinoma in chronic carriers of hepatitis B virus: incidence and prevalence of hepatocellular carcinoma in a North American urban population. Hepatology 1995; 22:432–8

Smith RA, Saslow D, Sawyer KA et al; American Cancer Society High-Risk Work Group; American Cancer Society Screening Older Women Work Group; American Cancer Society Mammography Work Group; American Cancer Society Physical Examination Work Group; American Cancer Society New Technologies Work Group; American Cancer Society Breast Cancer Advisory Group. American Cancer Society guidelines for breast cancer screening: update 2003. CA Cancer J Clin 2003; 53:141–69

Sobue T, Moriyama N, Kaneko M et al. Screening for lung cancer with low dose helical computed tomography: anti-lung cancer association project. J Clin Oncol 2002; 20:911–20

Staples CA, Muller NL, Miller RR et al. Mediastinal nodes in bronchogenic carcinoma: comparison between CT and mediastinoscopy. Radiology 1988; 167:367–72

Steinkamp HJ, Cornehl M, Hosten N et al. Cervical lymphadenopathy: ratio of long to short axis diameter as a predictor of malignancy. BJR 1995; 68:266–70

Tabár L, Vitak B, Chen HH et al. The Swedish two county trial twenty years later. Updated mortality results and new insights from long term to follow-up. Radiol Clin North Am 2000; 38:625–51

Tiguert R, Gheiler EL, Tefilli MV et al. Lymph node size does not correlate with the presence of prostate cancer metastasis. Urology 1999; 53:367–71

UK Trial of Early Detection of Breast Cancer Group. 16-year mortality from breast cancer in the UK trial of early detection of breast cancer. Lancet 1999; 353:1909–14 van Tinteren H, Hoekstra OS, Smit EF et al. Effectiveness of positron emission tomography in the preoperative assessment of patients with suspected non-small-cell lung cancer: the PLUS multicentre randomised trial. Lancet. 2002; 359:1388–93

Weissleder R, Rieumont M, Wittenberg J. Primer of diagnostic imaging, 2nd edn. Mosby, St Louis, 1997, p 1008

Williams AD, Cousins C, Soutter WP et al. Detection of pelvic lymph node metastases in gynecologic malignancy: comparison of CT, MRI and positron emission tomography. AJR 2001; 177:343–8

Yang WT, Lam WWM, Yu MY et al. Comparison of dynamic helical CT and dynamic MR imaging in the evaluation of pelvic lymph nodes in cervical carcinoma. AJR 2000; 175:759–66

Yee J. Screening CT colonography. Semin Ultrasound, CT MRI 2003; 24:12–22

Yoon YC, Lee KS, Shim YM et al. Metastasis to regional lymph nodes in patients with oesophageal squamous cell carcinoma: CT versus FDG PET. Radiology 2003; 227:764–70

Zardi EM, Uwechie V, Picardi A, Costantino S. Liver focal lesions and hepatocellular carcinoma in cirrhotic patients: from screening to diagnosis. Clinica Terapeutica 2001; 152:185–8

In-theatre Radiology

24

D. Walsh

Background

Imaging is used by surgeons in the operating theatre to assist with the accurate and efficient performance of surgical procedures. The imaging modalities of X-ray, ultrasound and MRI have all been used in theatre by surgeons. The most widely used in theatre imaging modality for general surgeons is X-ray, although ultrasound may surpass this in the near future. Operative MRI remains experimental and prohibitively expensive. This chapter focuses on the use of intraoperative X-ray, by exploring three common scenarios where in theatre radiology is employed:

- operative cholangiogram,
- localisation of foreign bodies and
- surgical insertion of central venous catheters for long-term vascular access.

THE RADIOLOGICAL INVESTIGATIONS

Specific issues with 'in-theatre' radiology

Traditionally, in-theatre radiology involved plain film X-rays, producing static images, after a delay for film processing and development. In most situations, image intensification is now considered superior, due to the ability to produce an immediate, onscreen image in real time. Image intensification comes at the cost of potentially increased radiation exposure, often with a lesser quality hardcopy image.

Efficient and safe in-theatre radiology is the surgeon's responsibility and requires expertise and planning. The safety of patient and staff must be the prime concern. Whereas most modern image intensification systems produce images with minimal radiation scatter, all in-theatre radiology must aim to reduce excessive radiation exposure to every member of the operating room team. In general terms, this means reducing the duration of screening or number of static images exposed. Planning the required imaging before radiation activation is pivotal. It is essential to understand the best method of obtaining quality imaging from the equipment. From the patient's perspective, radiation exposure can be minimised by appropriate shielding (often overlooked in theatre), consideration of unintentional organ exposure and adoption of a 'selective' rather than 'routine' policy for in theatre radiology procedures. Staff exposure can be reduced by routinely shielding all essential staff (lead gowns), the evacuation of unnecessary theatre staff during imaging and monitoring radiation exposure.

After the safety aspects, planning for the incorporation of radiological intervention during a particular surgical procedure must be thought through. Failure to consider these issues before commencing the procedure can compromise patient and staff safety, increase radiation exposure, prolong anaesthesia and operating times and produce unsatisfactory imaging, which may in turn lead to intense frustration amongst theatre personnel. Key questions that the surgeon must address include:

- Will the image intensification equipment be functional and available when it is required?
- Are trained staff available to use the equipment?
- How will hardcopy images be obtained?
- Is the operating table compatible with and positioned correctly for the available X-ray equipment?
- How will safe anaesthesia and monitoring be maintained during imaging? How will sterility be ensured?

Intraoperative imaging: the future of surgery?

At present intraoperative imaging is mainly restricted to fluoroscopy and ultrasound. Both of these modalities have limitations: fluoroscopy because of the radiation exposure to both patient and staff, and ultrasound because of its inability to penetrate bone or air-filled structures. In addition both modalities are uniplanar and produce images subject to considerable artefact.

CT has been used more extensively in an interventional capacity in recent years and has a role in abscess drainage and biopsy. Its usefulness in the intraoperative setting is limited due to logistical considerations and the exposure of both patient and staff to ionising radiation.

Intraoperative MRI is the most recent development in intraoperative imaging. It has the ability to assist accurate targeting of lesions, define tumour margins and detect intraoperative problems such as haemorrhage. Advances in guidance systems allow intraoperative MRI to be combined with potentially novel tumour ablation methods. It has the advantage of being a non-ionising image modality. MRI provides excellent soft tissue definition, can be used to provide multiplanar images and can detect heat changes in tissues. This last capability makes it an ideal means of monitoring thermal destruction modalities as it can reliably detect temperature changes of less than 1 degree Celcius, with a spatial resolution of 2 mm.

Logistic concerns have limited the use of intraoperative MRI until recently. One of the key problems has been the requirement to move the patient in and out of the magnetic field during the surgery. Conventional MRI scanners restrict access for the surgeon but newer machines have overcome this problem in novel ways: one example is the use of a magnet that swings out of the operative field, e.g. via a ceiling mount, but can be repositioned for imaging at any stage, another is the use of a 'double doughnut' magnet in which the operating team stand either side of the patient between the elements of the magnet. Monitors above the surgeon allow for viewing of the images whilst performing surgery.

MRI is considered safe but there is no evidence about possible adverse effects for theatre teams exposed on a regular basis over a long period of time. Surgical instruments must be compatible with MRI. Ferromagnetic instruments cannot be used within a 0.5 Gauss distance, as they have the potential to become missiles or be stuck in the magnet.

The cost of creating an intraoperative MRI facility will limit its use, and the sites that are being developed in the USA, Japan and Europe are likely to focus on its role in neurosurgery.

THE CLINICAL PROBLEMS

Operative cholangiography

Whether on not cholangiography is performed depends on the surgeon's adherence to the routine or selective school of thought. Approximately 12% of patients will have common bile duct stones at cholecystectomy; 90% of these patients will have some preoperative indication (e.g. a history of jaundice or abnormal liver function tests). There is no convincing evidence that routine cholangiography decreases the risk of bile duct injury, which is quoted at 1 in 300–1000 patients for open surgery and 3 in 1000 for laparoscopic cholecystectomy, although one study of over 1 million patients in the USA suggested that the risk of common bile duct injury was significantly higher when intraoperative cholangiography was not used.

Surgeons who advocate routine cholangiography maintain that this approach is efficient in terms of operative scheduling, detects unexpected biliary pathology (Figs 24.1 and 24.2) and reduces the impact of bile duct injury by detection during the initial procedure (Box 24.1). In one study unsuspected stones were detected in 3.9% of patients undergoing routine cholangiograms. In a further 0.8% it was felt that management would have been disadvantaged if intraoperative cholangiography had not been performed.

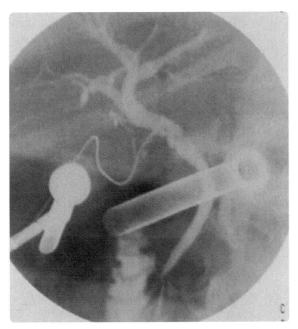

Fig. 24.1 A late sequence operative cholangiogram showing contrast in the biliary tree and duodenum. There has been good filling of the common bile duct, the common hepatic, right and left hepatic ducts and the larger intrahepatic branches. The ducts are of normal calibre and there are no filling defects.

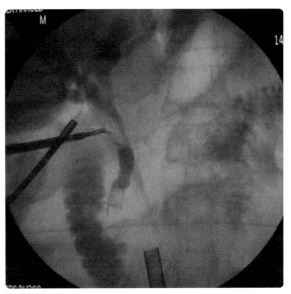

Fig. 24.2 A stone at the lower end of the common bile duct. This was an incidental finding during routine cholangiography. The common bile duct is only marginally dilated and there is unimpeded flow of contrast into the duodenum. The stone was removed by choledochotomy.

WHAT TO LOOK FOR Box 24.1

on the operative cholangiogram

- Identify the cystic duct and determine the point of insertion into the CBD
- Estimate the CBD diameter: beware of magnification, compare with known objects in the operative field
- Identify the right and left hepatic ducts
- Ensure there are no biliary tree filling defects or strictures (see Fig. 24.2)
- Ensure that the normal tapering of the distal CBD is present
- Ensure free flow of contrast into the duodenum
- Beware of contrast extravasation

Advocates of selective cholangiography argue that omission of the procedure saves time during cholecystectomy and any significant bile duct pathology should be anticipated preoperatively or can be dealt with by ERCP. The latter group would also point out that careful anatomical dissection is the key to preventing bile duct injury, and that if there are concerns regarding the operative findings, the options of cholangiography or open operative conversion are available. Table 24.1 summarises the main points made about cholangiography by the proponents of the routine and selective approaches.

Technical issues

Although a number of techniques for operative cholangiography have been described, most surgeons perform the procedure via the cystic duct. Thus the first step is to cannulate the cystic duct and to secure the catheter within the duct. This can be achieved either with a purpose-built cholangiogram forceps, or more cheaply using a ureteric catheter and surgical clip. The clip is applied sufficiently loosely to allow ease of flow

Table 24.1 A summary of the main arguments for and against routine cholangiography

Routine cholangiography	Selective cholangiography
Advantages	
Detects unsuspected bile duct pathology and choledocholithiasis	Reduces procedural time, organisational complexity and cost
Defines biliary anatomy	Unnecessary for most patients
May reduce incidence of bile duct injury (controversial)	Preoperative factors can select patients at risk of choledocholithiasis
Reduces impact of bile duct injury cholangiogram	Minimal 'false positive'
Prelude to more advanced laparoscopic biliary procedures	interpretations prompting unnecessary intervention
Predicts the need for surgical bile duct exploration or ERCP	
Disadvantages	
Additional procedural time, organisational complexity and cost	Unsuspected choledocholithiasis or biliary pathology missed
Additional radiation exposure to patients and staff	Increased incidence and impact of bile duct injuries (controversial)
Contrast allergies (rare)	Reduced training opportunities
'False positive' studies due to technical factors or errors in interpretation	When performed, the procedure is less efficient – technically, time factors, organisationally

into the cystic duct, yet firmly enough to prevent extravasation of contrast into the peritoneal cavity. This is checked when the catheter is flushed with saline, care being taken to exclude air bubbles from the system. Contrast can then be introduced into the cystic duct. The contrast usually used is an ionic, iodine-based contrast agent such as Urografin®. In patients with a history of iodine or contrast allergy, a non-ionic contrast should be used, which has a lower risk of reaction, even though the biliary tree is generally poorly absorbent of media. The image intensifier is now positioned over the region of Calot's triangle and scout images obtained to confirm correct positioning. Any superfluous instruments that might interfere with the quality of the image are removed from the field of view. The operating table is adjusted to allow the best position for imaging the bile duct. This usually involves rotating the table so that it is right side up and head level to avoid projection of the biliary tree over the spinal column. Contrast is then slowly injected to fill the biliary tree sequentially (see Fig. 24.1). Failure of

flow into the duodenum may be the result of sphincter of Oddi spasm and may be overcome by the administration of smooth muscle relaxants such as buscopan, glucagon, or nitrate preparations.

In interpreting operative cholangiograms, it is important to be aware of the common anatomical variants. A detailed assessment of anatomical variants is beyond the scope of this chapter but one of the more common pitfalls is to mistake a right hepatic branch for the cystic duct (Fig. 24.3).

Localisation of foreign bodies

The surgical removal of foreign bodies can be extremely difficult. Imaging has two roles in the localisation of soft tissue foreign bodies: (1) to confirm that a foreign body is present; (2) to aid in its removal. Although glass, metallic and stone objects may be visible on the preoperative plain film, plastics and vegetable material are less likely to be detected and may require ultrasonographic imaging.

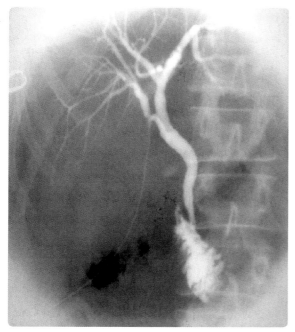

Fig. 24.3 Cannulation of the right hepatic duct. The cystic duct opened into the right hepatic duct. This abnormality of biliary anatomy was only realised when the cholangiogram was performed.

Plain X-rays performed preoperatively should include at least two views performed at right angles to each other. This will allow the determination of the position of the foreign body that is meaningful to an operative approach. It is prudent to mark the position of the entry point with a radio-opaque marker for similar reasons. Identifiable surface anatomical landmarks should be noted.

Intraoperatively, image intensification is most commonly employed. It is not a substitute for preoperative planning, adequate anaesthesia, knowledge of local anatomy, the use of ancillary aids such as limb tourniquets and of course surgical judgement. Increasingly, intraoperative ultrasound is being employed to help localise foreign bodies. Ultrasound has the advantage of avoiding ionising radiation, being movable throughout the operative field and can locate non radio-opaque foreign bodies.

Central venous access

Implanted central venous catheters or ports may be inserted in the operating theatre or in the radiology department (see Chapter 9). Image intensification greatly facilitates the former approach. In general the central catheter is placed over a guidewire, which is inserted so that the tip lies at the SVC/right atrial junction. The catheter may be placed into the subclavian vein, cephalic vein or via the internal jugular vein. Initially in-theatre radiology is used to confirm the correct position of the guidewire in the right heart system. Once the final catheter is inserted imaging can be used to adjust the final position, and if needed the length of catheter inserted can be adjusted. Angling of the patient position during the procedure and magnification can make the position of the catheter tip difficult to judge with image intensification. It may be helpful to identify surface landmarks such as the sternomanubrial joint with an instrument. Catheter tip movement can also be a guide to position. The tip moves in a uniphasic manner in the SVC and in a biphasic fashion in the right atrium. If a central venous catheter is positioned via the space between the first rib and clavicle, it must not be placed in a medial position such that compression between these two bones risks long-term catheter fracture. Image intensification can be used to image the catheter at this potential point of damage and ensure that catheter compression is not occurring.

Immediately following the procedure it is general practice to check the catheter position and to exclude complications such as pneumothorax or haemothorax associated with the insertion by performing a plain chest X-ray. Potential hazards of catheter insertion include inadvertent placement down the axillary vein or into the right atrium and progress of the catheter through the vein wall. In the latter instance the patient may get a pneumothorax or, if not recognised, a pleural effusion.

Further reading

Baillie J, Paulson EK, Vitellas KM. Biliary imaging: a review. Gastroenterology 2003; 124:1686–99

Cuschieri A, Shimi S, Banting S et al. Intraoperative cholangiography during laparoscopic cholecystectomy. Routine vs selective policy. Surg Endosc 1994; 8:302–5

Detry O, de Roover A, Detroz B, Honore P. The role of intraoperative cholangiography in detecting and preventing bile duct injury during laparoscopic cholecystectomy. Acta Chir Belg 2003; 103:161–2

Flum DR, Dellinger EP, Cheadle A et al. Intraoperative cholangiography and risk of common bile duct injury during cholecystectomy. JAMA 2003; 289:1639–44

Gluch L, Walker DG. Intraoperative magnetic resonance: the future of surgery. Aust N Z J Surg 2002; 72:426–36

Horton LK, Jacobson JA, Powell A et al. Sonography and radiography of soft-tissue foreign bodies. AJR 2001; 176:1155–9

Levy AD, Harcke HT. Handheld ultrasound device for detection of non-opaque and semi-opaque foreign bodies in soft tissues. J Clin Ultrasound 2003; 31:183–8

McEwan CN, Fukuta K. Recent advances in medical imaging: surgery, planning and simulation. World J Surg 1989; 13:343–8

Peters TM. Image-guided surgery: from X-rays to virtual reality. Comput Methods Biomech Biomed Engin 2000; 4:27–57

Imaging in Trauma

S.J. Neuhaus

Background

Radiology forms an important component in the assessment of trauma patients. It is essential that radiological investigations do not interfere with life-saving initial management. In a well-organised trauma unit, radiological facilities will be built-in and the team well practised, so that imaging investigations can be performed without disrupting ongoing patient resuscitation.

In the trauma setting a radiologist will rarely be available to review the initial films. It is essential that all images are examined systematically and thoroughly so that life-threatening injuries are not missed. This is particularly important as the stress and urgency of the trauma setting often lead to injuries being overlooked.

Equally, all films obtained in the trauma room must be formally reported as soon as possible and any unrecognised injuries followed up as part of the 'tertiary survey'. This chapter will focus on injuries sustained to the trunk and concentrate on the imaging investigations performed in the emergency room.

THE IMMEDIATE TRAUMA SERIES (SECONDARY SURVEY)

Protocols for the early management of severe trauma include cervical, chest and pelvic imaging as part of the secondary survey.

Cervical spine films

- Lateral (shoot through)
- Swimmer's
- AP C-spine
- Odontoid peg view.

Radiological evaluation of the cervical spine is normally included as part of the secondary survey (Box 25.1). Over 80% of cervical fractures can be identified using a combination of the above views. Evaluation of the cervical spine can be deferred until after necessary resuscitative efforts have taken place, provided the spine is immobilised and protected.

In addition to an AP view of the cervical spine, a lateral (shoot-through) film is normally obtained. It is usually necessary to pull down on the patient's shoulders to obtain an adequate film, i.e. one that visualises the skull base, the seven cervical vertebrae and T1. If it is not possible to view the lower vertebrae on the lateral film, a 'swimmer's view' (one arm extended

WHAT TO LOOK FOR   Box 25.1

on the C-spine films

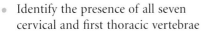

- Identify the presence of all seven cervical and first thoracic vertebrae
- Alignment:
  - There should be four uninterrupted curves formed by the anterior vertebral bodies, posterior vertebral bodies, posterior spinal canal (spinolaminar line) and tips of the spinous processes. Loss of alignment suggests cervical dislocation and/or fracture
  - The posterior vertebral body line is the most sensitive for dislocation as the anterior line may be disrupted by osteophytes
  - Narrowing of the vertebral canal is highly suspicious of spinal cord compression
  - The space between the anterior arch of C1 and the dens should be <2.5 mm (<5 mm in children) on the lateral view
  - On the PEG view the lateral margins C1 and C2 should be aligned
  - On the AP view the spinous processes should be aligned, remembering that cervical vertebrae have bifid spinous processes. Malalignment suggests unilateral locked facets
- Bones:
  - Reduction in vertebral height suggests a compression fracture
  - Check for protrusion posteriorly into the spinal canal
  - The pedicles, facets, laminae, transverse processes and spinous processes must all be assessed for evidence of fractures or dislocation
- Intervertebral disc spaces:
  - Loss of the intervertebral disc space may suggest a fracture of the vertebrae above or below
  - A narrowed disc with surrounding osteophytes is more likely to be degenerative

- Soft tissues:
  - Expansion of the prevertebral space occurs with haemorrhage accompanying a spinal cord injury. The prevertebral space is best assessed opposite the C3 vertebra and should be less than 5mm in diameter. Below this level it should be less than one vertebral body width. This sign is unreliable if the patient has been intubated
  - Loss of the prevertebral fat stripe indicates possible spinal injury
  - An increase in the distance between the spinous processes suggests a possible anterior spinal canal fracture with tearing of the interspinous ligaments

upwards, one arm pulled down) should be obtained. Approximately 70% of fractures will be detected using a combination of these two views alone. It is important to visualise all vertebrae as C1/2 and C5–7 are the most common sites of fracture.

An odontoid peg (open mouth) X-ray should be obtained in a conscious patient to further visualise the upper vertebrae and if there is any suspicion of a C1–C2 injury.

Associated injuries

Approximately 10% of patients with a cervical spine fracture will have a second fracture in the vertebral column. Therefore any patient with a cervical fracture must have imaging of the entire vertebral column.

Flexion/extension views

These do not form a part of the immediate assessment and evaluation of trauma patients and should only been undertaken in consultation with a spinal unit. The sensitivity of CT is such that it should be undertaken in preference to flexion/extension views.

Types of cervical fracture

- Atlanto-occipital dislocation
- C1 (Atlas) fracture
- C2 (Axis) fracture
- Fracture/dislocations of C3–7.

Atlanto-occipital dislocation This injury usually results from severe flexion with simultaneous head–body distraction. Most patients do not survive to reach the trauma room.

C1 (Atlas) fracture Fracture of C1 is uncommon and usually occurs in association with a C2 fracture. The most common pattern is a 'burst' (Jefferson) fracture resulting in disruption of both the anterior and posterior rings. There is commonly an associated disruption of the lateral mass. This fracture usually results from severe compressive trauma directed to the top of the head. On the PEG view the lateral masses of C1 are both displaced laterally with respect to C2. It is well defined on a CT scan. This is an unstable fracture and requires orthopaedic stabilisation.

C2 (Axis) fracture C2 fractures account for up to 20% of all cervical spine injuries. They can be classified as fractures of the odontoid peg or fractures of the posterior elements. Odontoid peg fractures are the most common variant and can usually be identified on a lateral (Fig. 25.1), AP or odontoid view. Fracture of the posterior elements (hangman's fracture) is less common and best visualised with CT.

Fractures of C3–7 Cervical fractures most commonly involve C5–6. Several patterns of fracture dislocation are possible but the most common are:

- vertebral body fracture (with or without subluxation)

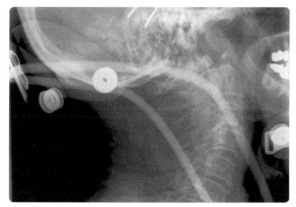

Fig. 25.1 A fracture involving C1 and C2 with displacement. The odontoid peg is fractured.

- subluxation of the articular processes
- fractures of the laminae, spinous processes, pedicles or lateral masses.

Facet dislocations are strongly predictive of neurological injury. In unilateral facet dislocation 80% of patients will have an associated neurological deficit and 30% will have complete spinal cord paralysis. On the AP film there is rotation of the vertebral bodies distal to the dislocation, with offset of the spinous processes. Bilateral facet injuries are associated with a significantly adverse prognosis with up to 85% complete paralysis. On the lateral film the vertebral body overrides the one below by at least 50%.

Common errors and pitfalls

- Failure to include T1 on the film:
  - inadequate 'pull down' on the arms
  - failure to perform a 'swimmers' view
- Inadequate visualisation of C1/2
- If all vertebrae cannot be seen a fracture cannot be excluded radiologically
- Normal variants.

CT of the cervical spine should be used to further assess any suspected injuries on plain X-ray, and to visualise areas which have not been adequately seen. In many centres, particularly in the USA, spiral CT of the entire cervical spine with multiplanar reconstruction is now performed routinely as part of the CT assessment of the multi-trauma patient.

Chest X-ray

A chest X-ray is mandatory in all patients with significant trauma, particularly if they have multiple injuries. If there is any suspicion of a tension pneumothorax this must be treated by drainage as an immediate priority and not delayed until radiological confirmation is made.

The approach to the trauma CXR is different from that of an elective film. Life-threatening abnormalities need to be detected promptly and acted on. The X-ray in the trauma room is normally taken in the supine position and some problems (e.g. haemothorax) can be missed if this different projection is not appreciated. It is imperative to be cognisant of, and recognise patterns of associated injury that may be suggested by particular CXR findings (Table 25.1).

Table 25.1 Summary of changes seen on a chest radiograph and the underlying injuries that need to be considered

Radiological changes	Possible underlying injury
Tracheobronchial tree	
Disruption of tracheal outline	Tracheobronchial disruption
Lungs	
Pneumothorax, haemothorax	Tracheobronchial disruption Oesophageal injury Pulmonary contusion
Diaphragm	
Diaphragmatic disruption or opacity	Diaphragmatic tear
Haemothorax/haemoperitoneum Subdiaphragmatic air	Perforated viscus
Mediastinum	
Widening of mediastinum Mediastinal air	Major vessel injury Tracheobronchial disruption Oesophageal injury
Thoracic skeleton	
Fracture upper ribs	Major airway or vessel injury Brachial plexus injury
Fracture lower ribs	Pneumothorax, haemothorax, Splenic, hepatic or renal injury
Flail segment	Major airway or vessel injury Pulmonary contusion
Scapular fracture	Brachial plexus injury
Sternal fracture	Cardiac contusion
Tubes and lines	
Nasogastric tube in the chest	Oesophageal perforation Ruptured diaphragm

Tracheobronchial injuries

Significant tracheobronchial disruption can often be clinically detected by the presence of a large pneumothorax with an ongoing air leak despite adequate drainage. Signs that may be visible on the CXR include:

- pneumomediastinum
- pneumothorax
- emphysema in the mediastinum, neck or subcutaneous tissues.

If a pneumomediastinum is suspected it may be visible as free air tracking up into the neck (Fig. 25.2). This can be difficult to see on a plain chest X-ray and may be better defined on a cervical spine view (Fig. 25.3) or on CT (see below).

Lungs

Pneumothorax and haemopneumothorax occur commonly in multiply injured patients. The features of a pneumothorax are discussed in Chapter 2. Because the trauma CXR is taken in a supine position, significant fluid collections can be underestimated. It is important to appreciate that a fluid level will not be present on the supine film as fluid layers posteriorly, producing a generalised increase in the density of the hemithorax. Likewise, free air will not accumulate superiorly and will be difficult to detect.

Pulmonary contusions are not normally visible on the immediate trauma CXR unless there has been a delay in presentation. Any patient with a significant chest injury should be suspected of having a significant contusion, especially in the presence of multiple

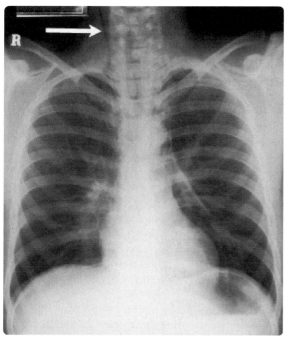

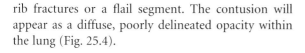

Fig. 25.2 Free gas (pneumomediastinum) seen tracking up into the neck (arrow).

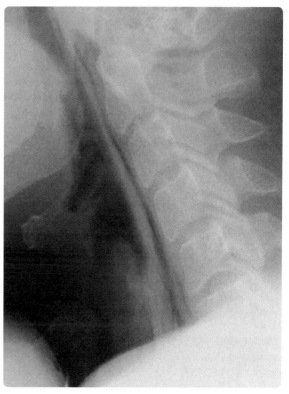

Fig. 25.3 Free gas from a ruptured bronchiole seen tracking up in the neck behind the oesophagus.

rib fractures or a flail segment. The contusion will appear as a diffuse, poorly delineated opacity within the lung (Fig. 25.4).

Mediastinum

Assessment of the cardiac outline is difficult as the films are taken in the AP projection with the patient supine, however a progressively increasing cardiac outline suggests bleeding within the pericardium. The cardinal sign suggesting a major vessel injury is widening of the mediastinum (Fig. 25.5), but this can be falsely increased on an AP film. Fractures of the first and second ribs are usually a guide to significant trauma and therefore a search should be made for other injuries.

Other signs of significant injury include:

- depression of the left main stem bronchus
- obliteration of the space between the pulmonary artery and the aorta (aortopulmonary window)
- obliteration of the aortic knob
- deviation of the trachea and oesophagus to the right indicated by the nasogastric tube.

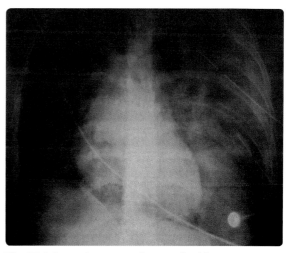

Fig. 25.4 Severe lung contusion sustained in a motor vehicle crash.

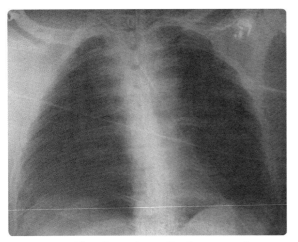

Fig. 25.5 A widened superior mediastinum secondary to blood tracking down from a ruptured subclavian artery.

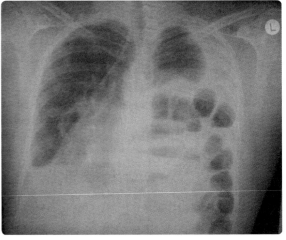

Fig. 25.6 Traumatic rupture of the left hemidiaphragm with colon herniated into the chest. The mediastinum has been shifted to the right.

Diaphragm

Diaphragmatic injuries are more common with left sided trauma. In the presence of diaphragmatic injury associated injuries, such as to liver and spleen, are common. Whereas initial plain radiographs will detect 60% of left-sided diaphragmatic ruptures, most right-sided ones will be missed. This is because the liver acts to prevent visceral herniation into the chest and what is detected on the radiograph is organ shift rather than the actual rent in the diaphragm. Signs of a diaphragmatic injury include:

- elevation, irregularity or obliteration of a hemidiaphragm
- presence of stomach, colon or nasogastric tube above the diaphragm (Fig. 25.6)
- pleural effusion
- contralateral mediastinal shift
- density above the diaphragm (may be due to herniation of a solid organ such as pancreas, spleen, liver).

Thoracic skeleton

The thoracic skeleton must be systematically examined for evidence of fractures. Whilst treatment of rib and/ or chest wall fractures alone is rarely required, such fractures can be important indicators of the degree of injury and associated injuries.

Thoracic spine fractures make up about 30% of all spine fractures, and carry a 60% risk of significant neurologic deficit. Most injuries are caused by hyper-flexion (motor vehicle crashes) and axial loading (falls). Fractures are often multiple and can be non-contiguous. Plain films of the thoracic spine in cases of multiple trauma are usually inadequate and difficult to interpret. Helical CT is more reliable than plain films in the detection of fractures of the thoracic spine, sternum and rib cage. Of those spinal fractures identified on CT scan, more than 60% are missed on plain film.

Rib fractures

Individual rib fractures may be difficult to visualise on the trauma CXR. Although all rib fractures are significant due to their effect on pain and inspiration, the significance of rib fractures is dependent on the level of the ribs involved and the extent of the fractures.

Rib fractures can be classified as:

- fracture of the upper ribs (1–4)
- fracture of the lower ribs (5–12)
- flail segment, i.e. fracture of several ribs in more than one place.

Fractures of ribs 1–4 usually indicates significant trauma and have a high correlation with other injuries such as:

- haemo-/pneumothorax
- major airway or vessel injury.

Fractures of the lower ribs are also associated with the possibility of:

- Haemo/pneumothorax
- Pulmonary contusion
- Subdiaphragmatic injury, e.g. splenic, liver and renal injuries

Fractures of the thoracic wall

A systematic survey should be carried out for fractures of the following:

- clavicle
- scapula (high association with other injury).

Sternal fractures

Sternal fractures require significant force and, if displaced, are associated with injuries such as cardiac contusion and major vessel injury. The AP film can be misleading so specific lateral sternal views are recommended if a sternal fracture is suspected.

Non-displaced sternal fractures have a low association with other injuries and the patient does not require cardiac monitoring if the trauma room ECG is normal.

Tubes and lines

The position of all tubes and lines should be checked on the CXR. This includes the placement of:

- endotracheal tubes
- nasogastric tubes (Fig. 25.7)
- central lines
- chest tubes.

Common pitfalls

- Delay in recognition and treatment of a tension pneumothorax due to waiting for CXR confirmation.
- Failure to recognise that a large haemothorax may be present without a characteristic fluid level due to the patient being supine.

AP pelvis

Major pelvic injuries are potentially life threatening and must be recognised promptly. An AP pelvic X-ray should be obtained in the trauma room as part of the secondary survey in all patients with multiple or severe abdominal trauma. Pelvic fractures are usually caused

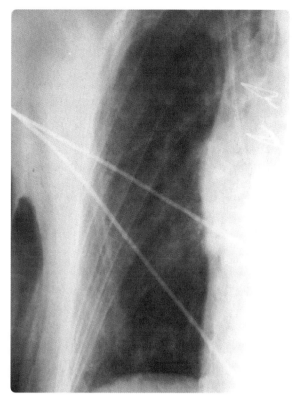

Fig. 25.7 Iatrogenic injury. Oesophageal rupture secondary to the passage of a Doppler probe for transoesophageal echography. The perforation was only detected when the nasogastric tube was seen coiled in the right chest.

by motor vehicle accidents, crush injuries or significant falls. The resulting forces can open the pelvic ring, and tear the sacral venous plexuses resulting in profuse haemorrhage. Clinical indicators of possible pelvic injury include unexplained hypotension, leg length discrepancy, a high riding prostate on rectal examination and progressive flank or perineal swelling.

An adequate film requires visualisation of the entire pelvic ring and both femoral heads (Box 25.2). It should be remembered that because the pelvic bones form a ring, a fracture at one point is usually accompanied by a second fracture elsewhere in the ring.

Patients with a pelvic fracture have a high risk of associated injury. Injuries that must be considered include:

- intra-abdominal injury
- retroperitoneal haematoma
- urethral, bladder, or rectal injury

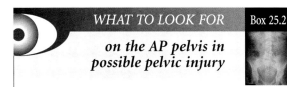

WHAT TO LOOK FOR   Box 25.2

on the AP pelvis in possible pelvic injury

- Any obvious fracture: usually identified as disruption of the symmetry of the pelvic ring
- Subtle fracture elsewhere in the ring once one fracture is discovered
- Widening of the sacroiliac joint
- Diastasis of the pubic symphysis
- Fracture/dislocation of the hip and/or femoral shaft

- sciatic nerve injury (with posterior hip dislocation).

OTHER RADIOLOGY IN THE TRAUMA ROOM

Other radiological investigations that may be used in the early management of trauma include the following:

- cystourethrogram
- emergency ultrasound (FAST scanning)
- 'the trauma CT'
- arch aortogram/CT aortogram.

Cystourethrogram

Urethrography is indicated in any patient suspected of urethral trauma, prior to attempting to insert a urinary catheter. Urethral trauma is usually associated with significant pelvic trauma and should be suspected in any patient with pelvic fractures.

Urethrography is best performed in the trauma department by the attending surgeon. A small-bore (14F) urethral catheter should be placed 1–2 cm into the fossa navicularis and then inflated with 1–2 mL water (just enough to achieve a snug fit without undue pressure). The patient is placed in a lateral position and iodinated contrast (Urografin® or equivalent) is then introduced in 10-mL increments. If dynamic image intensification is available, this is the preferred method of obtaining films. Alternatively, sequential static films can be taken in the lateral decubitus position.

Urethral rupture can be partial or complete. Injuries are classified as:

- Type I: urethral stretch injury, with no extravasation
- Type II: urethral disruption proximal to the genitourinary diaphragm
- Type III: urethral disruption both proximal and distal to the genitourinary diaphragm.

Emergency ultrasound (FAST scanning)

Blunt abdominal trauma

Diagnostic peritoneal lavage (DPL), emergency ultrasound and CT are complementary investigations in blunt abdominal trauma. Each has advantages and limitations with which the surgeon must be familiar.

Diagnostic peritoneal lavage is a non-specific investigation and carries a risk of iatrogenic injury. In addition it makes a subsequent CT scan more difficult to interpret due to the introduction of air and fluid into the peritoneal cavity.

Focused abdominal sonography in trauma (FAST) is a widely accepted diagnostic tool in the management of blunt abdominal trauma. It is quick, portable, non-invasive and can be performed in the resuscitation room by a radiographer/radiologist, a surgeon or an emergency medicine physician trained in the use of targeted ultrasound.

The purpose of FAST scanning is to detect free intraperitoneal fluid and demonstrate the presence or absence of a pericardial effusion. The abdomen is systematically examined looking for evidence of fluid around the liver (Morison's pouch), spleen (including the splenorenal recess), the paracolic gutters and the pelvis. Assessment of the pelvis is facilitated by clamping the urinary catheter to fill the bladder. This displaces bowel gas-filled loops and decreases the likelihood of missing a pelvic haematoma.

FAST scanning in experienced hands is a sensitive detector of peritoneal fluid with a sensitivity and specificity of up to 95%. Solid organs are not assessed as part of a standard FAST scan. The FAST examination cannot be used to assess the retroperitoneum or detect hollow organ injury and may miss other intraperitoneal injuries. Those most likely to have false negative studies include patients with fractures of the pelvis or thoraco-lumbar spine, lower rib fractures and haematuria. One of the advantages of FAST scanning is that it can be repeated, thereby detecting any ongoing accumulation of fluid in a clinically deteriorating patient.

FAST scanning is not indicated in haemodynamically stable patients, where CT is the investigation of choice. The main role of the FAST scan is in the unstable patient with multiple injuries, where the presence of intraperitoneal fluid is likely to be an indication for laparotomy. It should be considered an adjunct to clinical examination, not a definitive investigation.

Common pitfalls

- Limited access to a good acoustic window.
- Variable training of staff (sensitivity 36% after 6 hours of training and 20 scans, 94% for senior radiologist).
- Indirect method of detecting abdominal injuries so false negative results in visceral injuries without free intraperitoneal fluid are common (up to 30%).

'The trauma CT'

CT is an important component in the investigation of the trauma patient as it is able to examine many parts of the body in a short space of time (Box 25.3). It uses ionizing radiation and therefore should only be used if necessary, however in the severely injured patient the benefits clearly outweigh the risks.

CT is frequently used to help in the assessment of abdominal and pelvic injuries, with the addition of a

scan of the chest if there is clinical concern or an abnormal CXR (Fig. 25.8). Other components may include a scan of the brain if the patient has a decreased Glasgow Coma Score, base of skull if there is blood or CSF in the ear, or cervical spine if there has been inadequate visualisation or a suspected injury on plain film (Figs 25.9 and 25.10). If a head scan is performed this is usually done first prior to administration of intravenous contrast (see Chapter 4). In the case of a suspected aortic injury the scan parameters can be altered to obtain a CT aortogram. In patients who are haemodynamically unstable, it is usually more appropriate to take the patient directly to theatre, perhaps with the addition of a FAST ultrasound as described above.

CT with intravenous contrast is highly sensitive in detecting solid organ injuries, small volume pneumoperitoneum and free intra abdominal fluid. It may show active contrast extravasation indicating ongoing bleeding. In patients with penetrating injuries or gunshot wounds CT can show the tract and position of any indwelling foreign body, in particular its relation to vessels and organs. If there is concern regarding the renal system delayed scans can be performed of the kidneys or bladder. A delayed scan can be useful to assess renal drainage and provides an image similar to an intravenous urogram (see below).

Contusions of visceral organs manifest as areas of low density in the otherwise normally enhancing

---

WHAT TO LOOK FOR | Box 25.3

on the trauma CT

- Pneumothorax/haemothorax
- Mediastinal haematoma/aortic injury
- Lung contusion
- Rib fractures
- Tubes and lines
- Free gas/extraluminal oral contrast (intraperitoneal/retroperitoneal)
- Haemoperitoneum
- Visceral injury
- Mesenteric haematoma
- Bowel wall thickening
- Spinal or pelvic fractures

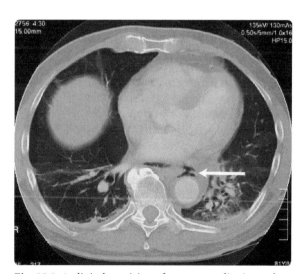

Fig. 25.8 A clinical suspicion of pneumomediastinum, but nothing visible on the plain chest radiograph. The CT shows a pocket of air anterior to the aorta (arrow).

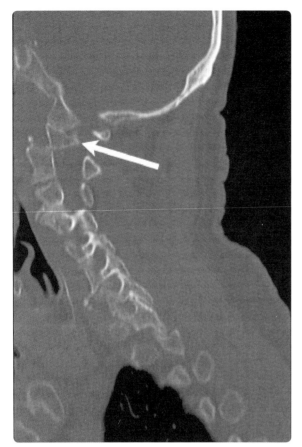

Fig. 25.9 A reconstructed sagittal view of the C1/2 fracture shown in Fig. 25.1. The view is not totally in the sagittal plane and thus the spinal canal is partially rotated out of the field of view. An arrow points to the displaced vertebral body.

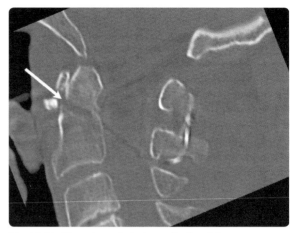

Fig. 25.10 There is a relatively undisplaced fracture through the odontoid peg (arrow) which can be seen on this reconstructed CT sagittal view.

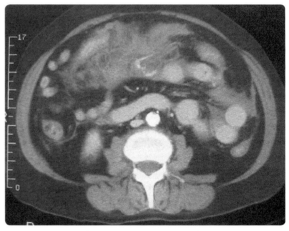

Fig. 25.11 Stranding in the mesentery of the transverse colon with extravasation of contrast in a patient with a traumatic haematoma.

parenchyma. If there is acute haematoma or acute contrast extravasation this will appear as an area of increased density. Subcapsular haematoma, for example around the spleen or kidneys, is a sign of injury. In extreme cases the organ may be shattered into several pieces. In mesenteric injuries focal haematoma or 'streakiness' of the fat may be visible (Fig. 25.11). Signs of bowel wall injuries range from wall thickening to focal perforation with free gas and/or oral contrast.

The use of oral contrast is debatable, and with the use of faster multislice CT scanners the visualisation of the bowel has been significantly improved. Recent studies suggest that the use of oral contrast is unnecessary, with similar sensitivity to bowel and mesenteric injuries both with and without oral contrast. The use of oral contrast will probably remain individual departmental preference in the immediate future.

Blunt splenic trauma

The spleen is the most frequently injured abdominal organ in blunt abdominal trauma. Over the last decade there has been an increasing trend towards splenic conservation in splenic trauma. This practice requires accurate identification of patients in whom non-operative management can be safely achieved. CT is an important component of this assessment and has been shown to be up to 98% accurate in the detection of blunt splenic injuries.

Although the decision to treat a patient conservatively or operatively must rely on a combination of clinical and radiological features, radiological grading of splenic injury is an important prognostic indicator. There are several systems of grading of splenic injury on CT. The most useful of these is the Buntain system (Table 25.2).

Low-grade splenic injuries in the haemodynamically stable patient are those most likely to be successfully managed conservatively (Fig. 25.12). CT has been reported to underestimate the injury found at surgery. This may be a true effect or be related to progression of bleeding between scanning and theatre. For this reason grade III and IV injuries are probably managed best with surgical intervention, despite the patient's haemodynamic status (see Chapter 10). Patients who demonstrate a 'vascular blush' on CT scan, suggesting active bleeding, should also be considered for immediate surgical intervention.

Blunt hepatic trauma

A similar trend to non-operative management exists in blunt hepatic trauma. It has been reported that up to 90% of patients with hepatic trauma can be managed in this way.

A system of CT grading for hepatic trauma was introduced by Mirvis in 1989. Although it is a useful classification of parenchymal damage, it correlates poorly with clinical outcome and is of more use in clinical research.

In general, lacerations of solid organs will appear as low attenuation areas within the normally enhancing parenchyma, unless there is high density haematoma or contrast extravasation (Box 25.4).

Renal trauma

The majority of renal trauma following blunt abdominal injury is superficial, consisting of small cortical lacerations, renal contusion and/or subcapsular haematoma (grade 1) (Box 25.5). Grade 2 injuries involve complete cortical laceration or fracture communicat-

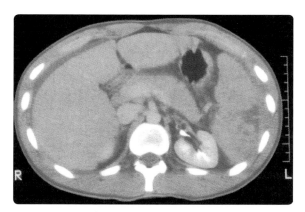

Fig. 25.12 A grade II splenic injury showing a laceration through the mid-body of the organ. This injury was managed conservatively.

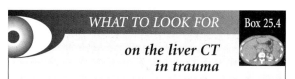

WHAT TO LOOK FOR   Box 25.4

on the liver CT in trauma

- Capsular tear
- Intraparenchymal fracture or laceration
- Subcapsular or intraparenchymal haematoma
- Active contrast extravasation
- Periportal tracking of blood
- Partial devascularisation due to vascular injury

Table 25.2 Buntain system of grading splenic injury

Grade	Description
I	Subcapsular haematoma or localized disruption without significant parenchymal injury
II	Capsular and parenchymal disruption not involving the hilar vessels
III	Fractures into the hilum and involving the hilar vessels
IV	Fragmentation of the spleen or avulsion of the hilum

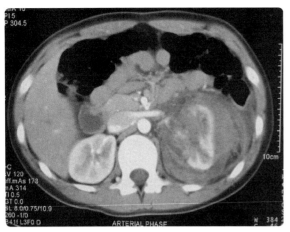

Fig. 25.13 A grade 3 renal injury. There has been partial disruption of the left kidney after a direct blow to that organ.

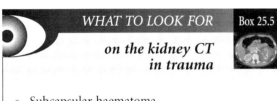

WHAT TO LOOK FOR — Box 25.5

on the kidney CT in trauma

- Subcapsular haematoma
- Contusion with area of non enhancement following contrast
- Extravasation of contrast
- Separation of renal poles
- Lack of renal enhancement

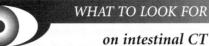

WHAT TO LOOK FOR — Box 25.6

on intestinal CT in trauma

- Free gas or extraluminal oral contrast (intraperitoneal or retroperitoneal)
- Focal bowel wall thickening > 3 cm
- Fluid or haematoma within the mesentery
- Streaky appearance of the mesenteric fat

CT FEATURES OF — Box 25.7

diaphragmatic rupture

- Direct discontinuity of hemidiaphragm
- Visceral herniation into chest
- 'Collar sign': waist-like constriction of viscus by diaphragm at site of rupture
- Dependent visceral sign: loss of posterior visceral support allowing organs to abut ribs posteriorly

ing with the calyceal system. Grade 3 injuries represent a shattered kidney, with injury to the renal vascular pedicle (Fig. 25.13).

Bowel and mesenteric injuries

These can be difficult to see on CT (Box 25.6), with or without the use of oral contrast. They include contusion, haematoma, and laceration of bowel wall. Injuries to the mesenteric vessels may lead to bowel ischemia and necrosis.

The CT scan and diaphragmatic injury

Between 0.8 and 8% of patients sustain diaphragmatic injuries following blunt trauma. As discussed above, these injuries can easily be missed on the initial plain radiograph. Fast acquisition scans and multislice CT

minimise motion artefacts and provide good definition of the diaphragms (Box 25.7).

Arch aortography/computed tomography aortogram

Traumatic aortic injury is usually associated with an acute deceleration. Only 10–20% of patients survive the initial injury. Of those arriving at hospital, rapid identification and treatment of the injury is required. Prompt diagnosis improves survival as 30% of untreated patients die within the first 6 hours and 40% within 24 hours.

It should be noted that:

- 90–95% of injuries occur at the isthmus, between the left subclavian and ligamentum arteriosum
- 5% involve the ascending aorta
- 2% involve the descending aorta.

Although up to 2% of patients with traumatic aortic injury have been reported to have a normal CXR on

CT SIGNS OF   Box 25.8

aortic injury

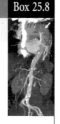

- Intimal flap
- Pseudoaneurysm
- Contour irregularity
- Contrast extravasation
- Mediastinal haematoma
- Abrupt calibre change in the aorta

arrival, most patients will demonstrate at least one major abnormality as discussed above. Any patient with a CXR with one of the following should undergo further imaging to exclude aortic injury:

- widening of the mediastinum
- aortic arch abnormalities
- opacification of the aortopulmonary window
- left or right apical capping.

Traditionally, arch aortography was considered the 'gold standard' for the diagnosis of aortic injury. However, it is an invasive procedure, is time and resource intensive and is usually available only in major trauma centres. The rapid improvement of helical CT technology now allows the performance of a highly sensitive CT angiogram on the trauma patient who is often already on the CT table (Box 25.8). The sensitivity of CT for detection of aortic injury is now as high as 96% with a specificity of 99% and it is becoming the accepted definitive diagnostic test for aortic injury in many centres with multi-slice helical CT technology.

Further reading

Allen TL, Mueller MT, Bonk RT et al. Computed Tomographic scanning without oral contrast solution for blunt bowel and mesenteric injuries in abdominal trauma. J Trauma 2004; 56:314–22

Bachulis BL, Long WB, Hynes GD, Johnson MC. Clinical indications for cervical spine radiographs in the traumatized patient. Am J Surg 1987; 153:473–78

Dyer DS, Moore EE, Mestek MF et al. Can chest CT be used to exclude aortic injury. Radiology 1999; 213:195–202

Helms CA. Fundamentals of skeletal radiology, 2nd edn. WB Saunders, Philadelphia, 1995

Hills MW, Thomas SG, McDougall PA et al. Traumatic thoracic aortic rupture: investigation determines outcome. Aust N Z J Surg. 1994; 64(5):312–18

Iochum S, Luidg T, Walter F et al. Imaging of diaphragmatic injury: a diagnostic challenge? Radiographics 2002; 22: S103–18

Lingawi SS, Buckley AR. Focussed abdominal US in patients with trauma. Radiology 2000; 217:426–29

Liu M, Lee CH, P'eng FK. Prospective comparison of diagnostic peritoneal lavage, computed tomographic scanning, and ultrasonography for the diagnosis of blunt abdominal trauma. J Trauma 1993; 35:267–70

Macdonald RL, Schwartz ML, Mirich D et al. Diagnosis of cervical spine injury in motor vehicle crash victims: how many x-rays are enough? J Trauma 1990; 30:392–7

McGahan JP, Richards J, Fogata ML. Emergency ultrasound in trauma patients. Radiol Clin N Am 2004; 42:417–25

Melton SM, Kerby JD, McGiffin D et al. The evolution of chest computed tomography for the definitive diagnosis of blunt aortic injury: a single-center experience. J Trauma. 2004; 56:243–50

Parmley LF, Manion WC, Mattingly TW, Jahenke EJ. Non-penetrating traumatic injury of the aorta. Circulation 1958; 17:1086–2101

Philipp MO, Kubin K, Hormann M, Metz VM. Radiological emergency room management with emphasis on multidetector-row CT. Eur J Radiol 2003; 48:2–4

Poletti P, Wintermark M, Schnyder P, Becker CD. Traumatic injuries: role of imaging in the management of the polytrauma victim. Eur Radiol 2002; 12:969–78

Rogers LF. Radiology of skeletal trauma, vol 2, 3rd edn. WB Saunders, Philadelphia, 2002

Sanders MN, Civil I. Adult splenic injuries: Treatment patterns and predictive indicators. Aust N Z J Surg 1999; 69:430–2

Scaglione M, Pinto A, Pinto F et al. Role of contrast-enhanced helical CT in the evaluation of acute thoracic injuries after blunt chest trauma. Eur Radiol 2001; 11(12):2444–8

Shapiro MJ, Krausz C, Durham RM, Mazuski JE. Overuse of splenic scoring and computed tomographic scans. J Trauma 1999; 47:651–8

Stafford RE, McGonigal MD, Weigelt JA, Johnson TJ. Oral contrast solution and computed tomography for blunt abdominal traumas: a randomized study. Arch Surg 1999; 134:622–6

Wintermark M, Wicky S, Schnyder P. Imaging of acute traumatic injuries of the thoracic aorta. Eur Radiol 2002; 12:431–42

Appendix

RADIATION PROTECTION AND PATIENT DOSES IN DIAGNOSTIC IMAGING

With the increased demand for procedures involving radiation, it is important that doctors and their patients understand something of the principles of radiation protection and the doses associated with the different procedures. There is evidence that even radiologists are unable to accurately estimate the comparative doses of CT and plain radiographs and that insufficient attention is paid to the provision of information to patients on the risks, benefits and radiation doses for a CT scan.

The degree of risk is determined by the sensitivity of the organ irradiated and the dose received. In many countries it is a legal requirement that the use of ionising radiation is justified to the person performing the examination, which is why including appropriate information on the clinical request form is so important. The dose to the patient should always be considered when ordering an investigation, and risk versus benefit considered. This is particularly important in children and females of reproductive age. It is necessary to ensure that a patient is not pregnant prior to any ionising radiation procedure. Table 1 lists the most common examinations, the dose and equivalent period of natural background radiation.

Radiation units

There are a number of measures of radiations dose:

- Gray (Gy) has replaced the now obsolete term, rad (1 Gy = 100 rad)
- Sieverts (Sv) are a measure of 'dose equivalence' or biological effect. The effective dose is the dose equivalent (Sv) multiplied by a tissue weighting factor, which is high for gonads, bone marrow and colon, and lowest for skin.

Biological effects of radiation

Radiation exposure induces both acute and chronic effects. Radiological investigations are now the most common source of exposure to manmade radiation. Diagnostic imaging contributes to approximately 20% of the general populations total radiation dose. Of this, CT is the major contributor, due to a combination of high dose and large examination numbers.

Acute effects

Acute effects occur at high dose levels, e.g. following radiotherapy or exposure to atomic radiation. Effects include skin ulceration, pulmonary fibrosis, marrow depletion, desquamation of endothelial surfaces, especially those of the gut with a high rate of tissue turnover. A dose of 100 Gy is fatal in hours due to CNS malfunction, whole-body exposure of 3–5 Gy leads to death in 1–2 months due to loss of bone marrow function.

Chronic effects

Doses below 1 Gy typically produce no acute effect. There is, however, an increased risk of development of a subsequent malignancy or genetic abnormalities in future offspring. There is a typical time lag of 10–25 years.

Specific risk considerations

Pregnancy

Irradiation of the fetus should be avoided whenever possible. If a woman of reproductive age cannot be

Table 1 Typical radiation doses for selected examinations

Examination	Dose (mSv)	Equivalent number of CXR	Equivalent period of natural background radiation (approx.)
X-ray			
Limb	<0.01	<0.5	<1.5 days
Chest	0.02	1	3 days
Skull	0.06	3	9 days
Hip	0.4	20	2 months
Pelvis	0.7	35	4 months
Thoracic spine	0.7	35	4 months
Abdomen	0.7	35	4 months
Lumbar spine	1	50	5 months
Contrast studies			
Barium swallow	1.5	75	8 months
Barium follow through	3	150	16 months
Barium enema	7.2	360	3.2 years
CT			
Brain	2	100	10 months
Chest	8	400	3.6 years
Abdomen or pelvis	10	500	4.5 years
Nuclear medicine			
Lung ventilation/perfusion	1.3	65	7.5 months
Bone scan	4	200	1.8 years
Whole-body PET	10	500	4.5 years

certain she is not pregnant, and her last menstrual period was >28 days ago, she should be asked to perform a pregnancy test or the test should be rebooked for after her next menstrual period. Any deleterious effect due to radiation at a gestation earlier than 8 weeks is most likely to lead to a spontaneous abortion.

The fetus is considered to be most at risk between 8 and 15 weeks gestation, with an increased risk of Down syndrome and a reduction in IQ. There is also a slight increased risk of fatal childhood malignancy. Data are at best uncertain and typically based on high-dose experiences. A current estimate is a 5% increased risk of fatal malignancy per 1 sievert of radiation. (This varies considerably, with the gut, lung and bone marrow at greater risk than the skin or thyroid). There

is thought to be a 2% per sievert risk of genetic effects in future offspring.

In all cases of imaging in pregnancy the referring clinician should perform a risk–benefit assessment on a case-by-case basis.

If a fetus has been inadvertently exposed to ionising radiation, the individual risk assessment should be assessed by a radiation physicist and the results discussed with the patient. The level of risk involved is not generally considered to be reason enough to terminate a pregnancy.

Paediatrics

In all areas of radiology it is the obligation of all concerned to reduce the dose to the patient as far as possible. This is particularly important in paediatrics, where the developing skeleton and organs are of greater sensitivity to radiation than in adults. In addition the small size of a baby, and the lack of cooperation by young children, may make appropriate gonad shielding difficult.

Patient radiation exposure and protection

Patient protection is best effected by:

- minimising the number of, especially high dose, examinations
- utilising modern equipment
- using alternative examinations that do not use ionising radiation, e.g. ultrasound or MRI.

Protection of staff

Staff receive a small radiation dose predominantly from secondary X-rays scattered from the patient. It is advisable to periodically or continuously monitor staff exposed to radiation. Thermoluminescent dosimeters (TLDs) are used in most centres. Due largely to technological improvements and a reduction in the number of fluoroscopic examinations performed, staff doses are now below detectable levels in most cases.

Factors that reduce the patient dose will also tend to reduce the amount of scatter to staff. There are three important factors that influence the dose received by staff:

Distance

The intensity of radiation is inversely proportional to the square of the distance from the source. Standing twice as far away from the patient therefore reduces the dose by 4.

Time

Other factors being equal the dose received is proportional to the duration of exposure. This applies both to fluoroscopy times for an individual case, and to the total number of cases over a period of time.

Shielding

Placing lead or other barriers between the patient/X-ray source and the staff will result in a dramatic reduction in dose, but only to the protected areas. The two means in common use are fixed screens and 'lead' gowns. A typical 'lead' gown will transmit 1–10% of the incident radiation.

Further reading

Lee CI, Haims AH, Monico EP et al. Diagnostic CT scans: assessment of patient, physician, and radiologist awareness of radiation dose and possible risks. Radiology 2004; 231:393–8

R.C.R. Working Party. Making the best use of a department of clinical radiology. Guidelines for Doctors (5th Ed) London. The Royal College of Radiologists, 2003

Index